Role of Nutraceuticals in Skin Health and Disease

Role of Nutraceuticals in Skin Health and Disease

Editor: Nydia Morand

AMERICAN
MEDICAL PUBLISHERS
www.americanmedicalpublishers.com

AMERICAN
MEDICAL PUBLISHERS
www.americanmedicalpublishers.com

Cataloging-in-Publication Data

Role of nutraceuticals in skin health and disease / edited by Nydia Morand.
p. cm.
Includes bibliographical references and index.
ISBN 978-1-63927-806-0
1. Skin--Care and hygiene. 2. Skin--Diseases--Treatment. 3. Functional foods.
4. Functional foods--Therapeutic use. 5. Nutrition. I. Morand, Nydia.
RL87 .R65 2023
646.726--dc23

American Medical Publishers,
41 Flatbush Avenue,
1st Floor, New York,
NY 11217, USA

ISBN 978-1-63927-806-0 (Hardback)

Contents

Preface

Every book is a source of knowledge and this one is no exception. The idea that led to the conceptualization of this book was the fact that the world is advancing rapidly; which makes it crucial to document the progress in every field. I am aware that a lot of data is already available, yet, there is a lot more to learn. Hence, I accepted the responsibility of editing this book and contributing my knowledge to the community.

Nutraceuticals are substances that are a food or a part of food, and provide medical or health benefits such as preventing and treating a disease. Alternatively, plant-derived pharmaceuticals are also called nutraceuticals. Nutritional and dietary factors play an important role in maintaining healthy skin. Some of the common types of nutraceuticals such as probiotics, phenolics and vitamins have the potential to prevent and help in medically managing or treating dermatological conditions. Nutritional factors are studied for their use in skin aging, acne, inflammation, and several chronic immune-mediated disorders such as atopic dermatitis, psoriasis, wounds, and various types of skin cancer. There are several ways by which nutraceuticals can inhibit adverse skin conditions. A diet rich in nutrients and vitamins (nutraceuticals and antioxidants), particularly those derived from fruits and vegetables help in maintaining healthy skin and also prevent disease progression. For instance, nutraceuticals with anti-oxidative or metal chelating properties are being actively examined as natural tools to modulate, prevent, or inhibit oxidative mechanisms. This book includes some of the vital pieces of works being conducted across the world, on various topics related to the role of nutraceuticals in prevention and treatment of skin disorders. Those in search of information to further their knowledge will be greatly assisted by it.

While editing this book, I had multiple visions for it. Then I finally narrowed down to make every chapter a sole standing text explaining a particular topic, so that they can be used independently. However, the umbrella subject sinews them into a common theme. This makes the book a unique platform of knowledge.

I would like to give the major credit of this book to the experts from every corner of the world, who took the time to share their expertise with us. Also, I owe the completion of this book to the never-ending support of my family, who supported me throughout the project.

Editor

1

Potential of Skin Microbiome, Pro- and/or Pre-Biotics to Affect Local Cutaneous Responses to UV Exposure

VijayKumar Patra [1,2], Irène Gallais Sérézal [3,4] and Peter Wolf [2,*]

1 Center for Medical Research, Medical University of Graz, 8010 Graz, Austria; vijaykumar.patra@medunigraz.at
2 Research Unit for Photodermatology, Department of Dermatology, Medical University of Graz, 8010 Graz, Austria
3 Department of Medicine, Unit of Rheumatology, Karolinska Institutet, 171 77 Solna, Sweden; igallaisserezal@chu-besancon.fr
4 Department of Dermatology, Besançon University Hospital, 25000 Besancon, France
* Correspondence: peter.wolf@medunigraz.at

Abstract: The human skin hosts innumerable microorganisms and maintains homeostasis with the local immune system despite the challenges offered by environmental factors such as ultraviolet radiation (UVR). UVR causes cutaneous alterations such as acute (i.e., sunburn) and chronic inflammation, tanning, photoaging, skin cancer, and immune modulation. Phototherapy on the other hand is widely used to treat inflammatory skin diseases such as psoriasis, atopic dermatitis, polymorphic light eruption and graft-versus-host disease (GvHD), as well as neoplastic skin diseases such as cutaneous T cell lymphoma, among others. Previous work has addressed the use of pro- and pre-biotics to protect against UVR through anti-oxidative, anti-inflammatory, anti-aging, anti-carcinogenic and/or pro-and contra-melanogenic properties. Herein, we discuss and share perspectives of the potential benefits of novel treatment strategies using microbes and pro- and pre-biotics as modulators of the skin response to UVR, and how they could act both for protection against UVR-induced skin damage and as enhancers of the UVR-driven therapeutic effects on the skin.

Keywords: ultraviolet radiation; skin inflammation; skin microbiome; probiotics; prebiotics; photobiology; photoimmunology

---

1. Introduction

1.1. Skin Microbiome

The healthy human skin harbors multitude of diverse and complex communities of bacteria, fungi, viruses, archaea, and mites, collectively called the skin microbiome [1–4]. The skin displays striking variation of microbial composition across body sites, shaped by their physical, chemical, and biological features [5–7]. Unlike the nutrient rich intestinal environment, the skin surface lacks many nutrients beyond basic proteins and lipids. In order to survive in this hostile environment, the resident microbes have to adapt and utilize available resources present in the stratum corneum (sphingolipids, amino acids, peptides, nitric oxide), sweat (NaCl, H_2O, HCO_3^+, glucose, amino acids, free fatty acids, urea, ammonia, lactate, vitamins, peptides, sterols, mucopolysaccharides) and sebum (free fatty acids, sterols, squalene, wax esters). In addition, the skin microbiome must maintain a constant interaction and healthy interplay with the skin's immune system for its survival. Studies using germ-free animals have shown a crucial role of skin microbiome in physiological and immunological functions. For example, *Staphylococcus epidermidis*, one of the dominant skin-associated bacteria produces several antimicrobial compounds and proteases that can limit the formation of biofilms by pathogenic species. Colonizing the skin with *Staphylococcus epidermidis* remodels the skin immunity by inducing IL-17a+ CD8+ T cells that migrate to the epidermis, enhances the immunity and limits pathogen invasion [5,8]. Numerous studies suggest that the skin microbiome is intricately involved in a wide range of molecular and cellular processes within the skin and beyond [9,10]. Thus, the nutrients that play an important role in shaping the individual differences in microbial signature ultimately contribute to health and diseases.

1.2. Ultraviolet Radiation (UVR)

UVR, especially UV-A (315–400 nm) and UV-B (290–315 nm) is one of the most prominent external factors affecting the skin. UV-A rays are either UV-A1 (340–400 nm) or UV-A2 (320–340 nm). The penetration of UV-A through the skin layers (epidermis and dermis) is about 5–10 times higher than that of UV-B [11], and UV-A (like UV-B) is known to play a more major role in skin aging, wrinkling (photoaging) and takes part in initiating and promoting skin cancers. This carcinogenic effect is due to the action of UV-A on various endogenous photosensitizers to produce reactive oxygen species (ROS), which can damage both the DNA and its cellular repair machinery. In contrast to UV-A, UV-B can only penetrate through the epidermis and not the dermis. UV-B exposure is biologically more active by causing sunburn and other physiological changes in the skin, which includes the delayed and more long-lasting tanning. The intensity of UV-B radiation (unlike UV-A) vastly varies depending upon geographic location, time, and season. One of the prominent targets of UV-B is cellular DNA, which can absorb UV-B radiation leading to the formation of cyclobutane pyrimidine dimers [12], (6-4) photoproducts [13] and other lesions in the DNA. In addition, UV-B causes significant adverse effects on organisms such as bacteria [14,15], cyanobacteria, phytoplankton, algae [16], plants [17], animals and humans [18]. Some organisms have evolutionary developed UV-absorbing pigments as the first line of defense, though they cannot prevent UVR completely from reaching the DNA in superficial tissues [19]. DNA repair systems, such as nucleotide excision repair, superoxide dismutase (SOD), catalase (CAT) and peroxidase (POD), and vitamins, such as B, C, D and E, play a protective role against UV-B [19]. Vitamin D3 (cholecalciferol) is mainly generated in the skin as a response to UVR and is further converted to the principal biologically active form 1, 25 $(OH)_2D_3$ with the help of various enzymes. Vitamin D is one of the most important nutrients for optimal health and wellbeing. It is known to have a variety of potential benefits such as prevention of cancers and autoimmune diseases [20,21], reduction of high blood pressure [22], positive regulation of immune system [23] and antimicrobial activity [24–26]. UVR also causes systemic effects such as increasing blood concentrations of inflammatory (IL1β, TNF-α) and metabolic (low/high density lipoproteins) factors [27,28]. UVR impacts the skin-brain axis by releasing neuro-endocrine-immune factors such as β-endorphin and corticotropin-releasing hormones from the skin into the blood circulation. Then, these factors exert endocrine and opioidergic effects on the central nervous system [29]. Indeed, behavioral effects of therapies using UVR are described. Psoralen used together with UV-A (PUVA) treatment in early-stage mycosis fungoides seems to have a positive impact on patient's quality of life and psychological wellbeing [30]. This opioidergic effect is thought be the result of UV-induced production of endorphins (which modulate itch, pain and reduce stress) by interacting with the neuroendocrine system [31–34]. Moreover, UVR is reported to induce the production of endocannabinoids in serum [35]. Together, those mediators may favor and support psychologic wellbeing. Furthermore, recent study shows a striking correlation between serum concentrations of 25(OH)D levels and abundance of various microbes in the gut, thereby suggesting an interplay between UVR exposure and the skin-gut axis [36]. Effects of UVR on the local and systemic levels have been very well reviewed elsewhere [29,37–39]. This article will focus on the potential of skin microbiome and pro- and prebiotics on local responses to UVR exposure.

2. Perspectives

2.1. UVR-induced Pigmentation and Antioxidation

Skin pigmentation has long been believed to be the most important photoprotective factor, with melanin (especially eumelanin) functioning both as broadband UVR absorbent (of 50–70% of UVR) and possessing antioxidant and radical scavenging properties [40]. The underlying regulatory mechanisms leading to pigmentation are not well understood. Extensive data, however, suggests that UVR-induced DNA damage initiates signals that increases the melanogenesis. Melanin is produced in dendritic melanocytes (in specific ovoid organelles knowns as melanosomes), which account for mere 1% of the epidermal cells. Melanogenesis is regulated via various mechanisms such as transcriptional regulation, intracellular signal transduction pathways with cAMP responsive element being the critical factor [41] and reaction substrates such L-tyrosine, L-dihydroxyphenylalanine (L-DOPA), which also serve as bioregulators of melanogenesis [42,43]. Interestingly, the melanin precursors L-tyrosine and L-DOPA serve an additional role as hormonelike bioregulators, which is governed by melanocytes [44]. Darker skin contains more eumelanin than fair skin and is better protected against UV-induced skin damage. Furthermore, the epidermis of the darker skin allows only 7.4% of UV-B and 17.5% of UV-A to penetrate, in contrast to 24% UV-B and 55% UV-A that passes through fair (white) skin [45,46]. The capacity of several microbial strains to produce melanin could be relevant for skin health [47]. For instance, melanin harvested from cultures of *Streptomyces glaucescens* [48] exhibits anti-proliferative effects on human fibroblasts [23]. Melanin or melanin-like pigments can also be produced by fungi, but as their melanin production goes together with tissue invasion, their transplantation onto the skin might trigger an infection [49,50]. Fungi from the malassezia genus could be an exception, as some species can cause pityriasis versicolor, a condition with hyper- or hypopigmented skin patches, depending on the background color of the skin, while some others colonize the skin without symptoms [51,52]. Bacteria and fungi produce melanin as protection against UVR, solar or gamma radiation. For instance, melanization protects fungi such as *Cladosporium* spp. [53], *Sporothrix Schenckii* [54] and *Cryptococcus neoformans* [55] from UVR. With increasing evidence of UV-induced damage to skin microbiome, one could envision to use melanin as photoprotection not only for the skin, but also for the resident cutaneous microbes. *Escherichia* and *Enterococcus* species can produce serotonin, which is involved in skin pigmentation [56,57]. Indeed, inducing the production of melanin or transferring this capacity to non-melanogenic microbes using genetic modification has been discussed [58]. Interestingly, recombinant strains of *Bacillus thuringiensis* and *Pseudomonas putida*, which could produce increased levels of melanin, showed higher survival rate and resistance to UVR exposure [59,60]. Such (recombinant) microbes capable of producing and/or inducing melanin could be used for preventing the damaging effects of UVR on the resident microbiome and beyond. Apart from melanin, microorganisms can produce other compounds such as a large array of antioxidants [61]. *Malassezia furfur*, a human skin saprophyte, can produce pityriacitrin, a UV-absorbing indole alkaloid that protects the colonies from UVR [62]. The skin colonization with selected malassezia strains optimized for pityriacitrin production could have a clinical benefit in term of UV protection. On the other hand, toxins of *Malassezia furfur* may also lead to loss of pigment in the skin by complex mechanisms, including production of toxins such as dicarboxylic acids and inflammatory response [63,64]. Lastly, on the more classical probiotic front, the topical use of *Lactobacillus helveticus* supernatant on the skin has antioxidant effects on rodents [65]. Therefore, a novel approach to safely modulate pigmentation by microbes, or utilizing their antioxidation properties, could be beneficial for cutaneous photoprotection and preventing skin cancers (Figure 1).

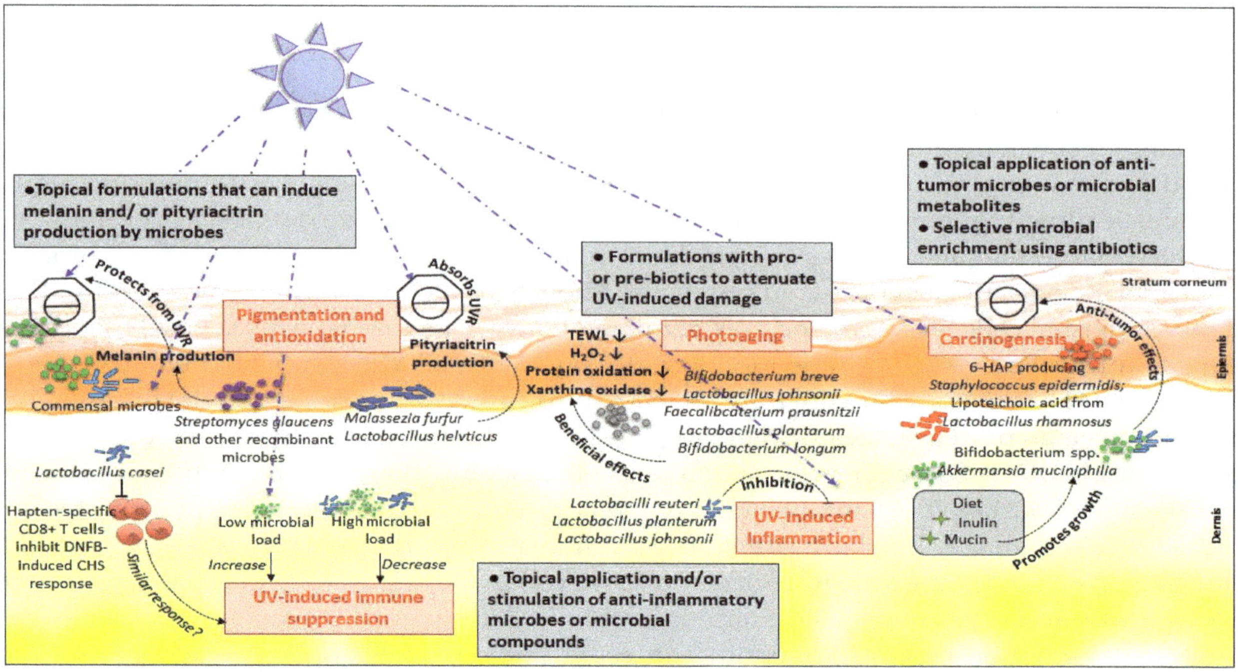

Figure 1. UV-induced effects on the skin and potential treatment strategies using microbes, pro- or pre-biotics. Topical formulations or application of recombinant microbes capable of inducing melanin and/or UV-absorbing compounds such as pityriacitrin could be used for pigmentation and antioxidation. Microbes or pro- or pre-biotics that can prevent and/or reduce UV-induced increase of transepidermal water loss (TEWL), hydrogen peroxide (H_2O_2) levels, oxidation of proteins and xanthine oxidase activity can have beneficial effects on photoaging. Novel strategies such as selective microbial enrichment using topical antibiotics, and/or application of anti-tumor, anti-inflammatory microbes or microbial metabolites/compounds could be beneficial to prevent UV-induced skin cancers and reduce UV-induced skin inflammation.

2.2. Protection from Photoaging

The skin consists of a complex network of cells and structures connecting cutaneous nerves, local neuroendocrine elements and the immune system [66,67]. UVR exposure accounts for 80% of the visible signs of skin aging, which includes dryness, scalping, wrinkling, disturbed pigmentation and solar freckles [67,68]. Multiple studies have shown that long-term exposure to UV-A leads to photoaging and free radical production, by damaging the dermis more significantly than UV-B [66,69]. The skin's response to external stress such as UVR involves coordination between various local and systemic responses, which are mediated by the skin neuroendocrine system [70,71]. Photoaging is known to correlate with cancer risk, as for instance shown in a study from Central Europe where subjects with early signs of wrinkling on the neck were over four times more susceptible to melanoma compared to subjects from general population. Furthermore, subjects with skin freckling on the back also showed over three times the risk of developing melanoma (compared to control population) [68]. The risk of developing melanoma is known to correlate with intermittent UV exposure [68,72]. That said, the skin microbiome is known to change overtime, and is largely influenced by chronological and physiological skin aging [73]. Moreover, UVR is known to cause local (skin) [74] and systemic (gut) [36,75] changes in the microbial landscape. With increasing understanding of multidirectional interplay between gut microbiome and neuroendocrine system (microbiome-gut-brain axis) [76], it is tempting to speculate on its role in photoaging.

Probiotics are emerging as potential therapeutic means to mitigate the damaging effects of UVR on the skin. Oral administration of *Bifidobacterium breve* in hairless mice prevented UVR-induced transepidermal water loss and suppressed UV-induced increase in hydrogen peroxide levels, oxidation of proteins and xanthine oxidase activity in the skin (Figure 1) [42]. Studies involving humans have also substantiated the role of probiotics in attenuating UV-induced skin damage. The probiotic *Lactobacillus johnsonii* was orally administered to UVR exposed-subjects and prevented the UVR-induced decrease in Langerhans cells and improved the recovery of immune homeostasis [77]. Other probiotics such as *Faecalibacterium prausnitzii* [45,46], *Lactobacillus plantarum* [47], *Bifidobacterium Breve Strain Yakult* [48], *Bifidobacterium longum* [47] and *Lactobacillus plantarum HY7714* [78] are known to have beneficial effects on photoaging in humans and mice. In depth reviews of probiotics in photoaging have been published elsewhere [72,79,80]. Moreover, orally administered prebiotics such as oligosaccharides are known to prevent transepidermal water loss, reduce erythema and prevent skin damage [81].

2.3. Anti-Tumor Effects of the Microbiome

UVR exposure has been associated with the development of different types of skin cancers. Chronic cumulative exposure is commonly associated with basal cell carcinoma (BCC) and squamous cell carcinoma (SCC). SCC can develop from actinic keratosis (AK), which is a typical lesion of photodamaged skin. Interestingly a recent study has shown higher relative abundances of commensal strains such as *Propionibacterium* and *Malassezia* in non-lesional skin compared to tissue of AK and SCC skin lesions. *Staphylococcus aureus* was significantly more abundant in lesional AK and SCC skin than non-lesional skin [53–55]. Moreover, *Staphylococcus aureus, Chlamydophila pneumoniae* and *Borrelia burgdorferi* have been associated with cutaneous T- or B-cell lymphoma [82,83]. Although studies on the role of skin microbiome in cancers is still in its infancy, initial reports, however, suggest an altered microbial landscape in cancerous skin that could be partly playing a role in disease pathogenesis and/or progression. Skin resident T cells play a role in the defense against formation and recurrence of skin neoplasia [84]. As the presence of bacteria on the skin surface can alter its T cell population [85], it is tempting to speculate that topical application of certain bacterial strains could act as secondary treatment against skin neoplasms. Skin exposure to UVR triggers inflammation [86] and studies suggests local (skin) and systemic (intestine) changes in microbial landscape after UVR exposure [36]. UVR-induced impairments of the immune system reduce the capacity of the host to reject skin cancers, and rather promote carcinogenesis. Moreover, microbial exposure plays a crucial role in cancer immunobiology by limiting chronic inflammation in early stages [87] and any disruptions of homeostatic skin microbiome could initiate inflammatory mechanisms that may lead to carcinogenesis. Overall, the response to UVR in the presence of microbiome on mice skin held in SPF conditions, compared to germ-free mice seem to be pro-inflammatory and protective [10]. Thus, the modification of certain strains could potentially be useful in fighting the development of cancerous cells locally. For instance, the colonization of mouse skin by strains of *S. epidermidis* that produce the antiproliferative agent 6-N-hydroxyaminopurine (6-HAP) diminishes the incidence of UV-induced skin neoplasms [88]. The systemic use of probiotics to control UV-B-induced immunosuppression has also gained interest, and oral intake of lipoteichoic acid from *Lactobacillus rhamnosus* decreased the number of UV-induced skin tumor in SKH-1 hairless mice [89]. Prebiotics, capable of inducing or limiting the growth of certain microbes, are now considered to modulate the growth of certain pathogenic skin microbes. Oral intake of prebiotics such as inulin and mucin have been reported to induce *Bifidobacterium* spp. [90] and *Akkermansia muciniphila* [91,92], which are involved in inhibiting melanoma growth [93]. Addition of inulin and mucin to the diet induces anti-tumor immune responses and inhibits subcutaneously implanted BRAF mutant melanoma in a syngeneic mouse model [94]. There is a growing body of evidence that microbiome enhances the effectiveness of chemotherapy, radiotherapy and immunotherapy [95,96]. However, the interplay between photo(chemo)therapy, used to treat various inflammatory diseases such as psoriasis, atopic eczema, lichen planus and graft-versus-host disease (GvHD) as well as neoplastic diseases such as cutaneous T cell lymphoma and other immunoproliferative conditions, and the local microbial environment needs to be addressed. Finally, recent reports have shown that antibiotic treatment or selective enrichment of certain microbial species in the gut can indeed limit the effectiveness of immune check point therapy in cutaneous melanoma [97,98]. Interestingly, a recent study demonstrated targeted depletion of bacteria from a mixed population by programmed inhibitor cells that can direct the antibacterial activity against specified target cells using the type VI secretion system (T6SS) [99]. Such an approach where topical treatment selectively enriches skin commensals or targets specified microbes (pathogenic), known to be involved in immune responses [100], could also be envisioned for modulating UVR-induced immune suppression and the efficacy of phototherapy (Figure 1).

2.4. Enhancement of the UVR-induced Immune Suppression

UVR has a profound effect on the skin's immune system, which can manifest both locally and systemically in a dose-dependent manner. The role of UVR in modulating adaptive immunity was shown in landmark studies by Kripke et al., where the mice exposed to sub-carcinogenic doses of UVR developed skin tumors due to further suppression of the anti-tumor immune response [101]. Several subsequent studies in mice and humans established that UVR-induced immune suppression was a result of activation of suppressor T cells (now called as regulatory T cells (Tregs)), modulation in the number and function of antigen presenting cells, activation and recruitment of neutrophils and increased expression of anti-inflammatory cytokines such as IL-4 and IL-10 [37]. The role of skin microbiome in UVR-induced immune suppression has also now been addressed. We have recently shown, using the contact hypersensitivity (CHS) model, that absence of microbiome enhanced UVR-induced immune suppression in mice lacking microbiome (germ-free), with predominant expression of anti-inflammatory cytokines such as IL-10, and increased numbers of monocytes/macrophages in the skin. In contrast, mice with a microbiome showed diminished UVR-induced immune suppression with higher expression of pro-inflammatory cytokines such as IL-1β, epidermal hyperplasia and neutrophilic infiltration [10]. Interestingly, administration of fermented milk containing *Lactobacillus casei* DN-114 001 in a CHS model reduced skin inflammation by inhibiting the hapten-specific CD8+ T cells [102], and enhancing the frequency of FoxP3+ regulatory T cells and IL-10 producing CD4+CD25+ effector T cells [103]. These studies in T cell-mediated allergic skin inflammation model demonstrate that certain microbes or pro-biotics can indeed reduce severity of the disease by regulating the immune response (Figure 1). Other skin commensals could show similar effects, which remains to be addressed.

2.5. Protection in UVR-induced Skin Inflammation

Several skin diseases are triggered by UVR, such as cutaneous lupus [104], or polymorphic light eruption (PLE) [105]. In cutaneous lupus, UVR exposure induces long-lasting molecular changes in keratinocytes, including increased inducible nitric oxide (NO) synthase (iNOS) and interferon-stimulated transcripts [106]. For these diseases, the use of topical anti-inflammatory probiotics could be beneficial. For instance, *Lactobacillus reuteri* showed anti-inflammatory properties on a reconstructed human epidermis upon UVR-induced inflammation [107]. Oral intake of fermented milk, exopolysaccharide or *Lactobacillus planterum* in mice reduced UVR-induced epidermal thickness and activity of metalloprotease [108]. That said, oral administration of probiotic supplements containing lycopene, beta-carotene and *Lactobacillus johnsonii* [109] or natural extracts from fern leaves, such as *Polypodium leucotomos*, has been previously described to prevent and/or diminish PLE symptoms [110,111]. Patients with PLE have been reported to have low levels of vitamin D, due to sun avoidance. UVR-induced vitamin D and its metabolites participate in various immune pathways [112], leading to immune suppression by influencing innate and adaptive immune cells [113]. High doses of vitamin D_3 can also alter the microbial composition in the gut [114]. Recently, it has been shown that exposure to narrow band UV-B increases serum vitamin D levels, which then modulates intestinal microbiome [36]. In this context, PLE pathogenesis, which is (hypothetically) linked with altered skin microbiome or microbial elements, could be treated/prevented using vitamin D supplements [105]. A clinical study has in fact shown that topical pre-treatment with a 1,25-dihydroxyvitamin D_3 analogue (calcipotriol) significantly reduced photo-provoked PLE symptoms [115]. Though the mechanism of this has remained elusive, this finding might be partly due to microbial modulation by calcipotriol and/or its metabolites. Moreover, UVR-induced vitamin D3 can help "program" the migration of T cells within the skin [25].

2.6. *Controlling Inflammatory Diseases in UV-exposed Skin Areas*

Acne, rosacea and seborrheic dermatitis are an interesting group of mostly facial diseases that occur in UVR-exposed skin, but in which no direct effect of UVR is proven in the pathophysiology. It is not known whether the UVR effects on skin possibly participate in an inappropriate immune response to local microbes. UV-B triggers inflammasome activation, which is potentialized by the presence of the antimicrobial peptide LL-37 [116]. LL-37 is produced by the skin following the exposure to *P. acnes* and *Malassezia* [117], and is induced by vitamin D in sebocytes [118], which could be a mechanism through which saprophytes might become proinflammatory on UV-exposed areas. In this context, microbes with anti-inflammatory effect could be of interest. In mice, the application of the short chain fatty acid (succinic acid) produced by *S. epidermidis* onto ears injected with *P. acnes* decreases local inflammation [119]. In humans, the scarcity of randomized controlled trials of pre- and probiotics in facial dermatosis makes it difficult to draw any conclusions. Among the few randomized trials, the local application of *Vitreoscilla filiformis* decreased the clinical score in seborrheic dermatitis in one trial [120]. In mice, this bacterium impacted dendritic cells and induced IL-10+ regulatory T cells and reduced AD-like inflammation [121]. In many other skin diseases, such as psoriasis and eczema, the exposure to natural light or to UVA/B is, however, used as a treatment. For these diseases, the question is merely if the use of anti-inflammatory pre- or probiotics could potentiate the benefit [122]. Hence, in the last decade, elegant mice data have shown that the skin microbiome has been able to modify local T cell population and poise its function [85,123]. As T cells can dwell and persist in the skin after infections [124,125], using anti-inflammatory bacteria to maintain the balance of local pool of cutaneous immune cells will hopefully open interesting perspectives for better protection against UVR (Figure 1). Moreover, skin microbiome transplantation (live-biotherapeutic approach) has been successfully demonstrated to reduce atopic dermatitis (AD) symptoms. Culturable gram-negative bacteria (*Roseomonas mucosa*) collected from healthy humans were associated with activating the innate immune system, enhanced the barrier function and controlled the growth of *S. aureus* in AD-like mouse model (MC903) [126]. This approach of topical application of live-biotherapeutics also successfully reduced AD disease severity and *S. aureus* burden in AD patients [127]. A similar approach of using live-biotherapeutics should be envisioned to control UV-induced inflammatory diseases.

3. Conclusions and Outlook

Overall, probiotics and prebiotics are promising in protecting the skin against UVR-induced skin damage. On the other side of the spectrum, pro- and prebiotics may also modulate the efficacy of phototherapy. With growing knowledge of the human microbiome and patients' unique microbial "fingerprint," personalized oral or skin care regimen should be envisioned using special formulations to promote commensal microbiome that can protects against UVR and suppress growth of pathogens. Using live microbes pose certain side effects such as infection, deleterious metabolic activity, excessive immune stimulation, and dysregulation in gene expression in susceptible individuals [128–130]. On the prebiotic front, although they are well tolerated, undesirable effects after oral administration may occur, with allergic reactions and abdominal discomfort, and even potential distant effects on the skin [129,131]. To succeed in using probiotics and prebiotics, many questions need to be answered: what is the best route of administration of a supplementation? Will a combination approach of pro- or prebiotic supplementation be most effective? Are live microbes more advantageous than using pro- or pre-biotics, and how do we successfully implant them without side-effects? To address these issues, further studies are warranted that will enhance our understanding of the potential of skin microbiome, pro- and pre-biotics and help in developing novel strategies to control the cutaneous interplay with UVR.

Author Contributions: Conceptualization, V.P. and I.G.S.; writing—original draft preparation, V.P and I.G.S.; writing—review and editing, P.W.; visualization, V.P.; All authors have read and agreed to the published version of the manuscript.

Acknowledgments: We thank Honnavara N. Ananthaswamy, Houston, TX, for critical reading and editing of the manuscript. Open Access Funding by the Austrian Science Fund (FWF).

References

1. Grice, E.A.; Kong, H.H.; Renaud, G.; Young, A.C.; Program, N.C.S.; Bouffard, G.G.; Blakesley, R.W.; Wolfsberg, T.G.; Turner, M.L.; Segre, J.A. A diversity profile of the human skin microbiota. *Genome Res.* **2008**, *18*, 1043–1050. [CrossRef]
2. Gilbert, J.A.; Blaser, M.J.; Caporaso, J.G.; Jansson, J.K.; Lynch, S.V.; Knight, R. Current understanding of the human microbiome. *Nat. Med.* **2018**, *24*, 392–400. [CrossRef]
3. Probst, A.J.; Auerbach, A.K.; Moissl-Eichinger, C. Archaea on human skin. *PLoS ONE* **2013**, *8*, e65388. [CrossRef]
4. Lacey, N.; Ni Raghallaigh, S.; Powell, F.C. Demodex mites–commensals, parasites or mutualistic organisms? *Dermatology* **2011**, *222*, 128–130. [CrossRef]
5. Byrd, A.L.; Belkaid, Y.; Segre, J.A. The human skin microbiome. *Nat. Rev. Microbiol.*. **2018**, *16*, 143–155. [CrossRef]
6. Costello, E.K.; Lauber, C.L.; Hamady, M.; Fierer, N.; Gordon, J.I.; Knight, R. Bacterial community variation in human body habitats across space and time. *Science* **2009**, *326*, 1694–1697. [CrossRef]
7. Gao, Z.; Perez-Perez, G.I.; Chen, Y.; Blaser, M.J. Quantitation of major human cutaneous bacterial and fungal populations. *J. Clin. Microbiol.* **2010**, *48*, 3575–3581. [CrossRef]
8. Naik, S.; Bouladoux, N.; Linehan, J.L.; Han, S.J.; Harrison, O.J.; Wilhelm, C.; Conlan, S.; Himmelfarb, S.; Byrd, A.L.; Deming, C.; et al. Commensal-dendritic-cell interaction specifies a unique protective skin immune signature. *Nature* **2015**, *520*, 104–108. [CrossRef]
9. Meisel, J.S.; Sfyroera, G.; Bartow-McKenney, C.; Gimblet, C.; Bugayev, J.; Horwinski, J.; Kim, B.; Brestoff, J.R.; Tyldsley, A.S.; Zheng, Q.; et al. Commensal microbiota modulate gene expression in the skin. *Microbiome* **2018**, *6*, 20. [CrossRef]
10. Patra, V.; Wagner, K.; Arulampalam, V.; Wolf, P. Skin Microbiome Modulates the Effect of Ultraviolet Radiation on Cellular Response and Immune Function. *iScience* **2019**, *15*, 211–222. [CrossRef]
11. Hoffmann, K.; Kaspar, K.; Altmeyer, P.; Gambichler, T. UV transmission measurements of small skin specimens with special quartz cuvettes. *Dermatology* **2000**, *201*, 307–311. [CrossRef] [PubMed]
12. Setlow, R.B.; Carrier, W.L. Pyrimidine dimers in ultraviolet-irradiated DNA's. *J. Mol. Biol.* **1966**, *17*, 237–254. [CrossRef]
13. Mitchell, D.L.; Nairn, R.S. The biology of the (6–4) photoproduct. *Photochem. Photobiol.* **1989**, *49*, 805–819. [CrossRef]
14. Peak, M.J.; Peak, J.G. Single-strand breaks induced in Bacillus subtilis DNA by ultraviolet light: Action spectrum and properties. *Photochem. Photobiol.* **1982**, *35*, 675–680. [CrossRef]
15. Peak, M.J.; Peak, J.G.; Moehring, M.P.; Webb, R.B. Ultraviolet action spectra for DNA dimer induction, lethality, and mutagenesis in Escherichia coli with emphasis on the UVB region. *Photochem. Photobiol.* **1984**, *40*, 613–620. [CrossRef]
16. Rozema, J.; Bjorn, L.O.; Bornman, J.F.; Gaberscik, A.; Hader, D.P.; Trost, T.; Germ, M.; Klisch, M.; Groniger, A.; Sinha, R.P.; et al. The role of UV-B radiation in aquatic and terrestrial ecosystems–an experimental and functional analysis of the evolution of UV-absorbing compounds. *J. Photochem. Photobiol. B* **2002**, *66*, 2–12. [CrossRef]
17. Quaite, F.E.; Sutherland, B.M.; Sutherland, J.C. Quantitation of pyrimidine dimers in DNA from UVB-irradiated alfalfa (*Medicago sativa* L.) seedlings. *Appl. Theor. Electrophor.* **1992**, *2*, 171–175.

18. Sinha, R.P.; Hader, D.P. UV-induced DNA damage and repair: A review. *Photochem. Photobiol. Sci.* **2002**, *1*, 225–236. [CrossRef]
19. Xie, Z.; Wang, Y.; Liu, Y.; Liu, Y. Ultraviolet-B exposure induces photo-oxidative damage and subsequent repair strategies in a desert cyanobacterium Microcoleus vaginatus Gom. *Eur. J. Soil Boil.* **2009**, *45*, 377–382. [CrossRef]
20. Ponsonby, A.L.; Lucas, R.M.; van der Mei, I.A. UVR, vitamin D and three autoimmune diseases–multiple sclerosis, type 1 diabetes, rheumatoid arthritis. *Photochem. Photobiol.* **2005**, *81*, 1267–1275. [CrossRef]
21. Grant, W.B.; Garland, C.F.; Holick, M.F. Comparisons of estimated economic burdens due to insufficient solar ultraviolet irradiance and vitamin D and excess solar UV irradiance for the United States. *Photochem. Photobiol.* **2005**, *81*, 1276–1286. [CrossRef] [PubMed]
22. Pilz, S.; Tomaschitz, A.; Ritz, E.; Pieber, T.R. Vitamin D status and arterial hypertension: A systematic review. *Nat. Rev. Cardiol.* **2009**, *6*, 621–630. [CrossRef] [PubMed]
23. Bell, E. Vitamin D3 promotes immune function in the skin. *Nat. Rev. Immunol.* **2007**, *7*, 174–175. [CrossRef]
24. Liu, P.T.; Stenger, S.; Li, H.; Wenzel, L.; Tan, B.H.; Krutzik, S.R.; Ochoa, M.T.; Schauber, J.; Wu, K.; Meinken, C.; et al. Toll-like receptor triggering of a vitamin D-mediated human antimicrobial response. *Science* **2006**, *311*, 1770–1773. [CrossRef]
25. Sigmundsdottir, H.; Pan, J.; Debes, G.F.; Alt, C.; Habtezion, A.; Soler, D.; Butcher, E.C. DCs metabolize sunlight-induced vitamin D3 to 'program' T cell attraction to the epidermal chemokine CCL27. *Nat. Immunol.* **2007**, *8*, 285–293. [CrossRef]
26. Schauber, J.; Dorschner, R.A.; Coda, A.B.; Buchau, A.S.; Liu, P.T.; Kiken, D.; Helfrich, Y.R.; Kang, S.; Elalieh, H.Z.; Steinmeyer, A.; et al. Injury enhances TLR2 function and antimicrobial peptide expression through a vitamin D-dependent mechanism. *J. Clin. Investig.* **2007**, *117*, 803–811. [CrossRef]
27. Banerjee, S.; Leptin, M. Systemic response to ultraviolet radiation involves induction of leukocytic IL-1beta and inflammation in zebrafish. *J. Immunol.* **2014**, *193*, 1408–1415. [CrossRef]
28. Gorman, S.; de Courten, B.; Lucas, R.M. Systematic Review of the Effects of Ultraviolet Radiation on Markers of Metabolic Dysfunction. *Clin. Biochem. Rev.* **2019**, *40*, 147–162. [CrossRef]
29. Slominski, A.T.; Zmijewski, M.A.; Plonka, P.M.; Szaflarski, J.P.; Paus, R. How UV Light Touches the Brain and Endocrine System Through Skin, and Why. *Endocrinology* **2018**, *159*, 1992–2007. [CrossRef]
30. Graier, T.; Fink-Puches, R.; Porkert, S.; Lang, R.; Pöchlauer, S.; Ratzinger, G.; Tanew, A.; Selhofer, S.; Sator, P.-G.; Hofer, A.; et al. Quality of life, anxiety and depression in patients with early-stage mycosis fungoides and the effect of oral psoralen plus UV-A (PUVA) photochemotherapy on it. *Front. Med.* **2020**, *7*, 330. [CrossRef]
31. Jozic, I.; Stojadinovic, O.; Kirsner, R.S.F.; Tomic-Canic, M. Skin under the (Spot)-Light: Cross-Talk with the Central Hypothalamic-Pituitary-Adrenal (HPA) Axis. *J. Investig. Dermatol.* **2015**, *135*, 1469–1471. [CrossRef] [PubMed]
32. Fell, G.L.; Robinson, K.C.; Mao, J.; Woolf, C.J.; Fisher, D.E. Skin beta-endorphin mediates addiction to UV light. *Cell* **2014**, *157*, 1527–1534. [CrossRef] [PubMed]
33. Tejeda, H.A.; Bonci, A. Shedding "UV" light on endogenous opioid dependence. *Cell* **2014**, *157*, 1500–1501. [CrossRef] [PubMed]
34. Bigliardi, P.L.; Dancik, Y.; Neumann, C.; Bigliardi-Qi, M. Opioids and skin homeostasis, regeneration and ageing—What's the evidence? *Exp. Dermatol.* **2016**, *25*, 586–591. [CrossRef]
35. Felton, S.J.; Kendall, A.C.; Almaedani, A.F.; Urquhart, P.; Webb, A.R.; Kift, R.; Vail, A.; Nicolaou, A.; Rhodes, L.E. Serum endocannabinoids and N-acyl ethanolamines and the influence of simulated solar UVR exposure in humans in vivo. *Photochem. Photobiol. Sci.* **2017**, *16*, 564–574. [CrossRef]
36. Bosman, E.S.; Albert, A.Y.; Lui, H.; Dutz, J.P.; Vallance, B.A. Skin Exposure to Narrow Band Ultraviolet (UVB) Light Modulates the Human Intestinal Microbiome. *Front. Microbiol.* **2019**, *10*, 2410. [CrossRef]
37. Bernard, J.J.; Gallo, R.L.; Krutmann, J. Photoimmunology: How ultraviolet radiation affects the immune system. *Nat. Rev. Immunol.* **2019**, *19*, 688–701. [CrossRef]
38. Yu, Z.; Wolf, P. How It Works: The Immunology Underlying Phototherapy. *Dermatol. Clin.* **2020**, *38*, 37–53. [CrossRef]
39. Vieyra-Garcia, P.A.; Wolf, P. From Early Immunomodulatory Triggers to Immunosuppressive Outcome: Therapeutic Implications of the Complex Interplay Between the Wavebands of Sunlight and the Skin. *Front. Med.* **2018**, *5*, 232. [CrossRef]

40. Brenner, M.; Hearing, V.J. The protective role of melanin against UV damage in human skin. *Photochem. Photobiol.* **2008**, *84*, 539–549. [CrossRef]
41. Romero-Graillet, C.; Aberdam, E.; Biagoli, N.; Massabni, W.; Ortonne, J.P.; Ballotti, R. Ultraviolet B radiation acts through the nitric oxide and cGMP signal transduction pathway to stimulate melanogenesis in human melanocytes. *J. Biol. Chem.* **1996**, *271*, 28052–28056. [CrossRef]
42. Slominski, A.; Paus, R. Towards defining receptors for L-tyrosine and L-dopa. *Mol. Cell Endocrinol.* **1994**, *99*, C7–C11. [CrossRef]
43. Slominski, A.; Tobin, D.J.; Shibahara, S.; Wortsman, J. Melanin pigmentation in mammalian skin and its hormonal regulation. *Physiol. Rev.* **2004**, *84*, 1155–1228. [CrossRef] [PubMed]
44. Slominski, A.; Paus, R. Are L-tyrosine and L-dopa hormone-like bioregulators? *J. Theor. Biol.* **1990**, *143*, 123–138. [CrossRef]
45. Heymann, W.R. Skin cancer in African Americans. *J. Am. Acad. Dermatol.* **2005**, *53*, 485–486. [CrossRef] [PubMed]
46. Halder, R.M.; Bridgeman-Shah, S. Skin cancer in African Americans. *Cancer* **1995**, *75*, 667–673. [CrossRef]
47. Rastogi, R.P.; Incharoensakdi, A. Analysis of UV-absorbing photoprotectant mycosporine-like amino acid (MAA) in the cyanobacterium Arthrospira sp. CU2556. *Photochem. Photobiol. Sci.* **2014**, *13*, 1016–1024. [CrossRef]
48. El-Naggar, N.E.; El-Ewasy, S.M. Bioproduction, characterization, anticancer and antioxidant activities of extracellular melanin pigment produced by newly isolated microbial cell factories Streptomyces glaucescens NEAE-H. *Sci. Rep.* **2017**, *7*, 42129. [CrossRef]
49. Chongkae, S.; Nosanchuk, J.D.; Pruksaphon, K.; Laliam, A.; Pornsuwan, S.; Youngchim, S. Production of melanin pigments in saprophytic fungi in vitro and during infection. *J. Basic Microbiol.* **2019**, *59*, 1092–1104. [CrossRef]
50. Youngchim, S.; Pornsuwan, S.; Nosanchuk, J.D.; Dankai, W.; Vanittanakom, N. Melanogenesis in dermatophyte species in vitro and during infection. *Microbiology* **2011**, *157*, 2348–2356. [CrossRef]
51. Morishita, N.; Sei, Y.; Takiuchi, I.; Sugita, T. Examination of the causative agent of pityriasis versicolor. *Nihon. Ishinkin Gakkai Zasshi* **2005**, *46*, 169–170. [CrossRef] [PubMed]
52. Findley, K.; Program, N.I.S.C.C.S.; Oh, J.; Yang, J.; Conlan, S.; Deming, C.; Meyer, J.A.; Schoenfeld, D.; Nomicos, E.; Park, M.; et al. Topographic diversity of fungal and bacterial communities in human skin. *Nature* **2013**, *498*, 367–370. [CrossRef] [PubMed]
53. Zhdanova, N.N.; Gavriushina, A.I.; Vasilevskaia, A.I. Effect of gamma and UV irradiation on the survival of Cladosporium sp. and Oidiodendron cerealis. *Mikrobiol. Zhurnal* **1973**, *35*, 449–452.
54. Romero-Martinez, R.; Wheeler, M.; Guerrero-Plata, A.; Rico, G.; Torres-Guerrero, H. Biosynthesis and functions of melanin in Sporothrix schenckii. *Infect. Immun.* **2000**, *68*, 3696–3703. [CrossRef]
55. Wang, Y.; Casadevall, A. Decreased susceptibility of melanized Cryptococcus neoformans to UV light. *Appl. Environ. Microbiol.* **1994**, *60*, 3864–3866. [CrossRef]
56. Cryan, J.F.; Dinan, T.G. Mind-altering microorganisms: The impact of the gut microbiota on brain and behaviour. *Nat. Rev. Neurosci.* **2012**, *13*, 701–712. [CrossRef]
57. Lee, H.J.; Park, M.K.; Kim, S.Y.; Park Choo, H.Y.; Lee, A.Y.; Lee, C.H. Serotonin induces melanogenesis via serotonin receptor 2A. *Br. J. Dermatol.* **2011**, *165*, 1344–1348. [CrossRef]
58. Martinez, L.M.; Martinez, Á.; Gosset, G. Production of Melanins With Recombinant Microorganisms. *Front. Bioeng. Biotechnol.* **2019**, *7*, 285. [CrossRef]
59. Ruan, L.; Yu, Z.; Fang, B.; He, W.; Wang, Y.; Shen, P. Melanin pigment formation and increased UV resistance in Bacillus thuringiensis following high temperature induction. *Syst. Appl. Microbiol.* **2004**, *27*, 286–289. [CrossRef]
60. Nikodinovic-Runic, J.; Martin, L.B.; Babu, R.; Blau, W.; O'Connor, K.E. Characterization of melanin-overproducing transposon mutants of Pseudomonas putida F6. *FEMS Microbiol. Lett.* **2009**, *298*, 174–183. [CrossRef]
61. Peyrat, L.A.; Tsafantakis, N.; Georgousaki, K.; Ouazzani, J.; Genilloud, O.; Trougakos, I.P.; Fokialakis, N. Terrestrial Microorganisms: Cell Factories of Bioactive Molecules with Skin Protecting Applications. *Molecules* **2019**, *24*, 1836. [CrossRef] [PubMed]
62. Mayser, P.; Schafer, U.; Kramer, H.J.; Irlinger, B.; Steglich, W. Pityriacitrin—An ultraviolet-absorbing indole alkaloid from the yeast Malassezia furfur. *Arch. Dermatol. Res.* **2002**, *294*, 131–134. [CrossRef] [PubMed]

63. Inamadar, A.C.; Palit, A. The genus Malassezia and human disease. *Indian J. Dermatol. Venereol. Leprol.* **2003**, *69*, 265–270. [PubMed]
64. Gupta, P.; Bansal, A.; Singh, A. Resurvey of symptomatics of the Jaipur district population and suggestion for alternative diagnostic criteria of asthma for epidemiological surveys. *Pigment. Int.* **2014**, *1*, 32–35. [CrossRef] [PubMed]
65. Rong, J.; Shan, C.; Liu, S.; Zheng, H.; Liu, C.; Liu, M.; Jin, F.; Wang, L. Skin resistance to UVB-induced oxidative stress and hyperpigmentation by the topical use of Lactobacillus helveticus NS8-fermented milk supernatant. *J. Appl. Microbiol.* **2017**, *123*, 511–523. [CrossRef]
66. Bocheva, G.; Slominski, R.M.; Slominski, A.T. Neuroendocrine Aspects of Skin Aging. *Int. J. Mol. Sci.* **2019**, *20*, 2798. [CrossRef] [PubMed]
67. Grant, W.B. The effect of solar UVB doses and vitamin D production, skin cancer action spectra, and smoking in explaining links between skin cancers and solid tumours. *Eur. J. Cancer* **2008**, *44*, 12–15. [CrossRef]
68. Wendt, J.; Schanab, O.; Binder, M.; Pehamberger, H.; Okamoto, I. Site-dependent actinic skin damage as risk factor for melanoma in a central European population. *Pigment. Cell Melanoma Res.* **2012**, *25*, 234–242. [CrossRef]
69. Marionnet, C.; Tricaud, C.; Bernerd, F. Exposure to non-extreme solar UV daylight: Spectral characterization, effects on skin and photoprotection. *Int. J. Mol. Sci.* **2014**, *16*, 68–90. [CrossRef]
70. Slominski, A.; Wortsman, J. Neuroendocrinology of the skin. *Endocr. Rev.* **2000**, *21*, 457–487. [CrossRef]
71. Slominski, A.T.; Zmijewski, M.A.; Skobowiat, C.; Zbytek, B.; Slominski, R.M.; Steketee, J.D. Introduction. In *Sensing the Environment: Regulation of Local and Global Homeostasis by the Skin's Neuroendocrine System*; Springer: Berlin/Heidelberg, Germany, 2012; pp. 1–6. [CrossRef]
72. Amaro-Ortiz, A.; Yan, B.; D'Orazio, J.A. Ultraviolet radiation, aging and the skin: Prevention of damage by topical cAMP manipulation. *Molecules* **2014**, *19*, 6202–6219. [CrossRef] [PubMed]
73. Shibagaki, N.; Suda, W.; Clavaud, C.; Bastien, P.; Takayasu, L.; Iioka, E.; Kurokawa, R.; Yamashita, N.; Hattori, Y.; Shindo, C.; et al. Aging-related changes in the diversity of women's skin microbiomes associated with oral bacteria. *Sci. Rep.* **2017**, *7*, 10567. [CrossRef]
74. Burns, E.M.; Ahmed, H.; Isedeh, P.N.; Kohli, I.; Van Der Pol, W.; Shaheen, A.; Muzaffar, A.F.; Al-Sadek, C.; Foy, T.M.; Abdelgawwad, M.S.; et al. Ultraviolet radiation, both UVA and UVB, influences the composition of the skin microbiome. *Exp. Dermatol.* **2019**, *28*, 136–141. [CrossRef] [PubMed]
75. Ghaly, S.; Kaakoush, N.O.; Lloyd, F.; Gordon, L.; Forest, C.; Lawrance, I.C.; Hart, P.H. Ultraviolet Irradiation of Skin Alters the Faecal Microbiome Independently of Vitamin D in Mice. *Nutrients* **2018**, *10*, 1069. [CrossRef] [PubMed]
76. Farzi, A.; Frohlich, E.E.; Holzer, P. Gut Microbiota and the Neuroendocrine System. *Neurotherapeutics* **2018**, *15*, 5–22. [CrossRef] [PubMed]
77. Gueniche, A.; Philippe, D.; Bastien, P.; Blum, S.; Buyukpamukcu, E.; Castiel-Higounenc, I. Probiotics for photoprotection. *Dermatoendocrinol* **2009**, *1*, 275–279. [CrossRef] [PubMed]
78. Kim, H.M.; Lee, D.E.; Park, S.D.; Kim, Y.T.; Kim, Y.J.; Jeong, J.W.; Jang, S.S.; Ahn, Y.T.; Sim, J.H.; Huh, C.S.; et al. Oral administration of Lactobacillus plantarum HY7714 protects hairless mouse against ultraviolet B-induced photoaging. *J. Microbiol. Biotechnol.* **2014**, *24*, 1583–1591. [CrossRef]
79. Ouwehand, A.C.; Tiihonen, K.; Lahtinen, S. The Potential of Probiotics and Prebiotics for Skin Health. In *Textbook of Aging Skin*; Farage, M.A., Miller, K.W., Maibach, H.I., Eds.; Springer: Berlin/Heidelberg, Germany, 2010; pp. 799–809. [CrossRef]
80. Kober, M.M.; Bowe, W.P. The effect of probiotics on immune regulation, acne, and photoaging. *Int. J. Womens Dermatol.* **2015**, *1*, 85–89. [CrossRef]
81. Hong, K.B.; Jeong, M.; Han, K.S.; Hwan Kim, J.; Park, Y.; Suh, H.J. Photoprotective effects of galacto-oligosaccharide and/or Bifidobacterium longum supplementation against skin damage induced by ultraviolet irradiation in hairless mice. *Int. J. Food Sci. Nutr.* **2015**, *66*, 923–930. [CrossRef]
82. Mirvish, J.J.; Pomerantz, R.G.; Falo, L.D., Jr.; Geskin, L.J. Role of infectious agents in cutaneous T-cell lymphoma: Facts and controversies. *Clin. Dermatol.* **2013**, *31*, 423–431. [CrossRef]
83. Nguyen, V.; Huggins, R.H.; Lertsburapa, T.; Bauer, K.; Rademaker, A.; Gerami, P.; Guitart, J. Cutaneous T-cell lymphoma and Staphylococcus aureus colonization. *J. Am. Acad. Dermatol.* **2008**, *59*, 949–952. [CrossRef] [PubMed]

84. Malik, B.T.; Byrne, K.T.; Vella, J.L.; Zhang, P.; Shabaneh, T.B.; Steinberg, S.M.; Molodtsov, A.K.; Bowers, J.S.; Angeles, C.V.; Paulos, C.M.; et al. Resident memory T cells in the skin mediate durable immunity to melanoma. *Sci. Immunol.* **2017**, *2*, eaam6346. [CrossRef] [PubMed]
85. Naik, S.; Bouladoux, N.; Wilhelm, C.; Molloy, M.J.; Salcedo, R.; Kastenmuller, W.; Deming, C.; Quinones, M.; Koo, L.; Conlan, S.; et al. Compartmentalized control of skin immunity by resident commensals. *Science* **2012**, *337*, 1115–1119. [CrossRef] [PubMed]
86. Hruza, L.L.; Pentland, A.P. Mechanisms of UV-induced inflammation. *J. Investig. Dermatol.* **1993**, *100*, 35S–41S. [CrossRef]
87. Gallimore, A.M.; Simon, A.K. Positive and negative influences of regulatory T cells on tumour immunity. *Oncogene* **2008**, *27*, 5886–5893. [CrossRef]
88. Nakatsuji, T.; Chen, T.H.; Butcher, A.M.; Trzoss, L.L.; Nam, S.J.; Shirakawa, K.T.; Zhou, W.; Oh, J.; Otto, M.; Fenical, W.; et al. A commensal strain of Staphylococcus epidermidis protects against skin neoplasia. *Sci. Adv.* **2018**, *4*, eaao4502. [CrossRef]
89. Friedrich, A.D.; Campo, V.E.; Cela, E.M.; Morelli, A.E.; Shufesky, W.J.; Tckacheva, O.A.; Leoni, J.; Paz, M.L.; Larregina, A.T.; Gonzalez Maglio, D.H. Oral administration of lipoteichoic acid from Lactobacillus rhamnosus GG overcomes UVB-induced immunosuppression and impairs skin tumor growth in mice. *Eur. J. Immunol.* **2019**, *49*, 2095–2102. [CrossRef]
90. Fehlbaum, S.; Prudence, K.; Kieboom, J.; Heerikhuisen, M.; van den Broek, T.; Schuren, F.H.J.; Steinert, R.E.; Raederstorff, D. In Vitro Fermentation of Selected Prebiotics and Their Effects on the Composition and Activity of the Adult Gut Microbiota. *Int. J. Mol. Sci.* **2018**, *19*, 3097. [CrossRef]
91. Everard, A.; Belzer, C.; Geurts, L.; Ouwerkerk, J.P.; Druart, C.; Bindels, L.B.; Guiot, Y.; Derrien, M.; Muccioli, G.G.; Delzenne, N.M.; et al. Cross-talk between Akkermansia muciniphila and intestinal epithelium controls diet-induced obesity. *Proc. Natl. Acad. Sci. USA* **2013**, *110*, 9066–9071. [CrossRef]
92. Singh, A.; Zapata, R.C.; Pezeshki, A.; Reidelberger, R.D.; Chelikani, P.K. Inulin fiber dose-dependently modulates energy balance, glucose tolerance, gut microbiota, hormones and diet preference in high-fat-fed male rats. *J. Nutr. Biochem.* **2018**, *59*, 142–152. [CrossRef]
93. Li, Y.; Tinoco, R.; Elmen, L.; Segota, I.; Xian, Y.; Fujita, Y.; Sahu, A.; Zarecki, R.; Marie, K.; Feng, Y.; et al. Gut microbiota dependent anti-tumor immunity restricts melanoma growth in Rnf5(-/-) mice. *Nat. Commun.* **2019**, *10*, 1492. [CrossRef] [PubMed]
94. Li, Y.; Elmen, L.; Segota, I.; Xian, Y.; Tinoco, R.; Feng, Y.; Fujita, Y.; Segura Munoz, R.R.; Schmaltz, R.; Bradley, L.M.; et al. Prebiotic-Induced Anti-tumor Immunity Attenuates Tumor Growth. *Cell Rep.* **2020**, *30*, 1753–1766. [CrossRef] [PubMed]
95. Alexander, J.L.; Wilson, I.D.; Teare, J.; Marchesi, J.R.; Nicholson, J.K.; Kinross, J.M. Gut microbiota modulation of chemotherapy efficacy and toxicity. *Nat. Rev. Gastroenterol. Hepatol.* **2017**, *14*, 356–365. [CrossRef] [PubMed]
96. Iida, N.; Dzutsev, A.; Stewart, C.A.; Smith, L.; Bouladoux, N.; Weingarten, R.A.; Molina, D.A.; Salcedo, R.; Back, T.; Cramer, S.; et al. Commensal bacteria control cancer response to therapy by modulating the tumor microenvironment. *Science* **2013**, *342*, 967–970. [CrossRef] [PubMed]
97. Gopalakrishnan, V.; Helmink, B.A.; Spencer, C.N.; Reuben, A.; Wargo, J.A. The Influence of the Gut Microbiome on Cancer, Immunity, and Cancer Immunotherapy. *Cancer Cell* **2018**, *33*, 570–580. [CrossRef]
98. Gopalakrishnan, V.; Spencer, C.N.; Nezi, L.; Reuben, A.; Andrews, M.C.; Karpinets, T.V.; Prieto, P.A.; Vicente, D.; Hoffman, K.; Wei, S.C.; et al. Gut microbiome modulates response to anti-PD-1 immunotherapy in melanoma patients. *Science* **2018**, *359*, 97–103. [CrossRef]
99. Ting, S.Y.; Martinez-Garcia, E.; Huang, S.; Bertolli, S.K.; Kelly, K.A.; Cutler, K.J.; Su, E.D.; Zhi, H.; Tang, Q.; Radey, M.C.; et al. Targeted Depletion of Bacteria from Mixed Populations by Programmable Adhesion with Antagonistic Competitor Cells. *Cell Host Microbe* **2020**. [CrossRef]
100. Belkaid, Y.; Hand, T.W. Role of the microbiota in immunity and inflammation. *Cell* **2014**, *157*, 121–141. [CrossRef]
101. Kripke, M.L.; Fisher, M.S. Immunologic aspects of tumor induction by ultraviolet radiation. *Natl. Cancer Inst. Monogr.* **1978**, *50*, 179–183.
102. Chapat, L.; Chemin, K.; Dubois, B.; Bourdet-Sicard, R.; Kaiserlian, D. Lactobacillus casei reduces CD8+ T cell-mediated skin inflammation. *Eur. J. Immunol.* **2004**, *34*, 2520–2528. [CrossRef] [PubMed]

103. Hacini-Rachinel, F.; Gheit, H.; Le Luduec, J.B.; Dif, F.; Nancey, S.; Kaiserlian, D. Oral probiotic control skin inflammation by acting on both effector and regulatory T cells. *PLoS ONE* **2009**, *4*, e4903. [CrossRef] [PubMed]
104. Jatwani, S.; Hearth Holmes, M.P. *Subacute Cutaneous Lupus Erythematosus*; StatPearls: Treasure Island, FL, USA, 2020.
105. Patra, V.; Wolf, P. Microbial elements as the initial triggers in the pathogenesis of polymorphic light eruption? *Exp. Dermatol.* **2016**, *25*, 999–1001. [CrossRef] [PubMed]
106. Katayama, S.; Panelius, J.; Koskenmies, S.; Skoog, T.; Mahonen, K.; Kisand, K.; Bondet, V.; Duffy, D.; Krjutskov, K.; Kere, J.; et al. Delineating the Healthy Human Skin UV Response and Early Induction of Interferon Pathway in Cutaneous Lupus Erythematosus. *J. Investig. Dermatol.* **2019**, *139*, 2058–2061. [CrossRef] [PubMed]
107. Khmaladze, I.; Butler, E.; Fabre, S.; Gillbro, J.M. Lactobacillus reuteri DSM 17938-A comparative study on the effect of probiotics and lysates on human skin. *Exp. Dermatol.* **2019**, *28*, 822–828. [CrossRef] [PubMed]
108. Ra, J.; Lee, D.E.; Kim, S.H.; Jeong, J.W.; Ku, H.K.; Kim, T.Y.; Choi, I.D.; Jeung, W.; Sim, J.H.; Ahn, Y.T. Effect of oral administration of Lactobacillus plantarum HY7714 on epidermal hydration in ultraviolet B-irradiated hairless mice. *J. Microbiol. Biotechnol.* **2014**, *24*, 1736–1743. [CrossRef]
109. Marini, A.; Jaenicke, T.; Grether-Beck, S.; Le Floc'h, C.; Cheniti, A.; Piccardi, N.; Krutmann, J. Prevention of polymorphic light eruption by oral administration of a nutritional supplement containing lycopene, beta-carotene, and Lactobacillus johnsonii: Results from a randomized, placebo-controlled, double-blinded study. *Photodermatol. Photoimmunol. Photomed.* **2014**, *30*, 189–194. [CrossRef]
110. Tanew, A.; Radakovic, S.; Gonzalez, S.; Venturini, M.; Calzavara-Pinton, P. Oral administration of a hydrophilic extract of Polypodium leucotomos for the prevention of polymorphic light eruption. *J. Am. Acad. Dermatol.* **2012**, *66*, 58–62. [CrossRef]
111. Caccialanza, M.; Percivalle, S.; Piccinno, R.; Brambilla, R. Photoprotective activity of oral polypodium leucotomos extract in 25 patients with idiopathic photodermatoses. *Photodermatol. Photoimmunol. Photomed.* **2007**, *23*, 46–47. [CrossRef]
112. Hart, P.H.; Norval, M.; Byrne, S.N.; Rhodes, L.E. Exposure to Ultraviolet Radiation in the Modulation of Human Diseases. *Annu. Rev. Pathol.* **2019**, *14*, 55–81. [CrossRef]
113. Clark, A.; Mach, N. Role of Vitamin D in the Hygiene Hypothesis: The Interplay between Vitamin D, Vitamin D Receptors, Gut Microbiota, and Immune Response. *Front. Immunol.* **2016**, *7*, 627. [CrossRef]
114. Bashir, M.; Prietl, B.; Tauschmann, M.; Mautner, S.I.; Kump, P.K.; Treiber, G.; Wurm, P.; Gorkiewicz, G.; Hogenauer, C.; Pieber, T.R. Effects of high doses of vitamin D3 on mucosa-associated gut microbiome vary between regions of the human gastrointestinal tract. *Eur. J. Nutr.* **2016**, *55*, 1479–1489. [CrossRef] [PubMed]
115. Gruber-Wackernagel, A.; Bambach, I.; Legat, F.J.; Hofer, A.; Byrne, S.N.; Quehenberger, F.; Wolf, P. Randomized double-blinded placebo-controlled intra-individual trial on topical treatment with a 1,25-dihydroxyvitamin D(3) analogue in polymorphic light eruption. *Br. J. Dermatol.* **2011**, *165*, 152–163. [CrossRef] [PubMed]
116. Salzer, S.; Kresse, S.; Hirai, Y.; Koglin, S.; Reinholz, M.; Ruzicka, T.; Schauber, J. Cathelicidin peptide LL-37 increases UVB-triggered inflammasome activation: Possible implications for rosacea. *J. Dermatol. Sci.* **2014**, *76*, 173–179. [CrossRef] [PubMed]
117. Bandholtz, L.; Ekman, G.J.; Vilhelmsson, M.; Buentke, E.; Agerberth, B.; Scheynius, A.; Gudmundsson, G.H. Antimicrobial peptide LL-37 internalized by immature human dendritic cells alters their phenotype. *Scand. J. Immunol.* **2006**, *63*, 410–419. [CrossRef] [PubMed]
118. Park, H.J.; Cho, D.H.; Kim, H.J.; Lee, J.Y.; Cho, B.K.; Bang, S.I.; Song, S.Y.; Yamasaki, K.; Di Nardo, A.; Gallo, R.L. Collagen synthesis is suppressed in dermal fibroblasts by the human antimicrobial peptide LL-37. *J. Investig. Dermatol.* **2009**, *129*, 843–850. [CrossRef] [PubMed]
119. Wang, Y.; Kuo, S.; Shu, M.; Yu, J.; Huang, S.; Dai, A.; Two, A.; Gallo, R.L.; Huang, C.M. Staphylococcus epidermidis in the human skin microbiome mediates fermentation to inhibit the growth of Propionibacterium acnes: Implications of probiotics in acne vulgaris. *Appl. Microbiol. Biotechnol.* **2014**, *98*, 411–424. [CrossRef]
120. Gueniche, A.; Cathelineau, A.C.; Bastien, P.; Esdaile, J.; Martin, R.; Queille Roussel, C.; Breton, L. Vitreoscilla filiformis biomass improves seborrheic dermatitis. *J. Eur. Acad. Dermatol. Venereol.* **2008**, *22*, 1014–1015. [CrossRef]

121. Volz, T.; Skabytska, Y.; Guenova, E.; Chen, K.M.; Frick, J.S.; Kirschning, C.J.; Kaesler, S.; Rocken, M.; Biedermann, T. Nonpathogenic bacteria alleviating atopic dermatitis inflammation induce IL-10-producing dendritic cells and regulatory Tr1 cells. *J. Investig. Dermatol.* **2014**, *134*, 96–104. [CrossRef]
122. Yu, Y.; Dunaway, S.; Champer, J.; Kim, J.; Alikhan, A. Changing our microbiome: Probiotics in dermatology. *Br. J. Dermatol.* **2020**, *182*, 39–46. [CrossRef]
123. Harrison, O.J.; Linehan, J.L.; Shih, H.Y.; Bouladoux, N.; Han, S.J.; Smelkinson, M.; Sen, S.K.; Byrd, A.L.; Enamorado, M.; Yao, C.; et al. Commensal-specific T cell plasticity promotes rapid tissue adaptation to injury. *Science* **2019**, *363*, eaat6280. [CrossRef]
124. Cheuk, S.; Wiken, M.; Blomqvist, L.; Nylen, S.; Talme, T.; Stahle, M.; Eidsmo, L. Epidermal Th22 and Tc17 cells form a localized disease memory in clinically healed psoriasis. *J. Immunol.* **2014**, *192*, 3111–3120. [CrossRef] [PubMed]
125. Gebhardt, T.; Wakim, L.M.; Eidsmo, L.; Reading, P.C.; Heath, W.R.; Carbone, F.R. Memory T cells in nonlymphoid tissue that provide enhanced local immunity during infection with herpes simplex virus. *Nat. Immunol.* **2009**, *10*, 524–530. [CrossRef] [PubMed]
126. Myles, I.A.; Williams, K.W.; Reckhow, J.D.; Jammeh, M.L.; Pincus, N.B.; Sastalla, I.; Saleem, D.; Stone, K.D.; Datta, S.K. Transplantation of human skin microbiota in models of atopic dermatitis. *JCI Insight* **2016**, *1*, e86955. [CrossRef] [PubMed]
127. Myles, I.A.; Earland, N.J.; Anderson, E.D.; Moore, I.N.; Kieh, M.D.; Williams, K.W.; Saleem, A.; Fontecilla, N.M.; Welch, P.A.; Darnell, D.A.; et al. First-in-human topical microbiome transplantation with Roseomonas mucosa for atopic dermatitis. *JCI Insight* **2018**, *3*, e120608. [CrossRef] [PubMed]
128. Borriello, S.P.; Hammes, W.P.; Holzapfel, W.; Marteau, P.; Schrezenmeir, J.; Vaara, M.; Valtonen, V. Safety of probiotics that contain lactobacilli or bifidobacteria. *Clin. Infect. Dis.* **2003**, *36*, 775–780. [CrossRef] [PubMed]
129. Marteau, P.; Seksik, P. Tolerance of probiotics and prebiotics. *J. Clin. Gastroenterol.* **2004**, *38*, S67–S69. [CrossRef]
130. Pfefferle, P.I.; Prescott, S.L.; Kopp, M. Microbial influence on tolerance and opportunities for intervention with prebiotics/probiotics and bacterial lysates. *J. Allergy Clin. Immunol.* **2013**, *131*, 1453–1463. [CrossRef]
131. Hungin, A.P.S.; Mitchell, C.R.; Whorwell, P.; Mulligan, C.; Cole, O.; Agreus, L.; Fracasso, P.; Lionis, C.; Mendive, J.; Philippart de Foy, J.M.; et al. Systematic review: Probiotics in the management of lower gastrointestinal symptoms—an updated evidence-based international consensus. *Aliment. Pharmacol. Ther.* **2018**, *47*, 1054–1070. [CrossRef]

2

Importance of Redox Equilibrium in the Pathogenesis of Psoriasis—Impact of Antioxidant-Rich Diet

Anna Winiarska-Mieczan [1], Tomasz Mieczan [2,*] and Grzegorz Wójcik [3]

1 Department of Bromatology and Food Physiology, University of Life Sciences in Lublin, 20-950 Lublin, Poland; anna.mieczan@up.lublin.pl
2 Department of Hydrobiology and Protection of Ecosystems, University of Life Sciences in Lublin, 20-262 Lublin, Poland
3 Department of Inorganic Chemistry, Maria Curie-Sklodowska University, 20-031 Lublin, Poland; g.wojcik@poczta.umcs.lublin.pl
* Correspondence: tomasz.mieczan@up.lublin.pl

Abstract: Psoriasis is a common, chronic, hyperproliferative, inflammatory skin disease occurring in most ethnic groups in the world. The disease is hereditary but the process of its inheritance is complex and still not fully understood. At the same time, it has been observed that psoriatic lesions may be triggered by certain prooxidative external factors: using narcotics, smoking, drinking alcohol, physical and mental stress, as well as bacterial infections and injury. Since the main physiological marker of psoriasis relates to disorders in the organism's antioxidative system, it is necessary to develop a well-balanced combination of pharmaceuticals and dietary antioxidants to facilitate the effective treatment and/or prevention of the disease. The dietary sources of antioxidants must be adequate for chronic use regardless of the patient's age and be easily available, e.g., as ingredients of regular food or dietary supplements. Diet manipulation is a promising therapeutic approach in the context of modulating the incidence of chronic diseases. Another potentially viable method entails the use of nutrigenomics, which guarantees a multiaspectual approach to the problem, including, in particular, analyses of the genetic profiles of psoriasis patients with the view to more accurately targeting key problems. The present paper pertains to the significance of redox equilibrium in the context of psoriasis. Based on information published in worldwide literature over the last decade, the impact of dietary exogenous antioxidants on the course of this chronic disease was analysed.

Keywords: psoriasis; exogenous antioxidants; diet; prevention; perspectives

---

1. Introduction

Psoriasis is a common, chronic, hyperproliferative, inflammatory skin disease occurring in most ethnic groups worldwide, occurring in approximately 2–3% of the population [1,2]. Psoriasis affects both male and female patients, in approximately 75% of the cases developing before the age of 40. The primary underlying cause of psoriasis stems from genetic predispositions [1,3]. Nonetheless, other factors have also been observed to impact the development of the disease, including dermal and systemic overexpression of proinflammatory cytokines, particularly interleukins (IL), tumour necrosis factor (TNF), and interferon-γ (IFN-γ), as well as complex molecular interactions between epidermal keratinocytes, mononuclear leukocytes, neutrophils, dendritic cells, and activated T-cells [2].

Psoriasis is a hereditary condition but the process of its inheritance is complex and still not fully understood. Over 60 genes have been identified as factors conditioning the disease, with a particular focus on the pathogenic contribution of genes related to the activation of Th17 cells [4]. A number of genes take part in the inheritance process and yet, even in the presence of the particular gene combination, psoriasis may not develop. At the same time, it has been observed that psoriatic lesions can be triggered by certain external factors—e.g., using narcotics, smoking, drinking alcohol, physical and mental stress, as well as bacterial infections or injury—due to the resulting gene–environment reactions [2,3]. The mentioned factors are common causes of strong oxidative stress [3,5–7], which leads to the conclusion that a disturbance of the organism's oxidative balance constitutes one of the primary causes of psoriasis in people with certain genetic predispositions. Moreover, activation of nicotinic pathways can increase the production of cytokines such as IL-12, IL-2, TNF, INF-α, and factors stimulating the formation of granulocyte colonies [8].

Oxidative stress can be a direct or indirect risk factor related to various disorders and diseases. It is also known to exacerbate already existing conditions. There is evidence to suggest that excessive amounts of reactive oxygen species (ROS) intermediating the emergence of oxidative stress, take part in numerous biological reactions that trigger DNA modifications and enhance lipid peroxidation and production of inflammatory cytokines [2,9]. Due to the upset process of terminal keratinocyte differentiation, psoriatic epidermis is unable to properly stratify; usually, the granular layer is absent while the stratum corneum contains nucleated cells [10]. T-cells and dendric cells infiltrate into the resulting lesions and produce proinflammatory cytokines. The interaction between activated T-lymphocytes and keratinocytes triggers chronic inflammation. The oxidative stress emerging in undifferentiated keratinocytes leads to the formation of abnormal stratum corneum as a result of inflammation, which increases the antioxidative activity and overexpression of apoptotic receptors [11]. In the course of psoriasis, one observes elevated levels of myeloid dendric cells in the skin, likely forming in response to the release of alpha interferon (IFN-α) as well as other proinflammatory cytokines and chemokines [12,13]. Myeloid dendric cells produce a number of proinflammatory cytokines such as TNF or IL [10]. As the outermost protective layer of the organism, the skin is more susceptible to excessive UV exposure compared to other tissues. UV radiation additionally contributes to decomposition of oxygen molecules into free atoms which can subsequently react with other oxygen molecules producing ozone—a reactive oxygen species [14]. Due to excitation, highly reactive singlet oxygen is formed. ROS created through the skin's exposure to UV radiation can trigger inflammation leading to cell damage. It is estimated that the effects of UV radiation on skin are a major source of ROS, second only to respiratory chains [15]. This is one of the reasons why skin is particularly susceptible to the harmful effects of ROS [2]. At the same time, a therapy using controlled doses of UV can be used in psoriasis treatment [16]. It has been demonstrated that damage to the basal layer of epidermis affected by psoriatic lesions is likely related to defects of the α-1-antitrypsin inhibitor and the disturbed balance between tissue proteolytic enzymes and their inhibitors [17]. Increased levels of α-2-macroglobulin due to lowered oxygen metabolism have also been observed in the course of psoriasis [18]. The phenomenon can be explained by reduced inactivation of protease inhibitors in the blood serum caused by the increased generation of ROS. Moreover, pruritus experienced in the locations of psoriatic lesions suggests the emergence of neurogenic inflammation related to ROS, similarly to neurological inflammatory disorders [19].

Free radicals originate primarily from mitochondria where, in the process of aerobic metabolism, oxygen is reduced to water [20]. One of the primary means of metabolite exchange between mitochondria and cytoplasm is the VDAC (voltage-dependent anion selective channel) intermediating in the determination of the oxidoreductive status of cytosol [21]. Cytosol is an important factor controlling the synthesis level of, for example, proteins eliminating the superoxide anion radical [21]. Damage induced by reactive oxygen and nitrogen species within mitochondrial DNA (mtDNA) is the source of mitochondrial mutagenesis [22]. The high susceptibility of mtDNA to oxidative damage is due to the fact that it is found in close proximity to the main source of ROS, i.e., the respiratory chain, as well as to the lack of histone protection in mtDNA. This may stem from the absence of intones, which, given the simultaneously high density of information contained in mtDNA, means that damage can occur at any given point of the mitochondrial genome. At the same time, limited capacity was observed for repairing mtDNA and proteins damaged due to replication errors related to oxidative phosphorylation [20]. Studies suggest that some nutrients may offer protection against oxidative damage to mitochondria, including in particular ω3 fatty acids, vitamin C, vitamins from the B group, folic acid, as well as antioxidative minerals such as zinc or magnesium [23].

Psoriasis is an incurable disease; treatment can only reduce the severity of its symptoms. Although it has been fairly well characterised clinically and histologically, its pathogenesis has yet to be fully explained, which is necessary if effective treatment and prophylactics are to be developed. As the main physiological marker of psoriasis is related to functional disorders of the antioxidative system [2,24–26], the primary method of supporting pharmacological treatment ought to entail the use of exogenous antioxidants, particularly those suitable for long-term use irrespective of the patient's age, and be readily available, for example, being present in food or diet supplements. The paper analyses the significance of redox equilibrium in the context of psoriasis. Based on information available from global literature published in the last decade, the authors analyse the impact of exogenous antioxidants present in food products on the course of this chronic disease.

2. Systemic Oxidoreductive Balance

The production of ROS must remain under close control of the enzymatic and nonenzymatic antioxidative system. Should the system become inefficient and/or should excessive ROS production be observed, a cell may suffer from imbalance between pro- and antioxidative factors that is typically referred as oxidative stress [9]. ROS-induced oxidative stress triggers inflammatory response as well as NF-κB protein-dependent gene transcription for various inflammatory factors [27]. The key parameters describing oxidative stress include enzymes: superoxide dismutase (SOD), catalase (CAT), and glutathione peroxidase (GPX), as well as nonenzymatic antioxidants present in cells, primarily glutathione (GSH) [9]. SOD catalyses the reaction of superoxide anion radical ($O_2\bullet^-$) dismutation, which leads to the formation of hydrogen peroxide (H_2O_2) and molecular oxygen (O_2) as a result of the reactions of reduction and oxidation of metal ions contained in active SOD centres. In peroxisomes, hydrogen peroxide is subject to further enzymatic dismutation to water and oxygen with the participation of CAT [9]. GPX is a selenoenzyme catalysing the reduction of hydrogen peroxide by GSH. The reaction produces oxidised glutathione [28]. GSH, one of the main nonprotein thiols present in living organisms next to cysteine, not only serves the role of an intracellular redox buffer—the direct "scavenger" of ROS—but also constitutes a cosubstrate in the reactions of ROS inactivation and the detoxication of xenobiotics catalysed by GSH-dependent enzymes. The -SH group in glutathione is far more easily available for oxygen than the thiol groups in enzymes, hence GHS is capable of protecting bioactive protein [9,29]. Cysteine is a reductive factor as well as substrate in the biosynthesis of GHS and a precursor for metabolically reactive sulphonic sulphur. Cysteine residue present on the surface of proteins serves antioxidative purposes and can also undergo reversible oxidation to unstable sulphonic acids [30]. The concentration of advanced oxidation protein products (AOPP) is considered to be a permanent marker of in vivo oxidative protein damage not only in the context of various inflammatory conditions accompanied by oxidative stress but also in the course of many diseases [31]. In order to ensure the correct level of GHS, it is necessary to maintain the adequate concentration of reductive equivalents. Reduced form of nicotinamide adenine dinucleotide phosphate (NADPH) is the most important intracellular reductant produced in the pentose pathway in cellular cytosol [32]. The enzyme responsible for maintaining the correct concentration of NADPH is glucose-6-phosphate dehydrogenase (G6PDH) which participates in the pentose pathway. Together with glutathione reductase, G6PDH keeps GSH in the reduced form, thus protecting the organism against oxidative stress [33]. As such, the role of G6PDH is primarily protective in this context. G6PDH is in fact the only source of NADPH in red blood cells, which renders them more susceptible than other cells to oxidative stress damage due to oxidation of thiol groups in haemoglobin and molecular membranes [33].

3. The Organism's Antioxidative Status in Psoriasis

3.1. Blood and Serum

3.1.1. SOD, CAT and GPX Activity

Kadam et al. [34] reported a reduction of the antioxidative status in the blood serum of patients suffering from psoriasis ($n = 90$) compared to healthy subjects ($n = 30$), which resulted in reduced activity of SOD and CAT (Table 1). The study also revealed increased levels of nitric oxide (NO) in psoriasis patients, which, in the authors' opinion, may be due to the immunological response and inflammatory processes inherent in the aetiopathogenesis of this disease. Moreover, the less-than-optimum ratio of endogenic oxidants and antioxidants was observed to exacerbate the progress of psoriatic lesions. Kute et al. [35] observed lower SOD activity and higher malondialdehyde (MDA) levels in patients suffering from psoriasis as compared to healthy persons. Additionally, the authors emphasised that smoking and drinking alcohol can lead to further disturbance of systemic antioxidative balance, while alcohol consumption also enhances histamine synthesis, which also negatively affects skin condition. Wójcik et al. [36] studied the status of antioxidative equilibrium in the lymphocytes of patients suffering from regular psoriasis and psoriatic arthritis. The obtained results revealed an increase in prooxidative parameters (elevated ROS level, decreased CAT activity and lower GPX as compared to healthy subjects). In the cited study, the authors also observed elevated levels of transcription factor Nrf2 activators in lymphocytes. The authors concluded that differences in terms of the Nrf2 pathway may be responsible for the disturbed redox equilibrium in the lymphocytes of psoriasis patients. Lymphocytes are among the most important cells involved in the pathogenesis of the disease [36].

Table 1. Plasma antioxidant capacity and lipid peroxidation biomarkers in psoriasis.

Characteristic	Antioxidant Capacity	Lipid Levels	Peroxidation Biomarkers	References
Psoriasis $n = 26$ Control $n = 16$	≈ SOD		↑ MDA	[25]
Psoriasis $n = 90$ Control $n = 30$	↓ SOD; ↓ CAT; ↑ NO; ↓ TAS		↑ MDA	[34]
Psoriasis $n = 90$ Control $n = 90$	↓ vitamin E; ↓ CAT		↑ MDA	[37]
Psoriasis $n = 50$ Control $n = 50$	↓ SOD; ↓ GPX		↑ MDA	[35]
Psoriasis $n = 40$ Control $n = 40$		↑ TG; ↑ TC	↑ MDA	[38]
Psoriasis $n = 48$ Control $n = 16$	↑ NOX; ↑ ROS; ↓ CAT; ↓ GSH; ↓ vitamin E; ↓ GPX		↑ MDA	[36]
Psoriasis $n = 50$ Control $n = 50$	↓ SOD; ↓ vitamin E; ↓ vitamin A; ↓ Zn; ↓ Cu		↑ MDA	[39]
Psoriasis $n = 29$ Control $n = 30$	≈ native SH; ≈ total SH; ↑ SS; ≈ SS/total SH			[40]
Psoriasis $n = 80$ Control $n = 80$	≈ native SH; ↓ total SH; ≈ SS; ↑ SS/total SH			[41]
Psoriasis $n = 92$ Control $n = 71$	≈ native SH; ≈ total SH; ↑ SS; ↓ SS/total SH	↑ TC; ↑ TG; ≈ HDL-chol; ≈ LDL-chol		[42]
Psoriasis $n = 32$ Control $n = 34$	↓ G6PDH		↑ ESP	[43]
Psoriasis $n = 100$ Control $n = 100$	↓ SOD; ↓ CAT	↑ TC; ↑ LDL-chol; ↓ HDL-chol; ↑ ApoB; ↑ Lp(a); ↑ TG	↑ MDA; ↓ PON	[44]

Table 1. *Cont.*

Characteristic	Antioxidant Capacity	Lipid Levels	Peroxidation Biomarkers	References
Psoriasis $n = 93$ Control $n = 60$		↓ HDL-chol; ≈ LDL-chol; ≈ TG; ≈ TC; ↓ ox-LDL		[45]
Psoriasis $n = 150$ Control $n = 150$	↓ RGSH	↓ HDL-chol; ≈ LDL-chol; ↑ TG; ↑ TC; ↑ ox-LDL;	↑ MDA	[46]
Psoriasis $n = 50$ Control $n = 50$			↑ MDA	[47]
Psoriasis $n = 34$ Control $n = 30$	↓ SOD; ↑ CAT		↑ MDA	[48]
Psoriasis $n = 60$ Control $n = 60$	↓ GPX; ≈ CAT; ≈ SOD	↑ TG; ↑ TC; ↑ LDH-chol; ≈ HDL-chol	↑ MDA	[49]
Psoriasis $n = 30$ Control $n = 30$	↓ SOD; ↓ GPX		↑ MDA	[50]
Psoriasis $n = 70$ Control $n = 30$		↑ TG; ↑ TC; ↑ LDH-chol; ↑ VLDL-chol; ≈ HDL-chol	↑ MDA	[51]
Psoriasis $n = 23$ Control $n = 23$	↑ NO		↑ MDA	[52]
Psoriasis $n = 50$ Control $n = 50$	↓ SOD; ↓ GPX	↑ TG; ↑ TC; ↑ LDH-chol; ↓ HDL-chol; ↑ VLDL-chol	↑ MDA	[53]

↑—Increased concentration or activity in comparison to the control (healthy) group; ↓—decreased or inhibited concentration or activity in comparison to the control (healthy) group; ≈ no differences in comparison to the control (healthy) group; SS—disulfides; SH—thiol; TC—total cholesterol; HDL-chol—high-density lipoprotein cholesterol; LDL-chol—low-density lipoprotein cholesterol; VLDL-chol—very low-density lipoprotein; G6PDH—glucose-6-phosphate dehydrogenase; ESP—lipid peroxidation of erythrocytes; GSH—glutathione; SOD—superoxide dismutase; CAT—catalase; MDA—malondialdehyde; GPX—glutathione peroxidase; TG—triglycerides; ox-LDL—oxidised LDL; ApoB—apolipoprotein B; PON—paraoxonase; Lp(a)—lipoprotein(a); NO—nitric oxide; TAS—total antioxidant status; RGSH—reduced glutathione; NOX—NADPH oxidase; ROS—reactive oxygen species.

3.1.2. Antioxidant Vitamins

The levels of blood serum vitamin E in erythrocytes are lower in psoriasis patients as compared to healthy subjects [37]. Johnson et al. [54] suggested that the pathway of vitamin A synthesis may be altered in psoriasis patients, which they inferred from the elevated ($p < 0.05$) levels of vitamin A and α-carotene in the blood serum of the affected subjects ($n = 156$) as compared to healthy individuals ($n = 6104$). On the other hand, contrary results were reported by Alwasiti et al. [39] who observed decreased levels of vitamin A in the blood serum of psoriasis patients as compared to healthy subjects.

3.1.3. Thiol/Disulphide Balance

–SH groups, as constituents of compounds with antioxidative properties, are oxidised to –S–S– disulphide bridges, which reflects the loss of the compensation capacity of antioxidative mechanisms [29]. Studies conducted in a group of 29 patients suffering from psoriasis revealed a higher level of -SS disulphide bridges in their blood, as compared to healthy subjects, while the general thiol levels remained the same [40]. The results indicate disturbance of the thiol/disulphide balance as a result of oxidative stress and inflammation. The cited authors also observed that the –SS level did not show a clear correlation with the advancement of psoriasis measured with PASI (Psoriasis Area and Severity Index). In a study by Aksoy and Kirmit [41] conducted in a group of 80 psoriasis patients, the results indicated that the thiol–disulphide equilibrium was maintained, but the overall thiol level was lower ($p < 0.01$) in psoriasis patients as compared to healthy individuals, whereas the -SS levels revealed no statistically significant differences. In a study by Kilic et al. [42] lower levels of -SS and higher levels of native plasma thiol were reported for psoriasis patients ($n = 92$) as compared to healthy subjects, which is indicative of antioxidative imbalance in the organism.

3.1.4. Lipid Levels and Lipid Peroxidation Biomarkers

Fatty acids metabolism disorders are considered to be one of possible causes of psoriasis [55]. In the case of skin dryness caused by deficits or abnormalities in terms of fatty acids metabolism, epidermal keratinisation disorders (keratosis) are often observed. Prostaglandins are among the elements responsible for regulating said processes. Lipid peroxidation is a chain, free-radical process of lipid oxidation with the participation of ROS [55]. The continuous production of reactive carbonyl species (RCS), by way of lipid peroxidation in the processes of oxygen metabolism, means that they take part in cellular homeostasis. The intensified lipid peroxidation induced by free radicals activates the process of oxidative stress, leading to the breakdown of membrane polyunsaturated fatty acids (PUFA) and consequently structural modification of cellular membranes [9]. MDA is a product of lipid peroxidation characterised by the greatest biological significance, commonly used as a marker of oxidative stress. ROS-mediated lipid peroxidation is considered to be one of the main causes of cell damage in psoriasis [44].

Numerous authors have reported that elevated total cholesterol and triglyceride levels in the blood serum were observed in psoriasis patients as compared to healthy individuals (Table 1). Studies in a group of psoriasis patients also revealed disorders in terms of lipid metabolism in the blood [36]. Boda et al. [43] reported increased lipid peroxidation in erythrocytes (ESP) for psoriasis patients ($n = 32$) compared to the control ($n = 34$), which was generated by intensified ROS effects at the erythrocyte level. The results of MDA determinations conducted by Pawłowska et al. [25] and Kadam et al. [56] indicated significantly higher concentrations of this compound in both the plasma and erythrocytes of psoriasis patients, compared to healthy individuals. This could suggest that the excessive production and harmful effects of ROS as well as the process of lipid peroxidation play a significant role in the pathogenesis of psoriasis. The unaffected concentration of primary lipid peroxidation products reported in the cited study, accompanied by significant changes in the concentration of the secondary products of this process observed in psoriasis patients, suggests a significant severity of free radical-induced cell damage. Undoubtedly, the process of lipid peroxidation resulting from excessive ROS production and impairment of the antioxidative system is exacerbated in patients suffering from psoriasis, whose serum and erythrocytes show elevated content of MDA resulting from decreased β-carotene, GSH, and α-tocopherol levels as well as increased SOD activity in red blood cells [57]. Bacchetti et al. [58] conducted a study in a group of 23 psoriasis patients to determine whether it is possible to modulate the lipid profile and antioxidative status of the same with the use of NTF-α inhibitors. The study revealed no significant ($p < 0.01$) impact of the analysed factor on the patients' lipid profile, but a significant decrease in the degree of lipid peroxidation (LPO) was observed as well as improvement in terms of antioxidative status parameters: total antioxidative capacity (TAC) and paraoxonase (PON). Barygina et al. [59] also demonstrated a significant impact of the anti-TNF-α therapy on the redox equilibrium of psoriasis patients, most likely related to normalisation of NADPH oxidase activity in white blood cells. Additionally, the authors concluded that NADPH oxidase may constitute a leading source of ROS overproduction in the white blood cells of psoriasis patients. Pietrzak et al. [45], in a study on psoriasis patients ($n = 93$), observed lipid metabolism irregularities and oxidative balance disorders that may be due to chronic inflammation. Particularly high levels of oxidised LDL (ox-LDL) were observed in the serum of psoriasis patients where they were over five times higher than the corresponding control levels. The cited authors did not test for epidermal ox-LDL levels, but a study by Tekin et al. [60] revealed significantly elevated ox-LDL and anti-ox-LDL concentrations in patients suffering from psoriasis, particularly in the top epidermal layer, whereas the skin of healthy persons contained neither ox-LDL nor anti-ox-LDL. A study by Nemati et al. [44] conducted in a group of 100 psoriasis patients revealed that elevated lipid and lipoprotein levels (particularly TC, LDL, Lp(a), and ApoB) as well as reduced levels of antioxidants (SOD, CAT, PON1) may cause accumulation of ox-LDL and ROS in psoriasis patients, which in turn may play an important role in the context of immunological inflammatory states causing skin cell damage or arterial atherosclerosis in psoriasis patients. Furthermore, in a study by Asha et al. [46], psoriasis patients showed elevated levels of MDA, a marker of lipid peroxidation and ox-LDL, with the corresponding decreased levels of endogenous antioxidants. Increased concentration of MDA in the blood serum, as compared to healthy individuals, was also reported in a study by Kiran and Deedi [47] where the authors additionally observed elevated levels of alanine aminotransferase (ALT) in psoriasis patients, which indicated hepatotoxicity attributable to either oxidative stress or the effects of medicines administrated in the treatment of psoriasis. Moreover, research results indicate that LDL oxidation and an increase in ROS levels, apart from being markers of inflammation, may also play a role in inducing atherosclerosis in psoriasis patients [46]. Protein modifications by the products of lipid peroxidation and MDA promoted the proapoptotic pathway in lymphocytes, which led to the increased expression of proapoptotic caspases [36].

3.2. *Epidermal Cells*

Interesting results were also obtained by Portugal-Cohen et al. [61]. Contrary to most published studies, the cited authors concluded that psoriasis-affected epidermal cells actually showed higher antioxidant total scavenging capacity (TSC) as well as higher content of uric acid when compared to unaffected epidermal cells. Nonpathological cells originating from psoriasis patients returned lower levels of TSC and uric acid than those of healthy individuals. In the opinion of the cited authors, the same may suggest increased scavenging rates of overproduced ROS in cells affected by the disease. In a study by Abdel-Mawla et al. [48], the levels of CAT in the blood serum and erythrocytes were significantly ($p < 0.05$) higher in patients suffering from psoriasis as compared to healthy control, which, in the authors' opinion, suggests oxidative damage and imbalance of the organism's antioxidative system. On the other hand, Metta et al. [49] did not observe statistically significant differences in terms of CAT and SOD content in the blood serum of psoriasis patients and healthy individuals. Short-term exposure to oxidative stress increased the activity of exogenous antioxidants, which indicated activation of defence mechanisms and cell adaptive response, however, under long-term exposure, cellular activity became clearly reduced [9]. Another possible explanation could be that with the progression of inflammation in tissues and organs, including the epidermis and dermis, one of the SOD enzymes, SOD3, is expressed, although that expression is reduced in skin affected by psoriasis [62]. The skin is the organism's primary barrier against exogenous threats such as exposure to UV radiation, chemicals and pathogens, it therefore needs to have a suitable endogenous strategy for preventing inflammation. As the tissular distribution of SOD3 is closely related to its substrates and functional position of peroxide production, it likely naturally protects tissues that are particularly strongly exposed to ROS by, for example, deactivating NADPH oxidase.

3.3. *Saliva*

Skutnik-Radziszewska et al. [38] analysed the levels of antioxidants and oxidants in the saliva of psoriasis patients. The authors concluded that the subjects' antioxidative balance in the saliva and erythrocytes, evaluated on the basis of salivary peroxidase activity (PX), CAT, GPX, AOPP, advanced glycation end products (AGEP), MDA, and total lipid hydroperoxide (LOOH), was disturbed. In the saliva, the same resulted in elevated concentrations of oxidised biomolecules as compared to healthy individuals, with the highest sensitivity observed for secretions from submandibular glands.

4. Exogenous Antioxidants in the Diet of Psoriasis Patients

4.1. *Diet Structure*

Diet is an important factor in the treatment of many dermatological conditions. High consumption of fresh fruit and vegetables tends to correlate with lower incidence of psoriasis, while vegetarian diets have been observed to facilitate overall improvement in psoriasis patients [63–65]. The same is most likely due to the related high intake of antioxidants, which boosts the organism's antioxidative capacity and solidifies the related equilibrium. Persons following a vegetarian diet on a long-term basis have been observed to show higher levels of antioxidant compounds in the blood serum and better lipid rates [66], although consuming increased amounts of vegetables over only several weeks was found to have no significant impact on those parameters [67]. There is a significant positive correlation between the overall intake of antioxidants and the organism's antioxidative capacity [68]. Moreover, a vegetarian diet contains lower amounts of arachidonic acid responsible for stimulating the emergence of inflammatory eicosanoids [69]. A Brazilian study conducted in a group of 44 psoriasis patients revealed positive effects of supplementation with n-3 fatty acids on the organism's antioxidative status [70].

Interesting results were obtained by Solis et al. [71], who studied the dietary habits of 34 male psoriasis patients aged between 19 and 60 years. The authors observed that the consumption of fresh fruit and vegetables in this group of patients was too low, which suggested a reduced intake of exogenous antioxidants. The researchers analysed the intake of vitamin (A, C, E, B-complex) and minerals (manganese, zinc, selenium) in this group and concluded that, on average, it did not exceed 50% of the respective requirement. In a similar study conducted in Italy by Barrea et al. [72], psoriasis patients ($n = 62$) were found to consume fewer fruit and vegetables and more red and processed meat (arachidonic acid) than healthy individuals. A Brazilian study also suggested that psoriasis patients followed an unhealthy died that predisposed them for the emergence of chronic diseases related to obesity and exacerbation of psoriatic lesions [71,73]. In Japan, psoriasis patients were observed to consume more fish and shellfish, leguminous plants, green and yellow vegetables, sugar and sweeteners, vitamin B12 and vitamin D, as well as less meat than healthy subjects [74]. The cited authors also reported that affected patients ingested more β-carotene and vitamin A with their diet, which evidenced radically different dietary habits of said psoriasis patients as compared to those from other parts of the world. Moreover, the same study indicated that persons with high PASI tended to consume more sweets than other sick individuals. A study conducted in the USA by Afifi et al. [75] demonstrated, in a group of 1206 psoriasis patients, that such persons were generally willing (86%) to modify their dietary habits in the course of the treatment, the authors also observed improvement in terms of skin condition after eliminating alcohol (prooxidative effects) and increasing the intake of vegetables and vitamin D (antioxidants).

Wong et al. [65] described the case of a woman who, having unsuccessfully tried to pharmacologically treat psoriasis-related skin lesions for 14 years, switched to a diet based on fresh vegetables, with a radical reduction of meat consumption and complete elimination of fast food and sugar. Additionally, the patient used vitamin-rich diet supplements containing e.g., vitamin C. After only six months of following the diet, the psoriasis lesions disappeared completely, despite having been significantly exacerbated in the first month of the therapy. The effectiveness of vitamin C in psoriasis treatment was also confirmed in a study conducted in a group of patients undergoing UVB radiation treatment [76]. The blood serum of patients receiving 500 mg of vitamin C for 12 weeks was observed to show decreased MDA levels and increased levels of GSH and vitamin C.

Curcumin, a natural polyphenol and yellow pigment obtained from curcuma spice shows strong antioxidative, anti-inflammatory, and antibacterial properties, which makes it highly recommendable for psoriasis patients [77]. One of the challenges related to maximising the therapeutic potential of curcumin is its low bioavailability, limited solubility in water, and chemical instability [78]. It has been demonstrated that curcumin can be effectively used as supplementary treatment in regular psoriasis as it significantly reduces the serum levels of IL-22 [79]. Research results show that the use of curcumin facilitates the improvement of the total antioxidative status (TAS) and decrease of MDA levels in the blood serum of rats [80] as well as in human mesenchymal stem cells isolated from adipose tissue [81]. In a study by Chen et al. [82], a clear increase in the SOD, CAT, and GSH activity was observed as well as a reduction of MDA levels in psoriatic cells, both in isolated human HaCaT cells and in a BALB/c mice model, after the use of a mixture of natural plant extracts, including curcumin.

Unfortunately, the use of diet supplements with antioxidative properties is not always effective. This may be due to both the dosage of antioxidants and the duration of treatment—studies suggest that, in order to be effective, supplementation requires consistent and long-term administration of antioxidants [83]. Zinc (Zn) has not been observed to be effective in psoriasis treatment [64], despite the fact that it is known to reduce the production of free radicals in the organism due to its inhibition of the activity of NADPH oxidase, its presence in Cu,Zn-SOD, and facilitation of the stability of –SH groups in proteins [21]. However, the blood serum of persons suffering from psoriasis has been shown to contain significantly higher levels of both Zn and copper (Cu) as compared to healthy subjects [39]. Selenium (Se) levels in the blood serum of psoriasis patients are lower than those in healthy individuals [84]. Selenium can influence immunological response by affecting the expression of cytokines and their receptors or increasing the resistance of immune cells to oxidative stress. As an ingredient of selenocysteine, it is active in the redox centre, which reduces the risk of oxidative damage spreading to lipids, lipoproteins, and DNA [85]. In a study by Serwin et al. [86] conducted in a group of 37 psoriasis patients, it was demonstrated that selenium supplementation, safely dosed (at 200 μg Se daily in the form of selenomethionine) for four weeks, proved ineffective in patients suffering from psoriasis. At the same time, it has been demonstrated that selenium molecules can prevent in vivo release of proinflammatory cytokines induced by UVB by inhibiting mRNA in human keratinocytes [85]. Inconclusive results have also been reported in terms of using folic acid, a vitamin with strong antioxidative properties [87]. American researchers demonstrated that daily administration of folic acid dosed at 1–2 mg/day can trigger or exacerbate psoriatic lesions, whereas increasing the dosage by two to four times results in weakening PASI [88].

4.2. *Food Containing Antioxidant Compounds*

Phenolic compounds present in many plant products can reduce or inhibit free radicals by transferring hydrogen atoms from their hydroxyl groups. The mechanism of the reaction between a phenolic compound and a peroxide radical (ROO•) includes the coordinated transfer of a hydrogen cation from the phenol to the radical, thus creating a transitional state of the H-O bond with a single electron [9]. Given the strong antioxidative properties of polyphenols contained in some food products, it could be advisable to include them in the diet of psoriasis patients, even though the available literature does not evidence their beneficial effects in such cases. However, due to their conclusively demonstrated impact on the organism's antioxidative status, one can reasonably expect them to also benefit the antioxidative system of psoriasis patients.

4.2.1. Tea

The popularity of tea as a beverage is exceeded worldwide only by water. Due to its content of antioxidants, it meets the conditions for classification as functional food [89]. The antioxidative properties of tea are due to its high content of polyphenols, mainly catechins, including epigallocatechin-3-gallate (EGCG) present in green tea, quercetin, theaflavin, and thearubigin present in black tea, as well as tannic acid [9]. The particularly high antioxidative activity of EGCG stems from the presence in its structure of eight -OH groups [9]. The activity of catechins stems not only from the antioxidative processes of donating H, but most likely also from the mechanisms and pathways that directly or indirectly regulate the expression of enzymatic antioxidants [90]. The total polyphenol content in tea reaches 25–35% of leaf dry mass [91]. The highest content thereof (determined as tannic acid equivalent) is found in white tea (2668 mg/1000 mL), followed by green (2363 mg/1000 mL), black (1220 mg/1000 mL), and red varieties (996 mg/1000 mL) [83]. The increased activity of SOD, CAT, GST, and GPX observed in numerous studies, as well as elevated GSH content and reduced LPO and MDA levels in in the organs of animals and humans receiving tea solutions, indicates improvement of antioxidative mechanisms' efficiency thanks to the supply of exogenous antioxidants, which facilitates maintaining the equilibrium of redox reactions and prevents the onset of oxidative stress [9]. It has been demonstrated that the antioxidative potential in the blood serum is increased by 34% after drinking green tea and by 29% after drinking black tea [92]. Notably, green tea is characterised by higher antioxidative activity than white or black tea, as confirmed in vitro in a study conducted on isolated human erythrocytes [93].

The increase of blood plasma antioxidative activity after drinking tea is dependent on the dosage [94]. Numerous studies conducted on laboratory animals confirmed the positive impact of tea on the antioxidative status of organisms poisoned with prooxidative substances [9]. Wistar rats poisoned with prooxidative toxic metals showed an increase in SOD, CAT, and GPX activity in their organs after 12 weeks of receiving black, green, white, and red tea infusions [83] as well as tannic acid [95]. After intraperitoneal administration of catechin and epicatechin to rats, a decrease in MDA levels in urine and increased SOD concentration was observed [90]. Similarly, administering polyphenols isolated from green tea to mice (50, 100, or 200 mg/kg) resulted in an improvement of antioxidative parameters (SOD, CAT, GPX, MDA, LPO) in their blood serum [96]. The GPX reduction observed in the cited study (without an impact on TAC) may be due to the fact that catechins protect GSH (which is a substrate of GPX) against free radicals [97].

4.2.2. Coffee

Similarly to tea, coffee is among the most popular beverages worldwide. It is a source of antioxidants—research results suggest that drinking coffee may increase the level of GSH and facilitate protection against DNA damage, especially if consumed regularly [98]. The antioxidative activity of coffee is due to the presence of phenolic acids: chlorogenic, ferulic, caffeic, and n-coumaric, as well as caffeine and trigonelline [99]. In the process of roasting coffee beans, melanoidins (brown pigments) are synthesised which show strong antioxidative properties [99]. Phenylalanines and heterocyclic compounds formed in the roasting process also show strong antioxidant activity [100]. The total content of polyphenols in coffee is higher than in tea, with green coffee exceeding roast coffee in this respect [101,102]. Moreover, instant coffee contains more total polyphenols compared to the grain variety, it also shows higher antioxidant activity [103]. Nonetheless, the results of studies conducted on humans remain inconclusive, some indicate improvement in terms of antioxidative parameters, others an increase in MDA content, and yet others absence of any correlation whatsoever between drinking coffee and the levels of antioxidative parameters in blood serum or saliva [98,104,105]. Jung et al. [106] argue that coffee shows physiological antioxidative and anti-inflammatory properties and its effects are negatively correlated with the levels of grain roasting (light, medium, city, and French), which was demonstrated in experiments conducted on cellular models.

4.2.3. Herbs and Spices

Some herbs used in the kitchen or for therapeutic or treatment purposes also contain antioxidants. In the case of common marigold (*Calendula officinalis* L.) these include in particular flavonoids (flavonols and flavone glycosides), coumarins, sterols, and carotenoids [107]. St John's wort (*Hypericum perforatum* L.) contains flavonoids and phenolic acids, and in oregano (*Origanum vulgare*) we find a range of phenolic compounds including protocatechuic, caffeic, coumaric, and rosmarinic acid, as well as quercetin [107]. A study conducted on laying hens revealed that administration of flavonoids, including quercetin, statistically significantly reduced their MDA and increased SOD, GSH, and GST levels [108]. Similarly, administering water oregano solutions to rats resulted in a significant ($p < 0.05$) reduction of MDA and increase of CAT and SOD in the kidneys compared to animals not receiving the extracts; similar results were also reported for quercetin [109]. The addition of oregano oil to the fodder mixture consumed by pregnant and farrowing sows reduced the systemic oxidative stress observed during pregnancy [110]. Oregano oil was also fed to sheep, which led to a general improvement of oxidative stress parameters in their meat and livers [111].

The addition of thyme oil to the diet of Japanese quails resulted in an increase of antioxidant parameters (SOD, CAT, GSH) and reduction of MDA in the blood serum and livers, compared to birds receiving standard diet [112]. Similar results were obtained in other animals with the use of various forms of thyme: rats [113], broilers [114], and fish [115]. The strong antioxidative properties of thyme are due to its content of phenolic compounds, particularly carvacrol and thymol, as well as monoterpenes (e.g., p-cymene, α-pinene, β-pinene, α-terpinene, limonene, myrcene, terpene alcohols) [113,116,117]. The antioxidative effectiveness of thymol was demonstrated in a study on rats poisoned with CCL_4 [118]. Similar effects were reported when thymol and carvacrol were used in an in vivo study on human hepatic cancer cell lines HepG2 subjected to a strong dose of acetaminophen (APAP) [119].

Dill (*Anethum graveolens* L.) contains numerous volatile ingredients with antioxidative properties, e.g., 7-α-hydroxy-manool, l-carvone, limonene, epi-α-bisabolol, α-terpinene, and α-phellandrene [120]. In the cited study, the use of water dill extract (3 g 100 mL^{-1} pf water) for 30 days in rats receiving prooxidative paracetamol yielded an improvement in terms of parameters describing oxidative balance: TAC, CAT, and GPX. Thanks to its content of polyphenols and antioxidative vitamins, cistus (*Cistus incanus* L.) lowers MDA and AOPP levels in the blood serum of people drinking the infusion as early as after 6 weeks of use [121].

The use of water or alcohol cinnamon extract improved oxidative stress parameters (↓ MDA, ↑ SOD, ↑ CAT) in the livers of rats poisoned with prooxidative tetrachloromethane (CCl_4) [122]. Similarly, in another study conducted on rats, oral administration of a water solution of powdered cinnamon (75 mg/kg/day) resulted in an increase in the serum SOD, CAT, and GPX levels and decrease of MDA [123]. In rats receiving a high-fat diet, the inclusion of cinnamon lowered MDA and increased TAC, SOD, CAT, and GPX levels in the blood serum and/or liver, while at the same time no influence of cinnamon on the oxidative status of the control group animals was observed [124]. After 12 weeks of administering capsules containing a water extract of cinnamon to patients suffering from glucose metabolism disorders, an increase in the number of –SH groups and oxidative status was observed, as well as lowered plasma MDA levels [125]. However, in the cited study no impact of cinnamon on the activity of SOD or CAT in red blood cells was reported. The authors attributed the observed oxidative stress reduction to the content of antioxidative phenolic compounds in cinnamon. The most potent antioxidants present in cinnamon bark include polyphenols (flavonoids and tannins) as well as volatile phenolic oils [126]. Moreover, the cited authors mentioned that the highest antioxidant activity was observed for traditionally prepared cinnamon solutions. Cinnamon contains over 30 times the amount of total phenols and approximately three times the amount of polyphenols compared to, for example, garlic or curcuma [127]. Hence, its antioxidant activity, i.e., the ability to scavenge free radicals, is very high [128].

Garlic extract (*Allium sativum*) administered to rabbits poisoned with prooxidative carbon tetrachloride CCl_4 stimulated improvement of hepatic antioxidative parameters: MDA, GSH, CAT, SOD, as well as lipid parameters [129]. Also studies conducted on rats confirmed an improvement in terms of TAS levels after oral administration of garlic extract (600 mg kg^{-1}) for one month, as compared to control animals receiving distilled water [130]. A water extract of garlic can contain up to 129 mg of phenolic compounds in 1 g, including 101 mg of flavonoids and 94 mg of flavonols, which translates to very high antioxidative potential [131]. It has been shown that aged garlic obtained in the process of fermentation is characterised by even better antioxidative properties than its fresh counterpart and, as such, meets the criteria for classification as functional food [131]. Studies conducted on rats and mice with a water extract of aged garlic corroborated its beneficial effects on tissular redox status parameters (MDA, GPX, GSH, SOD, CAT, TBARs, –SH groups) [132,133]. During garlic fermentation, allicin is transformed into water-soluble antioxidants such as S-allyl-cysteine, tetrahydro-β-carbolines, and bioactive alkaloids. S-allyl-cysteine is the most important bioactive compound found in garlic and its content in aged garlic exceeds that found in the fresh variety [131].

4.2.4. Fruit

Many types of fruit provide valuable sources of phenolic compounds, primarily flavonoids (anthocyanins, flavanols, quercetin, rutin, resveratrol), condensed tannins (proanthocyanidins), tannins (ellagitannins, gallotannins, tannic acid), stilbenes, hydroxybenzoic acids (ellagic and gallic) and phenolic (caffeic, chlorogenic, ferulic), as well as well as antioxidative vitamins [134–137]. The most valuable types of fruit include berries (blueberries, blackberries, raspberries, cranberries, strawberries, grapes, and others) as well as plums, pomegranates, apples, and grapefruits [134]. Research results confirm that extracts from various berry varieties show antioxidant activity, e.g., the ability to scavenge hydroxyl radicals, singlet oxygen, hydrogen peroxide and superoxide radicals, inhibit lipid peroxidation and ROS generation, as well as boost thiol levels and the activity of antioxidative enzymes [134,138]. Consuming a mixture of various berries over a period of eight weeks resulted in an increase in the blood serum vitamin C level compared to the control, but had no significant impact on the overall oxidative capacity [139], whereas after two weeks of consuming 300 mL of antioxidant-rich red grape and lingonberry juice (80:20), researchers observed increased SOD and CAT levels and lowered blood serum MDA as compared to the control group [140]. Studies conducted on rats revealed that oral administration of dried ethanol plum extract (150 mg kg^{-1} body weight) improved the oxidative stress parameters (H_2O_2, MDA, GSH, SOD, CAT) in the bones compared to animals poisoned with dexamethasone, but had no impact on said parameters when compared to control group animals [141]. The use of a methanolic extract of polyphenols obtained from apples on adenomatous human stomach cells MKN 28 prevented oxidative damage to those cells, triggered a fourfold increase in intracellular antioxidative activity, and prevented subsequent decrease thereof and lipid peroxidation induced by xanthine oxidase [142]. The main phenolic constituents include catechins and chlorogenic acid [142]. Intraperitoneal injection of 1 mg resveratrol, a flavonoid present, e.g., in grape skin, to rats suffering from spinal cord ischaemia, elevated the levels of enzymatic and nonenzymatic antioxidants such as GSH, SOD and CAT, and decreased MDA [136]. Also the consumption of pomegranate juice rich in polyphenols has been found to improve antioxidative parameters (CAT, GPX, MDA) in the blood serum of persons practicing strength sports [143]. Studies conducted on rats receiving methotrexate, a prooxidative drug used in the treatment of psoriasis, showed an improvement in terms of antioxidative parameters (GPX, SOD, MDA) and the serum lipid profile (TC, HDL-chol, LDL-chol) after the oral administration of 500 mg per kg of pomegranate in the form of a methanol extract from seeds or peels [144,145]. All the parts of a pomegranate (peel, seeds, arils) contain polyphenols, particularly flavonols, flavonoids, gallic acid, quercetin, tannins and anthocyanins, as well as vitamins C and E and β-carotene, which means that the fruit is characterised by particularly strong antioxidative activity [146,147].

5. External Application of Antioxidants in Psoriasis

Flavonoids are natural compounds with strong anti-inflammatory and antioxidative properties. Luteolin inhibits TNF-induced phosphorylation, nuclear translocation and DNA binding the nuclear factor kappa B (NF-κB) usually involved in the transcription of an inflammation mediator [148]. It was also observed that luteolin reduces the TNF-induced mRNA expression of two genes (NFKB1 and RELA) coding two NF-κB subunits (respectively NF-κB p50 and NF-κB p65). Interestingly, the expression of RELA genes is elevated in psoriatic skin. Studies have revealed that in human psoriatic HaCaT cells, astilbin—a glycoside flavonoid isolated from the root of *Smilax glabra*, a plant used in traditional Chinese medicine in the treatment of autoimmunological diseases, can induce translocation of the Nrf2 nucleus, which contributes to the reduction of ROS accumulation, expression of the vascular endothelial growth factor (VEGF), and inhibition of HaCaT proliferation stimulated by IL-17 and TNF-α [149]. The cited authors demonstrated that positive effects could be obtained with as little as 50 μg of astilbin. The use of antioxidative balsacones isolated from balsam poplar (*Populus balsamifera* L) on human fibroblasts harvested from fragments of psoriatic skin reduced the cell growth rate and stabilised the expression of cells in involucrin and loricrin more effectively than methotrexate [150]. Local application of propolis, due to its content of flavonoids, helps to improve the condition of psoriatic skin by suppressing the activity of macrophages and production of ROS [151]. Positive results were also observed after applying resveratrol on psoriatic cells [152]. Local administration of EGCG in BALB/c mice with psoriatic lesions induced with the use of imiquimod led to increased SOD and CAT activity in the plasma, as well as lowered MDA, as compared to the control group mice [153]. Moreover, the treatment also resulted in reducing the extent of overall disease-related skin lesions by limiting the expression of the epidermal proliferating cell nuclear antigen (PCNA), alleviating dermatitis accompanied by reduced infiltration of T cells, and lowering the levels of proinflammatory interleukins IL-17A, IL-17F, IL-22, and IL-23. Positive effects have also been reported after external application of caffeine on psoriatic skin [154]. Caffeine metabolites show antioxidant properties, which helps to reduce the inflammation caused by lipid peroxidation, DNA damage, and damage to cellular organelle.

6. Clinical Studies

The use of exogenous antioxidants results in a lower likelihood of inducing oxidative damage due to the decreased antioxidative capacity of the organism's defence system. The activity of exogenous antioxidants can be threefold: (1) synergistic—i.e., scavenging oxygen and chelating compounds catalysing oxidation reactions; their activity entails donating hydrogen to phenoxy-radicals, which restores their original antioxidative properties, (2) disruption of radical reactions by donating hydrogen atoms or electrons, which stabilises the form of the radical, as well as (3) mixed reactions, such as electron transfer coupled with proton transfer, electron transfer preceded by deprotonation, or proton transfer preceded by electron transfer [21].

Clinical studies conducted on psoriasis patients revealed that antioxidative strategies may constitute viable therapeutic methods complementing pharmacological treatment. Cellular signal pathways such as protein kinase, κB nuclear factor, or Janus kinase signal transducers are susceptible to oxygenation, and it has been demonstrated that they contribute to the progression of psoriasis [2]. Since 1959, drugs containing dimethyl fumarate (DMF) have been used orally in the treatment of various stages of psoriasis with considerable success [2]. DMF acts by chemically modifying the repressor protein Keap 1 that allows stabilisation and transfer to the cell nucleus of the transcription factor Nrf2, which in turn results in the activation of a cascade of several pathways with cytoprotective and antioxidative properties [155]. Keap1 is among the most important intracellular markers of the redox state, sensitive to inorganic and organic hydroxides, peroxynitrites, and other electrophilic molecules forming under the conditions of oxidative stress and tissue damage [156]. The results of in vitro studies and experiments on animal models indicate that DMF mediates the increase of glutathione levels and NADPH induction [2].

Studies conducted on psoriasis patients corroborated the effectiveness of exogenous antioxidants as a supplementary therapy in the course of pharmacological psoriasis treatment. Madhulatha and Vijayabhaskar [157] demonstrated a significant decrease of MDA and increased total antioxidative capacity (TAC) in the blood serum of patients receiving pharmacological treatment already after eight weeks of therapy using a mixture of antioxidants (30 mg β-carotene + 27.5 mg zinc sulphate monohydrate + 0.2 mg monohydrated selenium dioxide + 2 mg manganese + 1 mg copper). In a study by Kharaeva at al. [158], 58 patients suffering from severe psoriasis or psoriatic arthritis underwent supplementary treatment entailing oral administration of a mixture of oxidants: Q10 coenzymes, vitamin E, and selenium. After a month of therapy, normalisation was observed in terms of CAT and SOD activity in granulocytes and epidermal cells affected by psoriasis, as compared to the control group of psoriasis patients receiving placebo. Also in a study conducted on isolated Colo-16 cells exposed to UVB radiation, a decrease in ROS levels and increased activity of SOD and CAT was observed after the use of vitamin C and E and Ginsenoside Panaxatriol [159]. At the same time, in a study by Abdel-Mawla et al. [48], a therapy using a mixture of antioxidants (100 μg selenium + 1500 IU vitamin A + 90 mg vitamin C + 30 mg vitamin E) administered orally in the form of pills to psoriasis patients proved ineffective when compared to patients not receiving antioxidants as it failed to improve their antioxidative parameters (MDA, SOD, CAT) and skin condition. The latter results are difficult to explain given the fact that numerous authors have reported improvement of the antioxidative parameters in psoriasis patients even when using considerably lower doses of antioxidants. For instance, Kharaeva et al. [158] administered a mixture of antioxidants containing

50 mg of vitamin E, 48 μg of selenium, and 50 mg of coenzyme Q10 to their patients and observed improvement of antioxidative parameters after 30–50 days of therapy (Table 2).

Table 2. Protective effects of dietary antioxidants on the antioxidative status in patients with psoriasis.

Antioxidant/Design	Duration of Therapy	Characteristic	Target Sites	Antioxidant Capacity	References
Tablet containing 100 μg selenium + 1500 IU vitamin A + 90 mg vitamin C + 30 mg vitamin E; once daily	4 weeks	Seven psoriatic patients, different severities	Plasma, erythrocytes	≈ MDA; ≈ CAT; ≈ SOD	[48]
Epigallocatechin-3-gallate EGCG glycerin solvent (3%, 30 mg/mL, glycerin solvent: 50% glycerin, 50% normal saline)	3 weeks	Imiquimod induced psoriasis-like BALB/c mice	Serum	↑ SOD; ↑ CAT; ↓ MDA	[153]
30 mg β-carotene + 27.5 mg zinc sulfate monohydrate + 0.2 mg monohydrated selenium dioxide + 2 mg manganese + 1 mg copper	8 weeks	33 patients, 20–60 years, chronic plaque psoriasis	Serum	↓ MDA; ↑ TAC	[157]
50 mg/d coenzyme Q10 (ubiquinone acetate) + 50 mg/d vitamin E (natural alpha-tocopherol) + 48 μg/d selenium (aspartate salt) dissolved in soy lecithin	30–35 days	58 patients, severe erythrodermic and arthropathic forms of psoriasis	Granulocytes, affected epidermis	↑ SOD; ↑ CAT	[158]
Nigella sativa ointment (20% w/w); *Nigella sativa* capsule (500 mg seeds powder)	12 weeks	60 patients, 3 groups: Group 1 (control)—methotrexate tablets; Group 2—*Nigella sativa* ointment 2 times daily + *Nigella sativa* capsule 3 times daily; Group 3—methotrexate tablets + *Nigella sativa* (ointment + capsule).	Serum	↓ MDA	[160]

↑—Increased concentration or activity in comparison to the control (untreated) group; ↓—decreased or inhibited concentration or activity in comparison to the control (untreated) group; ≈ no differences in comparison to the control (untreated) group; TAC—total antioxidant capacity; MDA—malondialdehyde; SOD—superoxide dismutase; CAT—catalase.

A study conducted in a group of 28 psoriasis patients revealed that methotrexate, an organic compound belonging to the group of folic acid antagonists and used as a cytostatic drug (thanks to the inhibition of the NF-κB transcription factor whose excessive transcription can lead to increased production of IL-6 and IL-8 interleukins in the skin), apart from slowing down the multiplication of quickly dividing cells, is also capable of improving oxidative stress parameters (↓ MDA, ↑ total antioxidant capacity TAC) as compared to patients not receiving the drug [43]. It was additionally observed that the use of methotrexate alleviates dermal symptoms of psoriasis measured with the PASI scale. In turn, Barygina et al. [161] concluded that low doses (10 fg per mL) of IL-4, IL-10, and IL-11 cytokines administered orally reduce oxidative stress in the primary fibroblasts of skin fragments affected by psoriasis. Dermal fibroblasts provide a vital microenvironment for the epidermal function of keratocytes, and upon infiltration of polymorphonuclear leukocytes they start to intensively produce peroxide and H_2O_2, disrupting the redox equilibrium in psoriatic skin. In a clinical study, the cited authors concluded that oral administration of cytokines also resulted in a significant reduction of the PASI index compared to psoriasis patients not receiving cytokines. Cytokines influence the growth, proliferation, and excitation of cells, apart from being involved in the organism's immune response, they also partake in pathological processes and show cytotoxic effects [162]. Moreover, some cytokines not only show antioxidative properties [43] but indeed their expression is affected by the cellular redox status [61], which is why it is vital to stabilise their levels in psoriasis patients. Interleukins IL-12 and IL-23 have been discovered to play a vital role in the pathogenesis of psoriasis through their participation in the interaction between immune system cells and proinflammatory cytokines [163]. They stimulate the differentiation of T lymphocytes into the subpopulation of Th1 and Th17, and subsequently their proliferation, which constitutes a source of other inflammatory mediators, e.g., TNF-α, IL-6, and IFN-γ, although currently, the greatest focus is on IL-17 and IL-22 [160].

A study conducted in a group of 60 psoriasis patients revealed that a 12-week treatment with the seeds of *Nigella sativa* in the form of ointment containing oil and/or small capsules taken orally resulted in a decrease in blood serum MDA and partial alleviation of skin lesions compared to patients receiving standard methotrexate treatment [164]. In the cited study, particularly spectacular effects were reported for the simultaneous use of the ointment and capsules. Also a study conducted on a rabbit model yielded increased GSH levels and lowered MDA in the blood serum and liver after 39 days of using a paste containing powdered *Nigella sativa* seeds, as compared to rabbits receiving methotrexate [165]. Nigella also shows antioxidative properties that exceed those of ascorbic acid and α-tocopherol [166,167], and its consumption facilities a better antioxidative capacity of the organism. The above properties stem from the content of numerous phenolic compounds [56].

The use of diatomic hydrogen molecules (H_2) has been found to be safe and effective due to their antioxidative and immunomodulating properties with negligible side effects [168,169]. Unlike other antioxidants unable to target specific organelles, H_2 can penetrate biomembranes and enter the cytosol, mitochondria and cell nuclei [168]. It has been proven to selectively eliminate ROS and show a positive impact on cytokine balance, particularly proinflammatory Th1 and Th2 [170]. H_2 inhibits the chain reaction producing lipid peroxides and generating oxidative stress markers related to exacerbation of psoriasis symptoms. Moreover, the peroxynitrite formed in the reaction between nitrogen oxide and peroxide activated the p38 MAPK pathways related to the production of inflammatory cytokines such as TNF-α, IL-6 and IL-8, which stimulates the development of dermal psoriatic lesions [170]. The available research results pertain to hydrogen water (solubilised H_2) administered orally and externally, as well as effective inhalation of hydrogen gas and injections of normal saline with H_2 [169]. Zhu et al. [170] put 41 psoriasis patients through a treatment supplementary to the standard therapy and entailing baths in hydrogen water, which yielded positive results as measured in terms of PASI. A study conducted in a group of three psoriasis patients with the use of H_2 in the form of saline injections (containing 1 ppm of H_2), 3% H_2 inhalations, and drinking water containing a high concentration of H_2 (5–7 ppm) corroborated the high effectiveness of the treatment employed, as assessed on the basis of PASI and inflammatory cytokine levels [19]. Of the three methods of H_2 administration, inhalation proved particularly effective, which may be due to the fact that H_2 is absorbed into arterial blood in the lungs, which allows it to circulate in the organism and be ultimately released through the skin. The cited authors concluded that the beneficial effects were due to the high antioxidative activity of H_2, as evidenced by the lowered serum levels of proinflammatory cytokines playing a key role in the pathogenesis of psoriasis, as compared to the pretreatment levels of the same. This suggests the participation of internally produced free radicals in the progression of psoriatic lesions, as well as the therapeutic potential of H_2. Administering H_2 reduces the expression of oxidative stress markers such as myeloperoxidase (MPO), MDA, 8-hydroxy-deoxyguanosine 8-OHdG, 8-iso-prostaglandin F2a and substances reactive with thiobarbituric acid in humans and animal models [171].

7. Perspectives

What can be inferred from the available literature is that the main research focus ought to be on effectively combining pharmacological therapy with the use of exogenous antioxidants in the treatment of psoriasis patients or persons predisposed for this disease. Nutrigenomics seems promising in this context as it guarantees a multiaspect approach to the question at hand. The focus of nutrigenomics is on the impact of food ingredients on the expression of genes, i.e., the functioning of cells [172]. Nutrients act as ligands for the receptors of transcription factors, serve as signalling particles and are metabolised in order to modify the concentrations of substrates or intermediates formed in the altered phenotype. Nutrigenomics is still a young science and its concepts are not easy to implement given the difficulty inherent in corroborating interaction between a given gene and a given nutrient in the course of clinical studies, primarily due to the chemical complexity of food and genetic diversity of humans resulting in different physiological response to particular food ingredients. Nonetheless, it has been demonstrated that dietary factors can affect the level of DNA methylation in humans [173]. Antioxidant-rich diets facilitate DNA demethylation by repairing enzymes, which was evidenced in an experiment where volunteers received a diet containing 300 g of vegetables and 25 mL of chestnut oil for a period of eight weeks [174]. Environmental and dietary factors, particularly isolated nutrients or bioactive compounds, can also control microRNA. It is a group of small, endogenous, single-strand, noncoding RNA with the length of 20–22 nucleotides, partaking in the regulation of gene expression at the post-transcription level by way of epigenetic changes, and identified as regulators of many metabolic processes [175]. MicroRNA molecules are usually involved in post-transcriptional gene silencing by inducing mRNA degradation or translational repression through binding with target informational RNA [176]. It has been demonstrated that they are involved in skin morphogenesis. The therapeutic effects of microRNA inhibition or overexpression have been observed on mice models [177]. Given the role thereof as the main triggers of complex cellular processes, they may potentially serve therapeutic purposes in inflammatory skin conditions.

Hawkes et al. [175] demonstrated incorrect expression in over 250 microRNA isolated from psoriasis-affected keratinocytes, adjacent healthy cells, and peripheral blood of patients. In the course of psoriasis, the balance between the respective types of microRNA is upset due to incorrect expression, which suggests that it may indeed constitute one of the primary causes of the disease [178,179]. It has also been observed that inflammatory processes and disruptions of the redox equilibrium stem from incorrect expression of microRNA, which suggests the influence of some substances present in food on the endogenic synthesis of microRNA under experimental conditions, both in vivo and in vitro. Numerous data corroborate the beneficial impact of antioxidants on the microRNA equilibrium. For instance, quercetin, a flavonoid present in fruit, effectively elevates the level of MiR-146a, which leads to a reduction of proinflammatory NF-κB and decreased expression of TNF-α, IL-6, and IL-17 [180,181]. In turn, vitamin D and quercetin modulate miR-125b, which regulates the transcription of NF-κB and expression of proinflammatory cytokines [178]. Studies conducted on mice receiving, for six weeks, a diet rich in quercetin dosed at 0.1 mg g^{-1} of feed, revealed reduced expression of proinflammatory miR-155, which resulted in inhibition of NF-κB activation [182]. Resveratrol, vitamin D, and curcumin cause a decrease in miR-21 and miR-155, which regulates anti-inflammatory mechanisms by reducing the production of proinflammatory cytokines, such as TNF-α, IL-1β, IL-6, and IL-8 [178,183,184]. In a study with the use of human monocytes, Tili et al. [185] demonstrated that resveratrol increased the level of anti-inflammatory miR-663 and lowered proinflammatory miR-155, which affected the expression of cytokines. Similar results with respect to proinflammatory miR-21 in human glioma cells were reported by Li et al. [183]. Hydroxytyrosol is a phenolic compound present in olive oil which has proven antioxidative properties. Its direct application on macrophages results in the reduction of proinflammatory miR-146a levels therein [186].

Diet manipulation may be a promising therapeutic approach in modulating the risk of chronic diseases. Therefore, it is advisable for psoriasis patients and persons predisposed for the disease to consume functional food, primarily containing high quantities of antioxidants. However, for this potential to be fulfilled, further consistent and intensive scientific scrutiny will be required.

8. Conclusions

One should first consider whether oxidative stress is a cause or effect of psoriasis (Figure 1). The emergence of disease symptoms under conditions of oxidative stress as well as the clear improvement of the redox status in patients receiving exogenous antioxidants as well as the observable improvement of their general condition seem to suggest that oxidative stress may indeed be a cause of psoriasis.

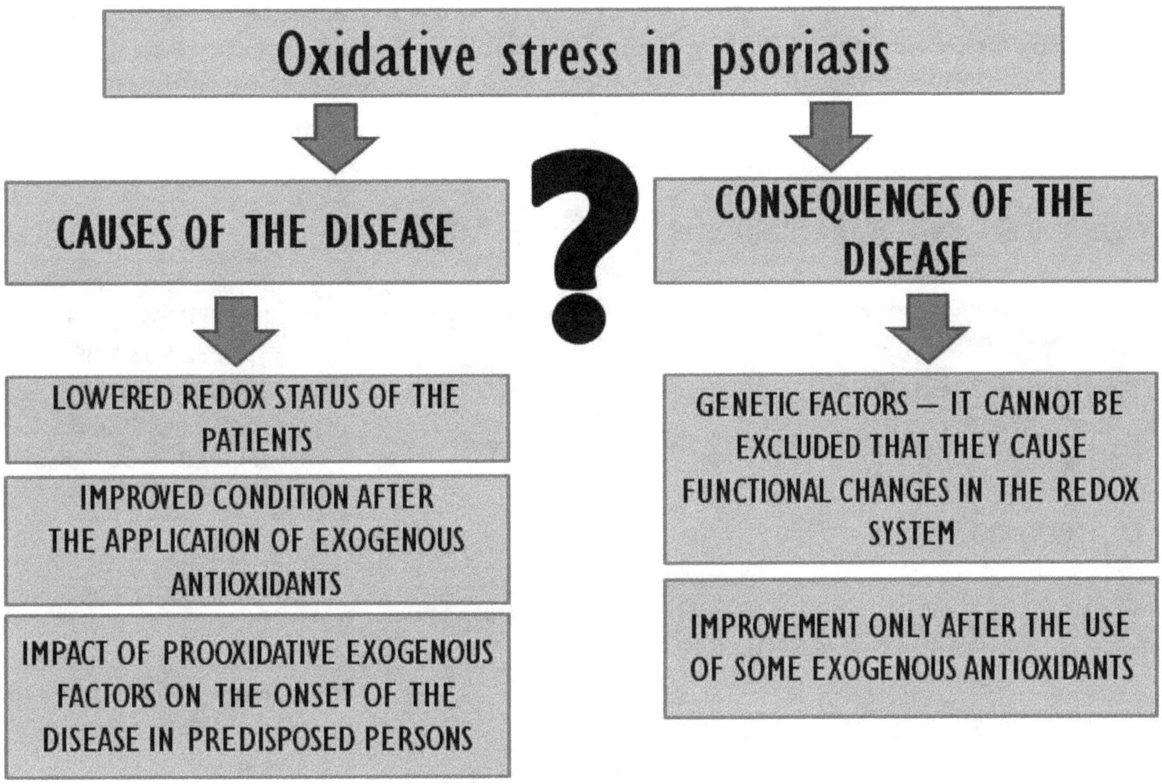

Figure 1. Oxidative stress in psoriasis—causes or consequences of the disease.

On the other hand, however, the fact that only some exogenous antioxidants prove effective despite the improvement in terms of the redox status as such would indicate that oxidative stress may be a consequence of the disease. Moreover, the available literature was found to lack data with regard to the redox status of persons genetically predisposed for but not suffering from psoriasis, it is therefore unclear whether the antioxidant levels in people whose genome includes genes responsible for the onset of the disease are imbalanced, and therefore whether the genes as such trigger functional changes in the redox system. In order to inactivate free radicals and stabilise cellular membranes, as well as to prevent further damage to the epidermis, one should consider the prophylactic consumption of antioxidants by genetically burdened persons and using the same to complement traditional therapy if the disease occurs. It is also worth considering certain lifestyle changes in the case of psoriasis patients, as research suggests that unhygienic habits (drug use, smoking, alcohol use) tend to increase the production of ROS in the organism and exacerbate the symptoms of psoriasis [35]. It is noteworthy that some ROS act only as signal messengers regulating a wide spectrum of physiological processes [187], which means that the perfect antioxidant ought to alleviate excessive oxidative stress but, at the same time, not interfere with redox homeostasis. Effective improvement of antioxidative parameters tends to be more viable with the use of a mixture of antioxidants as their respective effects will complement each other. It is necessary to develop a combination of pharmacological treatment and dietary antioxidant supplementation in psoriasis patients that would yield optimum results in the context of treatment and prevention. The results of numerous studies reveal that regular consumption of antioxidants in the diet can improve the organism's antioxidative capacity and stabilise the related equilibrium. High consumption of fresh fruit and vegetables correlates with lower incidence of the disease [63–65]. The diet of people suffering from or genetically predisposed for psoriasis should include antioxidative n-3 fatty acids, vitamins C, A, D, E, and B-complex, with a simultaneous minimization of sweets and alcohol consumption (Figure 2). They should be encouraged to follow a diet rich in polyphenolic compounds such as tea, coffee and a variety of herbs and spices. Unfortunately, the use of diet supplements with antioxidative properties does not always prove effective, which may be due to the dosage of antioxidants and the overall duration of treatment. Promising results have also been reported in the context of nutrigenomics, which guarantees a multiaspect approach to the discussed problem. Future directions may entail detailed studies of psoriasis patients' genetic profiles to allow more accurate targeting of therapeutic solutions.

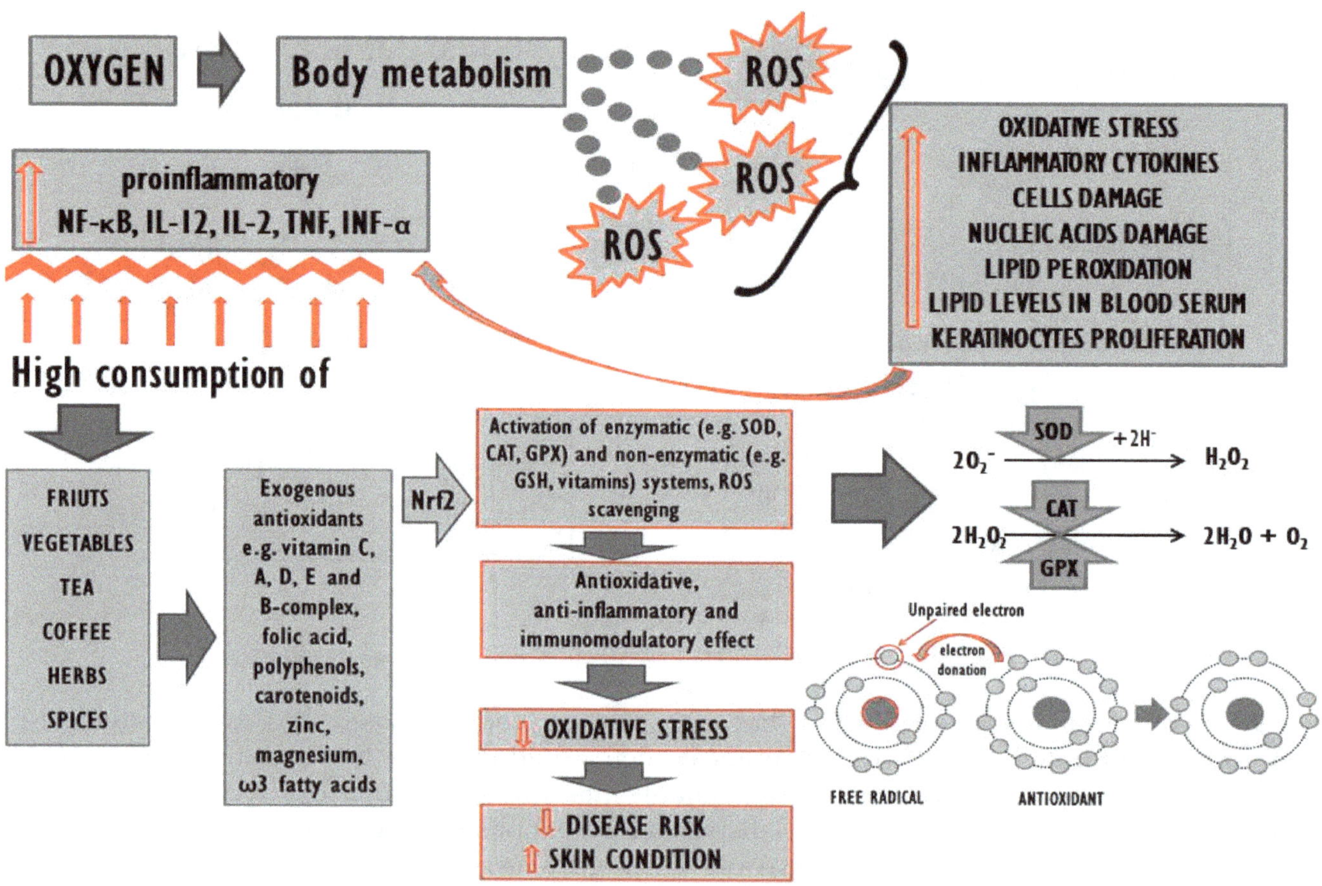

Figure 2. The effects of dietary supplementation with antioxidants in patients with psoriasis. Legends: ROS—reactive oxygen species; SOD—superoxide dismutase; CAT–catalase; GPX—glutathione peroxidase; GSH–glutathione; NF-κB—nuclear factor kappa B; IL–interleukins; TNF—tumour necrosis factor; IFN-α—alpha interferon; Nrf2—nuclear factor erythroid 2-related factor 2.

Author Contributions: Conceptualization, A.W.-M.; methodology, A.W.-M.; resources, A.W.-M., T.M. and G.W.; data curation, A.W.-M. and T.M.; writing—original draft preparation, A.W.-M.; writing—review and editing, T.M. and G.W.; visualization, T.M.; supervision, A.W.-M.; All authors have read and agreed to the published version of the manuscript reported.

References

1. Li, Y.; Liao, W.; Chang, M.; Schrodi, S.J.; Bui, N.; Catanese, J.J.; Poon, A.; Matsunami, N.; Callis-Duffin, K.P.; Leppert, M.F.; et al. Further genetic evidence for three psoriasis-risk genes: ADAM33, CDKAL1, and PTPN22. *J. Investig. Dermatol.* **2009**, *129*, 629–634. [CrossRef] [PubMed]
2. Zhou, Q.; Mrowietz, U.; Rostami-Yazdi, M. Oxidative stress in the pathogenesis of psoriasis. *Free Radic. Biol. Med.* **2009**, *47*, 891–905. [CrossRef] [PubMed]
3. Yin, X.Y.; Cheng, H.; Wang, W.J.; Wang, W.J.; Fu, H.Y.; Liu, L.H.; Zhang, F.Y.; Yang, S.; Zhang, X.J. TNIP1/ANXA6 and CSMD1 variants interacting with cigarette smoking, alcohol intake affect risk of psoriasis. *J. Dermatol. Sci.* **2013**, *70*, 94–98. [CrossRef]
4. Capon, F. The genetic basis of psoriasis. *Int. J. Mol. Sci.* **2017**, *18*, 2526. [CrossRef] [PubMed]
5. Deavall, D.G.; Martin, E.A.; Horner, J.M.; Roberts, R. Drug-induced oxidative stress and toxicity. *J. Toxicol.* **2012**, *2012*, 645460. [CrossRef] [PubMed]
6. López-Pedrajas, R.; Ramírez-Lamelas, D.T.; Muriach, B.; Sánchez-Villarejo, M.V.; Almansa, I.; Vidal-Gil, L.; Romero, F.J.; Barcia, J.M.; Muriach, M. Cocaine promotes oxidative stress and microglial-macrophage activation in rat cerebellum. *Front. Cell Neurosci.* **2015**, *9*, 279. [CrossRef]
7. Schiavone, S.; Jaquet, V.; Trabace, L.; Krause, K.H. Severe life stress and oxidative stress in the brain: From animal models to human pathology. *Antioxid. Redox Signal.* **2013**, *18*, 1475–1490. [CrossRef]
8. Roszkiewicz, M.; Dopytalska, K.; Szymańska, E.; Jakimiuk, A.; Walecka, I. Environmental risk factors and epigenetic alternations in psoriasis. *Ann. Agric. Environ. Med.* **2019**, 209184367, in press. [CrossRef]
9. Winiarska-Mieczan, A. Protective effect of tea against lead and cadmium-induced oxidative stress—a review. *Biometals* **2018**, *31*, 909–926. [CrossRef]
10. Partyka, A.; Czopek, A.; Stanisz-Wallis, K.; Zagórska, A. The use of biopharmaceuticals in the treatment of psoriasis. *Postepy Hig. Med. Dosw.* **2018**, *72*, 642–658. [CrossRef]
11. Shilov, V.N.; Sergienko, V.I. Oxidative stress in keratinocytes as an etiopathogenetic factor of psoriasis. *Bull. Exp. Biol. Med.* **2000**, *129*, 364–369. [CrossRef]
12. Baliwag, J.; Barnes, D.; Johnston, A. Cytokines in psoriasis. *Cytokine* **2015**, *73*, 342–350. [CrossRef] [PubMed]
13. Brembilla, N.C.; Senra, L.; Boehncke, W.H. The IL-17 family of cytokines in psoriasis: IL-17A and beyond. *Front. Immunol.* **2018**, *9*, 1682. [CrossRef]
14. de Gruijl, F.R.; van der Leun, J.C. Environment and health: 3. Ozone depletion and ultraviolet radiation. *Can. Med. Assoc. J.* **2000**, *163*, 851–855.
15. Oresajo, C.; Pillai, S.; Manco, M.; Yatskayer, M.; McDaniel, D. Antioxidants and the skin: Understanding formulation and efficacy. *Dermatol. Ther.* **2012**, *25*, 252–259. [CrossRef]
16. Zhang, P.; Wu, M.X. A clinical review of phototherapy for psoriasis. *Lasers Med. Sci.* **2018**, *33*, 173–180. [CrossRef] [PubMed]
17. Fattahi, S.; Kazemipour, N.; Hashemi, M.; Sepehrimanesh, M. Alpha-1 antitrypsin, retinol binding protein and keratin 10 alterations in patients with psoriasis vulgaris, a proteomic approach. *Iran. J. Basic Med. Sci.* **2014**, *17*, 651–655.
18. Rocha-Pereira, P.; Santos-Silva, A.; Rebelo, I.; Figueiredo, A.; Quintanilha, A.; Teixeira, F.J. The inflammatory response in mild and in severe psoriasis. *Brit. J. Dermatol.* **2004**, *150*, 917–928. [CrossRef]
19. Ishibashi, T.; Ichikawa, M.; Sato, B.; Shibata, S.; Hara, Y.; Naritomi, Y.; Okazaki, K.; Nakashima, Y.; Iwamoto, Y.; Koyanagi, S.; et al. Improvement of psoriasis-associated arthritis and skin lesions by treatment with molecular hydrogen: A report of three cases. *Mol. Med. Rep.* **2015**, *12*, 2757–2764. [CrossRef]
20. Mailloux, R.J.; Xiaolei, J.; Willmore, W.G. Redox regulation of mitochondrial function with emphasis on cysteine oxidation reactions. *Redox Biol.* **2014**, *2*, 123–139. [CrossRef]
21. Winiarska-Mieczan, A.; Baranowska-Wójcik, E.; Kwiecień, M.; Grela, E.R.; Szwajgier, D.; Kwiatkowska, K.; Kiczorowska, B. The role of dietary antioxidants in the pathogenesis of neurodegenerative diseases and their impact on cerebral oxidoreductive balance. *Nutrients* **2020**, *12*, 435. [CrossRef]
22. Mikhed, Y.; Daiber, A.; Steven, S. Mitochondrial oxidative stress, mitochondrial DNA damage and their role in age-related vascular dysfunction. *Int. J. Mol. Sci.* **2015**, *16*, 15918–15953. [CrossRef] [PubMed]

23. Du, J.; Zhu, M.; Bao, H.; Li, B.; Dong, Y.; Xiao, C.; Zhang, G.Y.; Henter, I.; Rudorfer, M.; Vitiello, B. The role of nutrients in protecting mitochondrial function and neurotransmitter signaling: Implications for the treatment of depression, ptsd, and suicidal behaviors. *Crit. Rev. Food Sci. Nutr.* **2016**, *56*, 2560–2578. [CrossRef] [PubMed]
24. Kizilyel, O.; Akdeniz, N.; Metin, M.S.; Elmas, Ö.F. Investigation of oxidant and antioxidant levels in patients with psoriasis. *Turk. J. Med. Sci.* **2019**, *49*, 1085–1088. [CrossRef] [PubMed]
25. Pawłowska, M.; Mila-Kierzenkowska, C.; Kwiatkowska, A.; Paprocki, J.; Sutkowy, P.; Woźniak, A. Evaluation of selected parameters of oxidative stress in patients with psoriasis. *Diagn. Lab.* **2016**, *52*, 101–106.
26. Priya, R.; Kumar, U.; Saran, A.; Kumari, R.; Koschore, C. Oxidative stress in psoriasis. *Biomed. Res.* **2013**, *25*, 132–134.
27. Giridharan, S.; Srinivasan, M. Mechanisms of NF-κB p65 and strategies for therapeutic manipulation. *J. Inflam. Res.* **2018**, *11*, 407–419. [CrossRef]
28. Li, S.; Yan, T.; Yang, J.Q.; Oberley, T.D.; Oberley, L.W. The role of cellular glutathione peroxidase redox regulation in the suppression of tumor cell growth by manganese superoxide dismutase. *Cancer Res.* **2000**, *60*, 3927–3939.
29. Ulrich, K.; Jakob, U. The role of thiols in antioxidant systems. *Free Radic. Biol. Med.* **2019**, *140*, 14–27. [CrossRef]
30. Ezerina, D.; Takano, Y.; Hanaoka, K.; Urano, Y.; Dick, T.P. N-acetyl cysteine functions as a fast-acting antioxidant by triggering intracellular H_2S and sulfane sulfur production. *Cell Chem. Biol.* **2018**, *25*, 447–459. [CrossRef]
31. Pouya, V.T.; Hashemy, I.; Shoeibi, A.; Tirkani, A.N.; Tavallaie, S.; Avval, F.Z.; Soukhtanloo, M.; Mashkani, B.; Alamdari, D.H. Serum pro-oxidant-antioxidant balance, advanced oxidized protein products (AOPP) and protein carbonyl in patients with stroke. *Razavi Int. J. Med.* **2016**, *4*, e38203.
32. Bradshaw, P.C. Cytoplasmic and mitochondrial NADPH-Coupled redox systems in the regulation of aging. *Nutrients* **2019**, *11*, 504. [CrossRef] [PubMed]
33. Ondei, L.S.; Silveira, L.M.; Leite, A.A.; Souza, D.R.S.; Pinhel, M.A.S.; Percário, S.; Ricci Júnior, O.; Bonini-Domingos, C.R. Lipid peroxidation and antioxidant capacity of G6PD-deficient patients with A-(202G>A) mutation. *Genet. Mol. Res.* **2009**, *8*, 1345–1351. [CrossRef] [PubMed]
34. Kadam, D.P.; Suryakar, A.N.; Ankush, R.D.; Kadam, C.Y.; Deshpande, K.H. Role of oxidative stress in various stages of psoriasis. *Indian J. Clin. Biochem.* **2010**, *25*, 388–392. [CrossRef]
35. Kute, P.K.; Muddeshwar, M.G.; Sonare, A.R. Pro-oxidant and anti-oxidant status in patients of psoriasis with relation to smoking and alcoholism. *J. Evol. Med. Dent. Sci.* **2019**, *8*, 2677–2680.
36. Wójcik, P.; Biernacki, M.; Wroński, A.; Łuczaj, W.; Waeg, G.; Žarković, N.; Skrzydlewska, E. Altered lipid metabolism in blood mononuclear cells of psoriatic patients indicates differential changes in psoriasis vulgaris and psoriatic arthritis. *Int. J. Mol. Sci.* **2019**, *20*, 4249. [CrossRef]
37. Pujari, V.M.; Ireddy, S.; Itagi, I.; Siddesh, K.H. The serum levels of malondialdehyde, vitamin E and erythrocyte catalase activity in psoriasis patients. *J. Clin. Diagn. Res.* **2014**, *8*, 14–16. [CrossRef]
38. Skutnik-Radziszewska, A.; Maciejczyk, M.; Fejfer, K.; Krahel, J.; Flisiak, I.; Kołodziej, U.; Zalewska, A. Salivary antioxidants and oxidative stress in psoriatic patients: Can salivary total oxidant status and oxidative status index be a plaque psoriasis biomarker? *Oxid. Med. Cell. Longev.* **2020**, *2020*, 9086024. [CrossRef]
39. Alwasiti, E.A.R.K.; Al-Rubayee, W.T.; Al-Tammimy, S.M. Serum copper, zinc and oxidative stress in patients with psoriasis. *Iraqi. J. Med. Sci.* **2011**, *9*, 137–142.
40. Üstüner, P.; Balevi, A.; Özdemir, M.; Olmusçelik, O.; Ülfer, G.; Yigitbasi, T. The role of thiol/disulfide homeostasis in psoriasis: Can it be a new marker for inflammation? *Turk. Arch. Dermatol. Venerol. Turkderm* **2018**, *52*, 120–125. [CrossRef]
41. Aksoy, M.E.; Kirmit, A. Thiol/disulphide balance in patients with psoriasis. *Adv. Dermatol. Allergol.* **2018**, *37*, 52–55. [CrossRef] [PubMed]
42. Kilic, A.; Yorulmaz, A.; Erdogan, S.; Cakmak, S.K.; Guney, E.; Sen, O.; Erel, O. An evaluation of thiol/disulphide homeostasis in patients with psoriasis. *Adv. Dermatol. Allergol.* **2017**, *5*, 464–467. [CrossRef]
43. Boda, D.; Negrei, C.; Nicolescu, F.; Bălălău, C. Assessment of some oxidative stress parameters in methotrexate treated psoriasis patients. *Farmacia* **2014**, *62*, 704–710.
44. Nemati, H.; Khodarahmi, R.; Sadeghi, M.; Ebrahimi, A.; Rezaei, M.; Vaisi-Raygani, A. Antioxidant status in patients with psoriasis. *Cell Biochem. Funct.* **2014**, *32*, 268–273.

45. Pietrzak, A.; Chabros, P.; Grywalska, E.; Kiciński, P.; Pietrzak-Franciszkiewicz, K.; Krasowska, D.; Kandzierski, G. Serum lipid metabolism in psoriasis and psoriatic arthritis—an update. *Arch. Med. Sci.* **2019**, *15*, 369–375. [CrossRef] [PubMed]
46. Asha, K.; Singal, A.; Sharma, S.B.; Arora, V.K.; Aggarwal, A. Dyslipidaemia & oxidative stress in patients of psoriasis: Emerging cardiovascular risk factors. *Indian J. Med. Res.* **2017**, *146*, 677–679.
47. Kiran, P.U.; Deedi, M.K. Study of MDA and SGPT levels in patients with psoriasis. *J. Evol. Res. Med. Biochem.* **2015**, *1*, 9–13.
48. Abdel-Mawla, M.Y.; Nofal, E.; Khalifa, N.; Abdel-Shakoor, R.; Nasr, M. Role of oxidative stress in psoriasis: An evaluation study. *J. Am. Sci.* **2013**, *9*, 151–155.
49. Metta, S.; Kumar, M.A.; Basalingappa, R.D.; Uppala, S.; Mohanty, S. Circulatory markers of oxidative stress and dyslipidemia in male patients of chronic plaque psoriasis. *Int. J. Med. Public Health* **2015**, *5*, 208–212.
50. Kaur, M.; Sharma, S.; Kukreja, S.; Kaur, J.; Bassi, R. Study of oxidative stress in patients of psoriasis. *Int. J. Res. Dermatol.* **2016**, *2*, 95–98. [CrossRef]
51. Altu'ma, F.J.; Al-Hassan, A.T.A.; Al-Da'amy, A.M.A. Correlation between malondialdehyde and dyslipidemia in psoriatic patients. *J. Contemp. Med. Sci.* **2016**, *2*, 56–58.
52. Şikar Aktürk, A.; Özdoğan, H.K.; Bayramgürler, D.; Çekmen, M.B.; Bilen, N.; Kıran, R. Nitric oxide and malondialdehyde levels in plasma and tissue of psoriasis patients. *J. Eur. Acad. Dermatol. Venereol.* **2012**, *26*, 833–837. [CrossRef] [PubMed]
53. Gupta, M.; Chari, S.; Borkar, M.; Chandankhede, M. Dyslipidemia and oxidative stress in patients of psoriasis. *Biomed. Res.* **2011**, *22*, 222–225.
54. Johnson, J.A.; Ma, C.; Kanada, K.N.; Armstrong, A.W. Diet and nutrition in psoriasis: Analysis of the National Health and Nutrition Examination Survey (NHANES) in the United States. *J. Eur. Acad. Dermatol. Venereol.* **2014**, *28*, 327–332. [CrossRef] [PubMed]
55. Bojarowicz, H.; Woźniak, B. Polyunsaturated fatty acids and their influence on skin condition. *Probl. Hig. Epidemiol.* **2008**, *89*, 471–475.
56. Kadam, D.; Lele, S.S. Extraction, characterization and bioactive properties of *Nigella sativa* seedcake. *J. Food Sci. Technol.* **2017**, *54*, 3936–3947. [CrossRef]
57. Kokcam, I.; Naziroglu, M. Antioxidants and lipid peroxidation status in the blood of patients with psoriasis. *Clin. Chim. Acta* **1999**, *289*, 23–31. [CrossRef]
58. Bacchetti, T.; Campanati, A.; Ferretti, G.; Simonetti, O.; Liberati, G.; Offidani, A.M. Oxidative stress and psoriasis: The effect of antitumour necrosis factor-α inhibitor treatment. *Br. J. Dermatol.* **2013**, *168*, 984–989. [CrossRef]
59. Barygina, V.; Becatti, M.; Lotti, T.; Taddei, N.; Fiorillo, C. Low dose cytokines reduce oxidative stress in primary lesional fibroblasts obtained from psoriatic patients. *J. Dermatol. Sci.* **2016**, *83*, 242–244. [CrossRef]
60. Tekin, N.S.; Tekin, I.O.; Barut, F.; Sipahi, E.Y. Accumulation of oxidized low-density lipoprotein in psoriatic skin and changes of plasma lipid levels in psoriatic patients. *Mediat. Inflamm.* **2007**, *2007*, 78454.
61. Portugal-Cohen, M.; Horev, L.; Ruffer, C.; Schlippe, G.; Voss, W.; Ma'or, Z.; Oron, M.; Soroka, Y.; Frušić-Zlotkin, M.; Milner, Y.; et al. Non-invasive skin biomarkers quantification of psoriasis and atopic dermatitis: Cytokines, antioxidants and psoriatic skin auto-fluorescence. *Biomed. Pharmacother.* **2012**, *66*, 293–299. [CrossRef] [PubMed]
62. Kwon, M.J.; Kim, B.; Lee, Y.S.; Kim, T.Y. Role of superoxide dismutase 3 in skin inflammation. *J. Dermatol. Sci.* **2012**, *67*, 81–87. [CrossRef] [PubMed]
63. Amin, S.S.; Adil, M.; Alam, M. Role of dietary intervention in psoriasis: A review. *Ind. J. Clin. Dermatol.* **2017**, *1*, 1–5.
64. Duarte, G.; Barbosa, L.O.; Rosa, M.E.A. The management of psoriasis through diet. *Psoriasis* **2012**, *2*, 45–53. [CrossRef]
65. Wong, A.P.; Kalinovsky, T.; Niedzwiecki, A.; Rath, M. Efficacy of nutritional treatment in patients with psoriasis: A case report. *Exp. Therap. Med.* **2015**, *10*, 1071–1073. [CrossRef]
66. Kim, M.K.; Cho, S.W.; Park, Y.K. Long-term vegetarians have low oxidative stress, body fat, and cholesterol levels. *Nutr. Res. Pract.* **2012**, *6*, 155–161. [CrossRef]
67. Peluso, I.; Raguzzini, A.; Catasta, G.; Cammisotto, V.; Perrone, A.; Tomino, C.; Toti, E.; Serafini, M. Effects of high consumption of vegetables on clinical, immunological, and antioxidant markers in subjects at risk of cardiovascular diseases. *Oxid. Med. Cell. Longev.* **2018**, *2018*, 5417165. [CrossRef] [PubMed]

68. Nälsén, C.; Basu, S.; Wolk, A.; Vessby, B. The importance of dietary antioxidants on plasma antioxidant capacity and lipid peroxidation in vivo in middle-aged men. *Scand. J. Food Nutr.* **2006**, *50*, 64–70. [CrossRef]
69. Araujo, M.L.; Burgos, M.G.; Moura, I.S. Nutritional influences in psoriasis. *An. Bras. Dermatol.* **2009**, *84*, 90–92. [CrossRef]
70. Mari, N.L.; Santos, L.F.R.F.; Alfieri, D.F.; Fauzino, T.; Lozovoy, M.A.B.; Martin, L.M.M.; Kipper, J.P.; Lena, C.P.; da Silva Taguti, P.; Colado Simão, A.N.; et al. Supplementation with fish oil improves life quality, and decreases inflammatory status and oxidative stress in psoriasis. *Clin. Res. Trials* **2018**, *4*, 1–7.
71. Solis, M.Y.; de Melo, N.S.; Macedo, M.E.; Carneiro, F.P.; Sabbag, C.Y.; Lancha Júnior, A.H.; Frangella, V.S. Nutritional status and food intake of patients with systemic psoriasis and psoriatic arthritis associated. *Einstein* **2012**, *10*, 44–52. [CrossRef] [PubMed]
72. Barrea, L.; Balato, N.; Di Somma, C.; Macchia, P.; Napolitano, M.; Savanelli, M.; Esposito, K.; Colao, A.; Savastano, S. Nutrition and psoriasis: Is there any association between the severity of the disease and adherence to the Mediterranean diet? *J. Translat. Med.* **2015**, *13*, 18. [CrossRef] [PubMed]
73. Leite, B.F.; Morimoto, M.A.; Gomes, C.; de Carvalho Klemz, B.N.; de Souza Genaro, P.; Teixeira Damasceno, N.R.; Szejnfeld, V.L.; de Medeiros Pinheiro, M. Higher bodily adiposity, fat intake, and cholesterol serum levels are associated with higher disease activity in psoriatic arthritis patients: Is there a link among fat and skin and joint involvement? *Lipids Health Dis.* **2020**, *19*, 21. [CrossRef]
74. Yamashita, H.; Morita, T.; Ito, M.; Okazaki, S.; Koto, M.; Ichikawa, Y.; Takayama, R.; Hoashi, T.; Saeki, H.; Kanda, N. Dietary habits in Japanese patients with psoriasis and psoriatic arthritis: Low intake of meat in psoriasis and high intake of vitamin A in psoriatic arthritis. *J. Dermatol.* **2019**, *46*, 759–769. [CrossRef] [PubMed]
75. Afifi, L.; Danesh, M.J.; Lee, K.M.; Beroukhim, K.; Farahnik, B.; Ahn, R.S.; Yan, D.; Singh, R.K.; Nakamura, M.; Koo, J.; et al. Dietary behaviors in psoriasis: Patient-reported outcomes from a U.S. national survey. *Dermatol. Ther.* **2017**, *7*, 227–242. [CrossRef] [PubMed]
76. Al-Katib, S.R.; Al-Wakeel, H.A.; Al-Rawaf, R.F. Role of vitamin C as antioxidant in psoriasis patients treated with NB-UVB phototherapy. *Indian J. Public Health Res. Dev.* **2018**, *9*, 375–380. [CrossRef]
77. Di Nardo, V.; Gianfaldoni, S.; Tchernev, G.; Wollina, U.; Barygina, V.; Lotti, J.; Daaboul, F.; Lott, T. Use of curcumin in psoriasis. *Maced. J. Med. Sci.* **2018**, *6*, 218–220. [CrossRef]
78. Panahi, Y.; Fazlolahzadeh, O.; Atkin, S.L.; Majeed, M.; Butler, A.E.; Johnston, T.P.; Sahebkar, A. Evidence of curcumin and curcumin analogue effects in skin diseases: A narrative review. *J. Cell. Physiol.* **2019**, *234*, 1165–1178. [CrossRef]
79. Antiga, E.; Bonciolini, V.; Volpi, W.; Del Bianco, E.; Caproni, M. Oral curcumin (Meriva) is effective as an adjuvant treatment and is able to reduce IL-22 serum levels in patients with psoriasis vulgaris. *BioMed Res. Int.* **2015**, *2015*, 283634. [CrossRef]
80. Moghadam, A.R.; Tutunchi, S.; Namvaran-Abbas-Abad, A.; Yazdi, M.; Bonyadi, F.; Mohajeri, D.; Mazani, M.; Marzban, H.; Łos, M.J.; Ghavami, S.; et al. Pre-administration of turmeric prevents methotrexate-induced liver toxicity and oxidative stress. *BMC Complement. Altern. Med.* **2015**, *15*, 246. [CrossRef]
81. Yousefi, F.; Lavi Arab, F.; Jaafari, M.R.; Rastin, M.; Tabasi, N.; Hatamipour, M.; Nikkhah, K.; Mahmoudi, M. Immunoregulatory, proliferative and anti-oxidant effects of nanocurcuminoids on adipose-derived mesenchymal stem cells. *EXCLI J.* **2019**, *18*, 405–421. [PubMed]
82. Chen, H.; Liu, H.; Lu, C.; Wang, M.; Li, X.; Zhao, H.; Yan, Y.; Yu, W.; Han, L.; Dai, Z. PSORI-CM02 formula increases CD4+ Foxp3+ regulatory T cell frequency and ameliorates imiquimod-induced psoriasis in mice. *Front. Immunol.* **2018**, *8*, 1767. [CrossRef] [PubMed]
83. Winiarska-Mieczan, A. The potential protective effect of green, black, red and white tea infusions against adverse effect of cadmium and lead during chronic exposure—A rat model study. *Regul. Toxicol. Pharmacol.* **2015**, *73*, 521–529. [CrossRef] [PubMed]
84. Al-Jebori, A.A. Serum selenium in psoriatic patients. *Iraqi J. Comm. Med.* **2007**, *20*, 409–413.
85. Nazıroğlu, M.; Yıldız, K.; Tamtürk, B.; Erturan, İ.; Flores-Arce, M. Selenium and psoriasis. *Biol. Trace Elem. Res.* **2012**, *150*, 3–9. [CrossRef] [PubMed]
86. Serwin, A.B.; Wasowicz, W.; Chodynicka, B. Selenium supplementation, soluble tumor necrosis factor-alpha receptor type 1, and C-reactive protein during psoriasis therapy with narrowband ultraviolet B. *Nutrition* **2006**, *22*, 860–864. [CrossRef]

87. Nga, N.T.T.; An, V.T.; Quang, D.D. Antioxidant properties of folic acid: A DFT study. *Viet. J. Sci. Technol.* **2018**, *56*, 39–45.
88. Aronson, P.J. Cases of psoriasis improved by lowering homocysteine using 4–7 mg folic acid, vitamins B6 and B12 previously worsened using 1–2 mg daily folic acid, B6 and B12 folic acid. *J. Transl. Sci.* **2017**, *3*, 1–6. [CrossRef]
89. Hicks, A. Current status and future development of global tea production and tea products. *AU JT* **2009**, *12*, 251–264.
90. Simos, Y.V.; Verginadis, I.I.; Toliopoulos, I.K.; Velalopoulou, A.P.; Karagounis, I.V.; Karkabounas, S.C.; Evangelou, A.M. Effects of catechin and epicatechin on superoxide dismutase and glutathione peroxidase activity in vivo. *Redox Rep.* **2012**, *17*, 181–186. [CrossRef]
91. Bharadwaz, A.; Bhattacharjee, C. Extraction of polyphenols from dried tea leaves. *J. Sci. Eng. Res.* **2012**, *3*, 1–5.
92. Serafini, M.; Ghiselli, A.; Ferro Luzzi, A. In vivo antioxidant effect of green and black tea in man. *Eur. J. Clin. Nutr.* **1996**, *50*, 28–32. [PubMed]
93. Gawlik, M.; Czajka, A. The effect of green, black and white tea on the level of α and γ tocopherols in free radical-induced oxidative damage of human red blood cells. *Acta Pol. Pharm.* **2007**, *64*, 159–164. [PubMed]
94. Sung, H.; Nah, J.; Chun, S.; Park, H.; Yang, S.E.; Min, W.K. In vivo antioxidant effect of green tea. *Eur. J. Clin. Nutr.* **2000**, *54*, 527–529. [CrossRef] [PubMed]
95. Winiarska-Mieczan, A. Protective effect of tannic acid on the brain of adult rats exposed to cadmium and lead. *Environ. Toxicol. Pharmacol.* **2013**, *36*, 9–18. [CrossRef] [PubMed]
96. Yi, R.; Wang, R.; Sun, P.; Zhao, X. Antioxidant-mediated preventative effect of Dragon-pearl tea crude polyphenol extract on reserpine-induced gastric ulcers. *Exp. Ther. Med.* **2015**, *10*, 338–344. [CrossRef]
97. Roychoudhury, S.; Agarwal, A.; Virk, G.; Cho, C.L. Potential role of green tea catechins in the management of oxidative stress-associated infertility. *Reprod. Biomed. Online* **2017**, *34*, 487–498. [CrossRef]
98. Martini, D.; Del Bo', C.; Tassotti, M.; Riso, P.; Del Rio, D.; Brighenti, F.; Porrini, M. Coffee consumption and oxidative stress: A review of human intervention studies. *Molecules* **2016**, *21*, 979. [CrossRef]
99. Yashin, A.; Yashin, Y.; Wang, J.Y.; Nemzer, B. Antioxidant and antiradical activity of coffee. *Antioxidants* **2013**, *2*, 230–245. [CrossRef]
100. Farah, A.; Donangelo, C.M. Phenolic compounds in coffee. *Braz. J. Plant Physiol.* **2006**, *18*, 23–36. [CrossRef]
101. Nebesny, E.; Budryn, G. Antioxidative activity of green and roasted coffee beans as influenced by convection and microwave roasting methods and content of certain compounds. *Eur. Food Res. Technol.* **2003**, *217*, 157–163. [CrossRef]
102. Natella, F.; Nardini, M.; Giannetti, I.; Dattilo, C.; Scaccini, C. Coffee drinking influences plasma antioxidant capacity in humans. *J. Agric. Food Chem.* **2002**, *50*, 6211–6216. [CrossRef]
103. Zujko, M.E.; Witkowska, A.M. Antioxidant potential and polyphenol content of beverages, chocolates, nuts, and seeds. *Int. J. Food Prop.* **2014**, *17*, 86–92. [CrossRef]
104. Agudelo-Ochoa, G.M.; Pulgarín-Zapata, I.C.; Velásquez-Rodriguez, C.M.; Duque-Ramírez, M.; Naranjo-Cano, M.; Quintero-Ortiz, M.M.; Lara-Guzmán, O.J.; Muñoz-Durango, K. Coffee consumption increases the antioxidant capacity of plasma and has no effect on the lipid profile or vascular function in healthy adults in a randomized controlled trial. *J. Nutr.* **2016**, *146*, 524–531. [CrossRef] [PubMed]
105. Teekachunhatean, S.; Tosri, N.; Sangdee, C.; Wongpoomchai, R.; Ruangyuttikarn, W.; Puaninta, C.; Srichairatanakool, S. Antioxidant effects after coffee enema or oral coffee consumption in healthy Thai male volunteers. *Hum. Exp. Toxicol.* **2012**, *31*, 643–651. [CrossRef]
106. Jung, S.; Kim, M.H.; Park, J.H.; Jeong, Y.; Ko, K.S. Cellular antioxidant and anti-inflammatory effects of coffee extracts with different roasting levels. *J. Med. Food* **2017**, *20*, 626–635. [CrossRef] [PubMed]
107. Danila, A.O.; Gatea, F.; Radu, G.L. Polyphenol composition and antioxidant activity of selected medicinal herbs. *Chem. Nat. Comp.* **2011**, *47*, 22–26. [CrossRef]
108. Iskender, H.; Yenice, G.; Dokumacioglu, E.; Kaynar, O.; Hayirli, A.; Kaya, A. The effects of dietary flavonoid supplementation on the antioxidant status of laying hens. *Braz. J. Poult. Sci.* **2016**, *18*, 663–668. [CrossRef]
109. Verma, P.K.; Raina, R.; Sultana, M.; Singh, M.; Kumar, P. Total antioxidant and oxidant status of plasma and renal tissue of cisplatin-induced nephrotoxic rats: Protection by floral extracts of *Calendula officinalis* Linn. *Ren. Fail.* **2016**, *38*, 142–150. [CrossRef] [PubMed]

110. Tan, C.; Wei, H.; Sun, H.; Ao, J.; Long, G.; Jiang, S.; Peng, J. Effects of dietary supplementation of oregano essential oil to sows on oxidative stress status, lactation feed intake of sows, and piglet performance. *Biomed. Res. Int.* **2015**, *2015*, 525218. [CrossRef]
111. Gümüş, R.; Erol, S.H.; İmik, H.; Halici, M. The effects of the supplementation of lamb rations with oregano essential oil on the performance, some blood parameters and antioxidant metabolism in meat and liver tissues. Kafkas Univ. *Vet. Fak. Derg.* **2017**, *23*, 395–401.
112. Gümüş, R.; Ercan, N.; Imik, H. The effect of thyme essential oil (*Thymus vulgaris*) added to quail diets on performance, some blood parameters, and the antioxidative metabolism of the serum and liver tissues. *Braz. J. Poult. Sci.* **2017**, *19*, 297–304. [CrossRef]
113. El-Nekeety, A.A.; Mohamed, S.R.; Hathout, A.S.; Hassan, N.S.; Aly, S.E.; Abdel-Wahhab, M.A. Antioxidant properties of Thymus vulgaris oil against aflatoxin-induce oxidative stress in male rats. *Toxicon* **2011**, *57*, 984–991. [CrossRef] [PubMed]
114. Abdel-Ghaney, D.M.; El-Far, A.H.; Sadek, K.M.; El-Sayed, Y.S.; Abdel-Latif, M.A. Impact of dietary thyme (*Thymus vulgaris*) on broiler chickens concerning immunity, antioxidant status, and performance. *Alex. J. Vet. Sci.* **2017**, *55*, 169–179.
115. Hoseini, S.M.; Yousefi, M. Beneficial effects of thyme (*Thymus vulgaris*) extract on oxytetracycline-induced stress response, immunosuppression, oxidative stress and enzymatic changes in rainbow trout (*Oncorhynchus mykiss*). *Aquacult. Nutr.* **2019**, *25*, 298–309. [CrossRef]
116. Gedikoğlu, A.; Sökmen, M.; Çivit, A. Evaluation of *Thymus vulgaris* and *Thymbra spicata* essential oils and plant extracts for chemical composition, antioxidant, and antimicrobial properties. *Food Sci. Nutr.* **2019**, *7*, 1704–1714. [CrossRef] [PubMed]
117. Cutillas, A.B.; Carrasco, A.; Martinez-Gutierrez, R.; Tomas, V.; Tudela, J. Thyme essential oils from Spain: Aromatic profile ascertained by GC-MS, and their antioxidant, anti-lipoxygenase and antimicrobial activities. *J. Food Drug. Anal.* **2018**, *26*, 529–544. [CrossRef]
118. Rašković, A.; Pavlović, N.; Kvrgić, M.; Sudji, J.; Mitić, G.; Čapo, I.; Mikov, M. Effects of pharmaceutical formulations containing thyme on carbon tetrachloride-induced liver injury in rats. *BMC Complement. Altern. Med.* **2015**, *15*, 442. [CrossRef]
119. Palabiyik, S.S.; Karakus, E.; Halici, Z.; Cadirci, E.; Bayir, Y.; Ayaz, G.; Cinar, I. The protective effects of carvacrol and thymol against paracetamol-induced toxicity on human hepatocellular carcinoma cell lines (HepG2). *Hum. Exp. Toxicol.* **2016**, *35*, 1252–1263. [CrossRef]
120. Ramadan, M.M.; Abd-Algader, N.N.; El-kamali, H.H.; Ghanem, K.Z.; Farrag, A.R.H. Volatile compounds and antioxidant activity of the aromatic herb *Anethum graveolens*. *J. Arab Soc. Med. Res.* **2013**, *8*, 79–88. [CrossRef]
121. Kuchta, A.; Konopacka, A.; Waleron, K.; Viapiana, A.; Wesołowski, M.; Dąbkowski, K.; Ćwiklińska, A.; Mickiewicz, A.; Śledzińska, A.; Wieczorek, E.; et al. The effect of *Cistus incanus* herbal tea supplementation on oxidative stress markers and lipid profile in healthy adults. *Cardiol. J.* **2019**, 30912576, in press. [CrossRef] [PubMed]
122. Moselhy, S.S.; Ali, H.K.H. Hepatoprotective effect of Cinnamon extracts against carbon tetrachloride induced oxidative stress and liver injury in rats. *Biol. Res.* **2009**, *42*, 93–98. [CrossRef]
123. Khaki, A. Effect of *Cinnamomum zeylanicumon* on spermatogenesis. *Iran Red. Crescent Med. J.* **2015**, *17*, e18668. [CrossRef] [PubMed]
124. Tuzcu, Z.; Orhan, C.; Sahin, N.; Juturu, V.; Sahin, K. Cinnamon polyphenol extract inhibits hyperlipidemia and inflammation by modulation of transcription factors in high-fat diet-fed rats. *Oxidative Med. Cell. Longev.* **2017**, *2017*, 1583098. [CrossRef] [PubMed]
125. Roussel, A.M.; Hininger, I.; Benaraba, R.; Ziegenfuss, T.N.; Anderson, R.A. Antioxidant effects of a cinnamon extract in people with impaired fasting glucose that are overweight or obese. *J. Am. Coll. Nutr.* **2009**, *28*, 16–21. [CrossRef] [PubMed]
126. Ervina, M.; Nawu, Y.E.; Esar, S.Y. Comparison of in vitro antioxidant activity of infusion, extract and fractions of Indonesian cinnamon (*Cinnamomum burmannii*) bark. *Int. Food Res. J.* **2016**, *23*, 1346–1350.
127. Settharaksa, S.; Jongjareonrak, A.; Hmadhlu, P.; Chansuwan, W.; Siripongvutikorn, S. Flavonoid, phenolic contents and antioxidant properties of Thai hot curry paste extract and its ingredients as affected of pH, solvent types and high temperature. *Int. Food Res. J.* **2012**, *19*, 1581–1587.

128. Gulcin, I.; Kaya, R.; Goren, A.C.; Akincioglu, H.; Topal, M.; Bingol, Z.; Cetin Çakmak, K.; Ozturk Sarikaya, S.B.; Durmaz, L.; Alwasel, S. Anticholinergic, antidiabetic and antioxidant activities of cinnamon (*Cinnamomum verum*) bark extracts: Polyphenol contents analysis by LC-MS/MS. *Int. J. Food Prop.* **2019**, *22*, 1511–1526. [CrossRef]
129. Naji, K.M.; Al-Shaibani, E.S.; Alhadi, F.A.; Al-Soudi, S.A.; D'souza, M.R. Hepatoprotective and antioxidant effects of single clove garlic against CCl4-induced hepatic damage in rabbits. BMC Complement. *Altern. Med.* **2017**, *17*, 411.
130. Zamani, A.; Ghiasvand, T.; Hadei, J.; Babaahmadi-Rezaei, H.; Pishdadian, A. Effect of garlic consumption on total antioxidant status and some biochemical and haematological parameters in blood of rats. *J. Sci. Food Agric.* **2009**, *89*, 1434–1437. [CrossRef]
131. Elosta, A.; Slevin, M.; Rahman, K.; Ahmed, N. Aged garlic has more potent antiglycation and antioxidant properties compared to fresh garlic extract in vitro. *Sci. Rep.* **2017**, *7*, 39613. [CrossRef] [PubMed]
132. Asdaq, S.M.B. Antioxidant and hypolipidemic potential of aged garlic extract and its constituent, S-allyl cysteine, in rats. *Evid.-Based Complement. Altern. Med.* **2015**, *2015*, 328545. [CrossRef] [PubMed]
133. Xiong, F.; Dai, C.H.; Hou, F.R.; Zhu, P.P.; He, R.H.; Ma, H.L. A study on the ageing method and anti-oxidant activity of black garlic residues. *Czech J. Food Sci.* **2018**, *36*, 88–97. [CrossRef]
134. Khurana, S.; Venkataraman, K.; Hollingsworth, A.; Piche, M.; Tai, T.C. Polyphenols: Benefits to the cardiovascular system in health and in aging. *Nutrients* **2013**, *5*, 3779–3827. [CrossRef] [PubMed]
135. Kim, S.N.; Kim, M.R.; Cho, S.M.; Kim, S.Y.; Kim, J.B.; Cho, Y.S. Antioxidant activities and determination of phenolic compounds isolated from oriental plums (Soldam, Oishiwase and Formosa). *Nutr. Res. Pract.* **2012**, *6*, 277–285. [CrossRef]
136. Fu, S.; Lv, R.; Wang, L.; Hou, H.; Liu, H.; Shao, S. Resveratrol, an antioxidant, protects spinal cord injury in rats by suppressing MAPK pathway. *Saudi J. Biol. Sci.* **2018**, *25*, 259–266. [CrossRef]
137. Han, X.; Shen, T.; Lou, H. Dietary polyphenols and their biological significance. *Int. J. Mol. Sci.* **2007**, *8*, 950–988. [CrossRef]
138. Olas, B. Berry phenolic antioxidants–implications for human health? *Front. Pharmacol.* **2018**, *9*, 78. [CrossRef]
139. Marniemi, J.; Hakala, P.; Maki, J.; Ahotupa, M. Partial resistance of low density lipoprotein to oxidation in vivo after increased intake of berries. *Nutr. Metab. Cardiovasc. Dis.* **2000**, *10*, 331–337.
140. Kuntz, S.; Kunz, C.; Herrmann, J.; Borsch, C.H.; Abel, G.; Fröhling, B.; Dietrich, H.; Rudloff, S. Anthocyanins from fruit juices improve the antioxidant status of healthy young female volunteers without affecting anti-inflammatory parameters: Results from the randomised, double-blind, placebo-controlled, cross-over ANTHONIA (ANTHOcyanins in Nutrition Investigation Alliance) study. *Br. J. Nutr.* **2014**, *112*, 925–936.
141. El-Wakf, A.M.; El-Komy, M.A.; Hassan, D.G. Preventive effect of dried plum extract against dexamethasone-induced osteoporosis in male rats through inhibiting cathepsin-K activity, lipogenesis and trabecular bone loss. *J. Innov. Pharmace. Biol. Sci.* **2019**, *6*, 52–61.
142. Graziani, G.; D'Argenio, G.; Tuccillo, C.; Loguercio, C.; Ritieni, A.; Morisco, F.; Del Vecchio Blanco, C.; Fogliano, V.; Romano, M. Apple polyphenol extracts prevent damage to human gastric epithelial cells in vitro and to rat gastric mucosa in vivo. *Gut* **2005**, *54*, 193–200. [CrossRef] [PubMed]
143. Ammar, A.; Turki, M.; Hammouda, O.; Chtourou, H.; Trabelsi, K.; Bouaziz, M.; Abdelkarim, O.; Hoekelmann, A.; Ayadi, F.; Souissi, N.; et al. Effects of pomegranate juice supplementation on oxidative stress biomarkers following weightlifting exercise. *Nutrients* **2017**, *9*, 819. [CrossRef] [PubMed]
144. Doostan, F.; Vafafar, R.; Zakeri-Milani, P.; Pouri, A.; Amini Afshar, R.; Mesgari Abbasi, M. Effects of pomegranate (*Punica granatum* L.) seed and peel methanolic extracts on oxidative stress and lipid profile changes induced by methotrexate in rats. *Adv. Pharm. Bull.* **2017**, *7*, 269–274. [CrossRef] [PubMed]
145. Doostan, F.; Abbasi, M.M.; Khordadmehr, M.; Fallah, F.; Behrouzy, A. Effects of pomegranate seed and peel methanolic extracts on methotrexate-induced hepatotoxicity in rats. *Pharm. Sci.* **2019**, *25*, 111–117. [CrossRef]
146. Abid, M.; Yaich, H.; Cheikhrouhou, S.; Khemakhem, I.; Bouaziz, M.; Attia, H.; Ayadi, M.A. Antioxidant properties and phenolic profile characterization by LC-MS/MS of selected Tunisian pomegranate peels. *J. Food Sci. Technol.* **2017**, *54*, 2890–2901. [CrossRef]
147. Anahita, A.; Asmah, R.; Fauziah, O. Evaluation of total phenolic content, total antioxidant activity, andantioxidant vitamin composition of pomegranate seed and juice. *Gen. Med.* **2015**, *3*, 1000164.

148. Weng, Z.; Patel, A.B.; Vasiadi, M.; Therianou, A.; Theoharides, T.C. Luteolin inhibits human keratinocyte activation and decreases NF-κB induction that is increased in psoriatic skin. *PLoS ONE* **2014**, *9*, e90739. [CrossRef]
149. Wang, W.; Wang, W.; Yuhai; Wang, H.; Bagenna, C. Astilbin reduces ROS accumulation and VEGF expression through Nrf2 in psoriasis-like skin disease. *Biol. Res.* **2019**, *52*, 49. [CrossRef]
150. Bélanger, A.; Grenier, A.; Simard, F.; Gendreau, I.; Pichette, A.; Legault, J.; Pouliot, R. Dihydrochalcone derivatives from *Populus balsamifera* L. buds for the treatment of psoriasis. *Int. J. Mol. Sci.* **2019**, *21*, 256. [CrossRef]
151. Skurić, J.; Orsolić, N.; Kolarić, D.; Dikić, D.; Benković, V.; Knezević, A.H.; Lisicić, D. Effectivity of flavonoids on animal model psoriasis—thermographic evaluation. *Period Biol.* **2011**, *113*, 457–463.
152. Kjær, T.N.; Thorsen, K.; Jessen, N.; Stenderup, K.; Pedersen, S.B. Resveratrol ameliorates imiquimod-induced psoriasis-like skin inflammation in mice. *PLoS ONE* **2015**, *10*, e0126599. [CrossRef] [PubMed]
153. Zhang, S.; Liu, X.; Mei, L.; Wang, H.; Fang, F. Epigallocatechin-3-gallate (EGCG) inhibits imiquimod-induced psoriasis-like inflammation of BALB/c mice. BMC Complement. *Altern. Med.* **2016**, *16*, 334.
154. Alashqar, M.B.; Goldstein, N. Caffeine in the treatment of atopic dermatitis and psoriasis: A review. *SKIN J. Cutan. Med.* **2019**, *3*, 59–71. [CrossRef]
155. Phillips, J.T.; Fox, R.J. BG-12 in multiple sclerosis. *Semin. Neurol.* **2013**, *33*, 56–65. [PubMed]
156. Brigelius-Flohé, R.; Flohé, L. Basic principles and emerging concepts in the redox control of transcription factors. *Antioxid. Redox Signal.* **2011**, *15*, 2335–2381. [CrossRef]
157. Madhulatha, M.; Vijayabhaskar, M. Evaluation of therapeutic efficacy of antioxidants in psoriatic cases. *Indian J. Med. Biochem.* **2019**, *23*, 167–169. [CrossRef]
158. Kharaeva, Z.; Gostova, E.; De Luca, C.; Raskovic, D.; Korkina, L. Clinical and biochemical effects of coenzyme Q(10), vitamin E, and selenium supplementation to psoriasis patients. *Nutrition* **2009**, *25*, 295–302. [CrossRef]
159. Jin, G.H.; Liu, Y.; Jin, S.Z.; Liu, X.D.; Liu, S.Z. UVB induced oxidative stress in human keratinocytes and protective effect of antioxidant agents. *Radiat. Environ. Biophys.* **2007**, *46*, 61–68. [CrossRef]
160. Mitra, A.; Fallen, R.S.; Lima, H. Cytokine-based therapy in Psoriasis. *Clin. Rev. Allergy Immunol.* **2012**, *44*, 173–182. [CrossRef]
161. Barygina, V.; Becatti, M.; Soldi, G.; Prignano, F.; Lotti, T.; Nassi, P.; Wright, D.; Taddei, N.; Fiorillo, C. Altered redox status in the blood of psoriatic patients: Involvement of NADPH oxidase and role of anti-TNF-a therapy. *Redox Rep.* **2013**, *18*, 100–106. [CrossRef] [PubMed]
162. Peplow, P.V.; Chatterjee, M.P. A review of the influence of growth factors and cytokines in in vitro human keratinocyte migration. *Cytokine* **2013**, *62*, 1–21. [CrossRef]
163. Zheng, Y.; Danilenko, D.; Valdez, P.; Kasman, I.; Eastham-Anderson, J.; Wu, J.; Ouyang, W. Interleukin-22, a TH17 cytokine, mediates IL-23-induced dermal inflammation and acanthosis. *Nature* **2007**, *445*, 648–651. [CrossRef] [PubMed]
164. Jawad, A.H.; Azhar, I.Y.; Khalil, A.H. Evaluation of efficacy, safety and antioxidant effect of *Nigella sativa* in patients with psoriasis: A randomized clinical trial. *J. Clin. Exp. Investig.* **2014**, *5*, 186–193.
165. Abbas, Y.M.; Ahmed, J.H.; Al-Haroon, S.S. A study of the effect of *Nigella sativa* (black seeds) on methotrexate induced hepatotoxicity in rabbits. *Int. J. Basic Clin. Pharmacol.* **2015**, *4*, 230–235. [CrossRef]
166. Bordoni, L.; Fedeli, D.; Nasuti, C.; Maggi, F.; Papa, F.; Wabitsch, M.; De Caterina, R.; Gabbianelli, R. Antioxidant and anti-inflammatory properties of *Nigella sativa* oil in human pre-adipocytes. *Antioxidants* **2019**, *8*, 51. [CrossRef]
167. Sicak, Y.; Erdoğan Eliuz, E.A. Chemical content and biological activity spectrum of *Nigella sativa* seed oil. *KSU J. Agric. Nat.* **2019**, *22*, 928–934.
168. Ohta, S. Molecular hydrogen as a novel antioxidant: Overview of the advantages of hydrogen for medical applications. *Methods Enzymol.* **2015**, *555*, 289–317.
169. Polovynkina, K.; Klonowska, J.; Grzyb, S. General characteristics of therapeutic molecular hydrogen. *Eur. J. Med. Technol.* **2019**, *3*, 38–43.
170. Zhu, Q.; Wu, Y.; Li, Y.; Chen, Z.; Wang, L.; Xiong, H.; Dai, E.; Wu, J.; Fan, B.; Ping, L.; et al. Positive effects of hydrogen-water bathing in patients of psoriasis and parapsoriasis en plaques. *Sci. Rep.* **2018**, *8*, 8051. [CrossRef]
171. Ge, L.; Yang, M.; Yang, N.N.; Yin, X.X.; Song, W.G. Molecular hydrogen: A preventive and therapeutic medical gas for various diseases. *Oncotarget* **2017**, *8*, 102653–102673. [CrossRef] [PubMed]

172. Jaros, J.; Katta, R.; Shi, V.Y. Dermatonutrigenomics: Past, present, and future. *Dermatology* **2019**, *235*, 164–166. [CrossRef] [PubMed]
173. Niculescu, M.D.; Zeisel, S.H. Diet, methyl donors and DNA methylation: Interactions between dietary folate, methionine and choline. *J. Nutr.* **2002**, *132*, 2333–2335. [CrossRef] [PubMed]
174. Switzeny, O.J.; Müllner, E.; Wagner, K.; Brath, H.; Aumüller, E.; Haslberger, A.G. Vitamin and antioxidant rich diet increases MLH1 promoter DNA methylation in DMT2 subjects. *Clin. Epigenet.* **2012**, *4*, 19. [CrossRef]
175. Hawkes, J.E.; Nguyen, G.H.; Fujita, M.; Florell, S.R.; Callis Duffin, K.; Krueger, G.G.; O'Connell, R.M. MicroRNAs in psoriasis. *J. Invest Dermatol.* **2016**, *136*, 365–371. [CrossRef]
176. Quintanilha, B.J.; Reis, B.Z.; Duarte, G.B.S.; Cozzolino, S.M.F.; Rogero, M.M. Nutrimiromics: Role of microRNAs and nutrition in modulating inflammation and chronic diseases. *Nutrients* **2017**, *9*, 1168. [CrossRef]
177. Bhardwaj, N. MicroRNAs in atopic dermatitis: A review. J. Transl. *Genet. Genom.* **2017**, *1*, 15–22.
178. Kocic, H.; Damiani, G.; Stamenkovic, B.; Tirant, M.; Jovic, A.; Tiodorovic, D.; Peris, K. Dietary compounds as potential modulators of microRNA expression in psoriasis. *Ther. Adv. Chronic Dis.* **2019**, *10*, 2040622319864805. [CrossRef]
179. Xiao, S.; Liu, X.; Wang, X.; Lv, H.; Zhao, J.; Guo, X.; Xian, F.; Ji, Y.; Zhan, G. Plasma microRNA expression profiles in psoriasis. *J. Immunol. Res.* **2020**, *2020*, 1561278. [CrossRef]
180. Lam, T.K.; Shao, S.; Zhao, Y.; Marincola, F.; Pesatori, A.; Bertazzi, P.A.; Caporaso, N.E.; Wang, E.; Landi, M.T. Influence of quercetin-rich food intake on microRNA expression in lung cancer tissues. *Cancer Epidemiol. Biomark. Prev.* **2012**, *21*, 2176–2184. [CrossRef]
181. Lovendorf, M.B.; Zibert, J.R.; Hagedorn, P.H.; Glue, C.; Ødum, N.; Røpke, M.A.; Skov, L. Comparison of microRNA expression using different preservation methods of matched psoriatic skin samples. *Exp. Dermatol.* **2012**, *21*, 299–301. [CrossRef] [PubMed]
182. Boesch-Saadatmandi, C.; Loboda, A.; Wagner, A.E.; Stachurska, A.; Jozkowicz, A.; Dulak, J.; Döring, F.; Wolffram, S.; Rimbach, G. Effect of quercetin and its metabolites isorhamnetin and quercetin-3-glucuronide on inflammatory gene expression: Role of miR-155. *J. Nutr. Biochem.* **2011**, *22*, 293–299. [CrossRef]
183. Li, H.; Jia, Z.; Li, A.; Jenkins, G.; Yang, X.; Hu, J.; Guo, W. Resveratrol repressed viability of U251 cells by miR-21 inhibiting of NF-κB pathway. *Mol. Cell. Biochem.* **2013**, *382*, 137–143. [CrossRef]
184. Reuter, S.; Gupta, S.C.; Park, B.; Goel, A.; Aggarwal, B.B. Epigenetic changes induced by curcumin and other natural compounds. *Genes Nutr.* **2011**, *6*, 93–108. [CrossRef] [PubMed]
185. Tili, E.; Michaille, J.-J.; Adair, B.; Alder, H.; Limagne, E.; Taccioli, C.; Ferracin, M.; Delmas, D.; Latruffe, N.; Croce, C.M. Resveratrol decreases the levels of miR-155 by upregulating miR-663, a microRNA targeting JunB and JunD. *Carcinogenesis* **2010**, *31*, 1561–1566. [CrossRef]
186. Bigagli, E.; Cinci, L.; Paccosi, S.; Parenti, A.; D'Ambrosio, M.; Luceri, C. Nutritionally relevant concentrations of resveratrol and hydroxytyrosol mitigate oxidative burst of human granulocytes and monocytes and the production of pro-inflammatory mediators in LPS-stimulated RAW264.7 macrophages. *Int. Immunopharmacol.* **2017**, *43*, 147–155. [CrossRef] [PubMed]
187. Bell, E.L.; Klimova, T.A.; Eisenbart, J.; Schumacker, P.T.; Chandel, N.S. Mitochondrial reactive oxygen species trigger hypoxia-inducible factor-dependent extension of the replicative life span during hypoxia. *Mol. Cell. Biol.* **2007**, *27*, 5737–5745. [CrossRef]

3

Possible Mechanisms of the Prevention of Doxorubicin Toxicity by Cichoric Acid—Antioxidant Nutrient

Agata Jabłońska-Trypuć [1,*], Rafał Krętowski [2], Monika Kalinowska [1], Grzegorz Świderski [1], Marzanna Cechowska-Pasko [2] and Włodzimierz Lewandowski [1]

1 Department of Chemistry, Biology and Biotechnology, Faculty of Civil Engineering and Environmental Engineering, Białystok University of Technology, Wiejska 45E Street, 15-351 Białystok, Poland; m.kalinowska@pb.edu.pl (M.K.); g.swiderski@pb.edu.pl (G.Ś.); w.lewandowski@pb.edu.pl (W.L.)

2 Department of Pharmaceutical Biochemistry, Medical University of Bialystok, 15-222 Białystok, Poland; r.kretowski@umb.edu.pl (R.K.); mapasko@gmail.com (M.C.-P.)

* Correspondence: a.jablonska@pb.edu.pl

Abstract: Skin is the largest organ in the human body, and which protects organism against unfavorable external factors e.g., chemicals, environment pollutants, allergens, microorganisms, and it plays a crucial role in maintaining general homeostasis. It is also an important target of oxidative stress due to the activity of oxygen reactive species (ROS), which are constantly generated in the fibroblasts in response to exogenous or endogenous prooxidant agents. An example of such compound with proved prooxidant activity is Doxorubicin (DOX), which is an effective anticancer agent belongs in anthracycline antibiotic group. Increasingly frequent implementation of various strategies to reduce undesirable DOX side effects was observed. Very promising results come from the combination of DOX with dietary antioxidants from the polyphenol group of compounds, such as cichoric acid (CA) in order to lower oxidative stress level. The aim of this work was to evaluate the influence of CA combined with DOX on the oxidative stress parameters in fibroblasts, which constitute the main cells in human skin. We also wanted to examine anti-apoptotic activity of CA in fibroblasts treated with selected concentrations of DOX. Results obtained from the combination of DOX with CA revealed that CA exhibits cytoprotective activity against DOX-induced damage by lowering oxidative stress level and by inhibiting apoptosis. The present finding may indicate that CA may serve as antioxidative and anti-apoptotic agent, active against DOX-induced damage.

Keywords: cichoric acid; doxorubicin; fibroblasts; skin; oxidative stress

---

1. Introduction

Skin is the largest organ in the human body. It protects the organism against unfavorable external factors e.g., chemicals, environment pollutants, allergens, microorganisms, and it plays a crucial role in maintaining general homeostasis [1]. Therefore, it is also an important target of oxidative stress due to the activity of reactive oxygen species (ROS), which are constantly generated in the fibroblasts and keratinocytes in response to exogenous or endogenous prooxidant agents [2]. Furthermore, ROS produced during normal skin metabolism, constitute a part of proper skin functionality and usually cause a little damage due to the activity of intracellular mechanisms, which reduce their harmful properties. It is worth noting that intensive or prolonged oxidative stress may overwhelm antioxidant defense mechanisms of the human skin and contribute to the skin disorders development, e.g.,: skin aging, dermatitis, allergic reactions or even skin neoplasms [3]. Main constituents of skin are fibroblasts, which arise during embryogenesis from embryonic mesenchyme. A certain amount of spindle-shaped mesenchymal cells differentiate into supporting cells—fibroblasts. They are usually elongated, spindle-shaped, with several projections lying in one plane. They have one cell nucleus, round or oval with distinct nucleoli. Sometimes several nucleoli within the nucleus can be observed. Fibroblasts are the main cells that build up the dermis. Skin consists of three layers: epidermis, dermis and subcutaneous tissue. The epidermis forms a surface layer that stays in contact with the external environment and is built principally of keratinocytes that synthesize keratin—a component of the stratum corneum of the epidermis. The skin is composed of two layers: papillary and reticular [4,5].

Free radicals as atoms or compounds, which have at least one unpaired electron in the outer orbit, are mainly produced in the mitochondria during electron flow through the mitochondrial respiratory chain, and they increase their reactivity through oxidation-reduction mechanisms. About 2% of oxygen consumed by the respiratory chain undergoes simultaneous reduction causing the formation of ROS. As a result of these processes, superoxide anion radicals are formed, that initiate a whole cascade of reactive oxygen species, such as hydroxyl radical, hydrogen peroxide and singlet oxygen. ROS are generated in cells in different ways, but their main source are mitochondria, which consume about 90% of the oxygen needed by the cells. Mitochondria are also most often damaged by ROS, and with age they degenerate fairly quickly. Under normal conditions ROS are permanently removed by a complex antioxidant system, but in pathological conditions there is an imbalance between prooxidants and antioxidants. This imbalance can lead to oxidative stress and subsequently overproduction of ROS, which modify cellular components such as DNA, proteins and lipids [6,7]. Oxidative stress largely affects the skin, which occupies the largest area of the human body and is a protective coating for the internal organs. The skin structure allows it to perform physical and biochemical protection functions. Due to its functions and localization in the human body, skin is the most exposed for oxidative stress tissue. It is most susceptible to oxidative damage, which results from the presence of potential biological targets for free radical reactions in its components.

Air pollution, naturally occurring airborne gases such as ozone or high concentrations of oxygen, ionizing and non-ionizing radiation, bacteria, viruses and various exogenous toxins and chemicals can be considered as exogenous sources of factors that promote oxidative stress in the skin. Oxidative stress can also be caused by physical damage to the skin, such as burns or injuries [8,9]. On the other hand, endogenous sources of oxidative damage are generated by enzymes involved in the autoxidation of endo- and exogenous compounds, as well as by lipoxygenases and cyclooxygenases during eicosanoid metabolism. Nitric oxide synthase is an example of an enzyme that produces NO (nitric oxide) radicals directly in the skin. The source of ROS may also be neutrophils activated by a bacterial invasion in which a respiratory burst is observed.

One of the classes of compounds, which activity in the human organism is based on the generation of oxidative stress, mainly in cancer cells, are anticancer drugs. An example of such compound with proved prooxidant activity is Doxorubicin (DOX). DOX is an effective anticancer agent from anthracycline antibiotic group, which has a large spectrum of activity and it is being used alone or in combination to treat a variety of tumors, both haematological and solid, such as breast cancer [10,11]. It inhibits cell proliferation, induces oxidative stress, inhibits topoisomerase II, and finally leads to the cell death mainly through apoptosis [12–14]. DOX tends to accumulate in mitochondria, causing changes in their structure and function. However, the main cause of DOX side effects observed in human is an extremely high level of oxidative stress within the cell, eventually causing apoptotic cell death [15,16]. A generation of free radicals caused by DOX can be described in two ways. The first one is an enzymatic mechanism consisting of the formation of semiquinone free radicals by the activity of NADPH-dependent reductases, which cause a one—electron reduction of DOX to DOX-semiquinone. Redox transformations of DOX-derived quinone/semiquinone provide superoxide radicals in the presence of oxygen [17,18]. The second mechanism has non-enzymatic background and it involves reaction with an iron (Fe^{3+}), which produces Fe^{2+}-doxorubicin free radical complex. This Fe-DOX complex is able to reduce oxygen to hydrogen peroxide and other free radicals. In our previous experiment regarding DOX influence on breast cancer cells we revealed that DOX-metal complexes are even more efficient than a parent drug [10,17].

Increasingly frequent implementation of various strategies to reduce undesirable DOX side effects was observed. Besides dose regulation, combined therapies with antioxidants, especially plant origin substances, are being used. Very promising results come from the combination of DOX with dietary antioxidants from the polyphenol group of compounds in order to lower oxidative stress level [19]. One of the antioxidative agents with promising properties is cichoric acid. Cichoric acid (CA), a dicaffeyltartaric acid, was identified in a variety of edible plants and vegetables, such as: iceberg lettuce, basil, *Cichorium intybus* L., dandelion, *Echinacea purpurea* and *Orthosiphon stamineus*. Many of above-mentioned plants are being used in folk medicine. CA exhibits many biological properties including anti-hyaluronidase activity, protection of collagen from possible free radical damage, antiviral activity, promoting phagocyte activity and free radical scavenger properties [20,21]. According to the literature, CA also inhibits HIV (human immunodeficiency virus) integrase, which is responsible for the HIV DNA copy integration with the DNA of the host cell [22]. It should be also mentioned that CA has the ability to influence an immune response in chronically stressed mice, causing a significant decrease in stress level [23,24]. In addition recent research revealed that CA enhances glucose uptake in muscle cells and subsequently stimulates Langerhans islets to the secretion of the insulin [25]. Despite so many beneficial activities of CA described in literature, no studies exist regarding its antioxidative properties against DOX-induced oxidative stress in normal human fibroblasts.

Several studies have shown that CA reveals its general antioxidative properties, which may counteract doxorubicin-induced cytotoxicity, but they were conducted on cancer cell lines and they have not clarified the mechanisms of its action. Therefore, with our study, we wanted to determine if CA acts as an antioxidant against doxorubicin—induced oxidative stress and if it acts via antioxidative and/or antiapoptotic pathway. We tested it in human normal fibroblasts cell line, because fibroblasts are very responsive to chemical signals and changes made to this signals can affect other cells. Fibroblasts constitute also main cell type of the skin, which is exposed for anticancer drugs side effects. Therefore strategies to attenuate the toxic effects of doxorubicin, such as combined therapy with dietary antioxidants (e.g., CA) are implemented.

2. Materials and Methods

2.1. Reagents

Dulbecco's modified Eagle's medium (DMEM), containing glucose at 4.5 mg/mL (25 mM), penicillin, streptomycin, trypsin–EDTA (ethylenediaminetetraacetic acid), FBS (Fetal Bovine Serum) and PBS (Phosphate-buffered saline) (without Ca and Mg) were provided by Gibco (San Diego, CA, USA), GSH/GSSG-Glo™ Assay kit, Caspase-Glo® 3/7 Assay kit, Caspase-Glo® 9 Assay kit were provided by Promega, Madison, WI, USA. MTT reagent was purchased from Sigma-Aldrich (St. Louis, MO, USA). Acridine orange and ethidium bromide were obtained from Sigma-Aldrich (St. Louis, MO, USA). Dichlorodihydrofluorescein diacetate assay (DCFH-DA) was provided by Sigma-Aldrich, St. Louis, MO, USA. SDS (Sodium dodecyl sulfate), TCA (Trichloroacetic acid), TBA (Thiobarbituric acid), Folin-Ciocalteu reagent were provided by Sigma-Aldrich and DTNB (Ellman's Reagent) (5,5-dithio-bis-(2-nitrobenzoic acid)) by Serva. Cichoric acid, chlorogenic acid, caffeic acid, quercetin, DPPH (2,2-diphenyl-1-picrylhydrazyl), trolox, H_2O_2, horseradish peroxidase, phosphate buffer pH = 7 were purchased from Sigma-Aldrich Co. and used without purification. Methanol was purchased from Merck (Darmstadt, Germany).

2.2. Anti-/Pro-Oxidant Activity

Antiradical activity was determined according to the DPPH assay described by [26]. The methanolic solutions of cichoric, chlorogenic and caffeic acids, quercetin and DPPH were prepared just before analysis. 1 mL of tested compound and 2 mL of DPPH was added to each tube, vortexed and incubated in the darkness for 1 h at 23 °C. The final concentrations of phenolic compounds were 8, 5, 1 and 0.5 μM, and DPPH was 40 μM. The absorbance of solutions was measured at 516 nm against methanol as the blank using Agilent Carry 5000 spectrophotometer (Agilent, Santa Clara, CA, USA). The control sample consisted of 2 mL of DPPH solution and 1 mL of methanol. The antiradical activity of phenolic compounds was calculated as the percent of DPPH inhibition according to the equation:

$$\%I = \frac{A^{516}_{control} - A^{516}_{sample}}{A^{516}_{control}} \times 100\%$$

where: %I—% inhibition of DPPH radical, A^{516}_{conrol}—absorbance of the control, A^{516}_{sample}—absorbance of the sample.

The pro-oxidant activity of tested compounds was determined as the rate of oxidation of trolox according to the procedure described by Zeraik et al. [27]. 100 μM trolox, 50 μM H_2O_2, 0.01 μM horseradish peroxidase in phosphate buffer (pH = 7) and 0.25 μM tested substances were incubated at 25 °C. The measurement was conducted at 272 nm using Agilent Carry 5000 spectrophotometer.

2.3. Cell Culture

The effect of CA, DOX and CA-DOX was examined in normal human skin fibroblast cell line (CRL1474), which was obtained from American Type Culture Collection (ATCC). Cells were maintained in DMEM (Gibco) supplemented with 10% FBS (Gibco), penicillin (100 U/mL), and streptomycin (100 μg/mL) at 37 °C in a humidified atmosphere of 5% CO_2 in air. The viability of cells was estimated at CA concentrations of: 0.5 μM, 1 μM, 10 μM, 50 μM, 100 μM, 200 μM and 300 μM; DOX concentrations of: 0.09 μM, 0.18 μM, 0.38 μM, 0.75 μM, 1.5 μM, 3 μM and 6 μM; mix of CA and DOX in concentrations: 0.5 μM CA + 3 μM DOX, 1 μM CA + 3 μM DOX, 10 μM CA + 3 μM DOX, 50 μM CA + 3 μM DOX, 100 μM CA + 3 μM DOX, 200 μM CA + 3 μM DOX and 300 μM CA + 3 μM DOX. Caspases 3/7 activity, caspase 9 activity, SH (thiol) group content, TBARS (Thiobarbituric acid reactive substances) content, GSH/GSSG (Glutathione/Oxidized Glutathione) ratio, ROS content and apoptosis were examined at CA concentrations of 300 μM, DOX concentration of 3 μM and the mixture of these two compounds (CA + DOX, concentrations: 300 μM + 3 μM, respectively). Fibroblasts were seeded in 96-well plates at a density 2 × 10^4 cells/well. The cells were cultured for 24 h and 48 h and were treated with DOX in a concentration of 3 μM, CA in a concentration of 300 μM and with a mixture of DOX and CA (3 μM + 300 μM, respectively). Cells were seeded in: (a) transparent plates for cytotoxicity tests; (b) white plates for determination of caspase 3/7 and 9 activity, determination of GSH/GSSG ratio; (c) black plates for intracellular ROS detection.

2.4. Chemical Treatment of Cells

CA was stored in a refrigerator at temperature 4 °C. CA was dissolved in TrisHCl buffer. The compound was added to the cultured cells for a final concentration in the range of 0.5 μM to 300 μM. DOX was stored in a freezer at temperature −20 °C. The compound was added to the culture cells for a final concentration in the range of 0.09 μM to 6 μM. CA and DOX were both added to the cultured cells in selected concentrations. The control cells were incubated without the tested compounds.

2.5. CA, DOX and CA-DOX Cytotoxicity

CA, DOX and CA-DOX cytotoxicity were measured according to the method of Carmichael using 3-(4,5-dimethylthiazol-2-yl)-2,5-diphenyltetrazolium bromide (MTT) [28]. The cells cultured for 24 h and 48 h were treated with: 1st—CA in the concentration range from 0.5 μM to 300 μM; 2nd—DOX in the concentration range from 0.09 μM to 6 μM; 3rd—CA combined with DOX: CA in the concentration range from 0.5 μM to 300 μM combined with DOX in the 3 μM concentration. After 24 h and 48 h cells were washed 3 times with PBS and subsequently incubated with 10 μL of MTT solution (5 mg/mL in

PBS) for 2 h at 37 °C in 5% CO_2 in an incubator. Subsequently, 100 μL of DMSO was added and cells were incubated in the dark for the next 2 h. The absorbance was measured at 570 nm in a microplate reader GloMax®-Multi Microplate Multimode Reader (Promega Corporation, Madison, WI, USA). The viability of fibroblast cells was calculated as a percentage of control cells, incubated without tested compounds. All the experiments were done in triplicates.

2.6. Determination of Caspase 3/7 Activity

After intended time of incubation medium was removed and Assay reagents were added to the wells. The activity of caspases 3/7 was measured using luminescent assay based on the substrate which contains the tetrapeptide sequence DEVD in a reagent optimized for caspase activity, luciferase activity and cell lysis. The cell lysis was followed by the caspase cleavage of the substrate and generation of the luminescent signal. The luminescence is proportional to the amount of caspase activity present in the sample. Assay is based on the thermostable luciferase activity, which generates stable, "glow-type" luminescent signal. The luminescence was measured in a microplate reader GloMax®-Multi Microplate Multimode Reader. All the experiments were done in triplicates.

2.7. Determination of Caspase 9 Activity

After intended time of incubation medium was removed and Assay reagents were added to the wells. The activity of caspase 9 was measured by using luminescent assay based on a luminogenic caspase-9 substrate in a buffer system provided for caspase activity, luciferase activity and cell lysis. The addition of a special Caspase-Glo® 9 Reagent results in cell lysis, followed by caspase cleavage of the substrate, and generation of a "glow-type" luminescent signal. The signal generated is proportional to the amount of caspase activity present in the sample. The assay is based on thermostable luciferase, which generates the stable "glow-type" luminescent signal. The luminescence was measured in a microplate reader GloMax®-Multi Microplate Multimode Reader (Promega Corporation, Madison, WI, USA). All the experiments were done in triplicates.

2.8. Total Protein Content in Cells

Fibroblasts (1×10^5 cells/mL) were incubated in 2 mL of culture medium with tested compounds in tissue culture 6-well plates. The determination of protein concentration was performed spectrophotometrically as per Lowry et al. (1951) as described previously [29]. All the experiments were done in triplicates.

2.9. Determination of SH Groups

SH-groups were measured using the method of Rice-Evans (1991) as described previously [29]. Fibroblasts (1×10^5 cells/mL) were incubated in 2 mL of culture medium with tested compounds in tissue culture 6-well plates. All the experiments were done in triplicates.

2.10. Determination of TBA Reactive Species (TBARS) Levels

The method of Rice-Evans (1991) was applied in order to measure the level of membrane lipid-peroxidation products (TBARS), as described previously [29]. Fibroblasts (1×10^5 cells/mL) were incubated in 2 mL of culture medium with test compounds in tissue culture 6-well plates. All the experiments were done in triplicates.

2.11. Determination of GSH/GSSG

Total glutathione and GSH/GSSG ratio were each assayed in triplicate via GSH/GSSG-Glo™ kit (Promega, Madison, WI, USA) following manufacturer's instructions. Prior to the assay growth media were removed and cells washed with PBS. Assay is based on a luminescence measurement and detects and quantifies total glutathione (GSH + GSSG), GSSG and GSH/GSSG ratios in cultured cells. Stable luminescent signals are correlated with either the GSH or GSSG concentration of a sample. In this method GSH-dependent conversion of a GSH probe, Luciferin-NT, to luciferin by a glutathione S-transferase enzyme is coupled to a firefly luciferase reaction. Light from luciferase depends on the amount of luciferin formed, which in turn depends on the amount of GSH present. Thus, the luminescent signal is proportional to the amount of GSH. GSH/GSSG ratios are calculated directly from luminescence measurements.

2.12. Intracellular ROS Detection

The intracellular ROS level was measured according to Kręttowski R. et al. [30]. After diffusion through the cell membrane, DCFH-DA is deacetylated by cellular esterases to a non-fluorescent compound, which is later oxidized by intracellular ROS into a fluorescent 2′,7′–dichlorofluorescein (DCF). After 24 h, the medium was removed, the cells were stained with 10 μM of DCFH-DA in 200 μL PBS at 37 °C, 5% CO_2 incubator, for 45 min. Next, the dye was removed and replaced with DOX in a concentration of 3 μM, CA in a concentration of 300 μM and with a mixture of DOX + CA (3 μM + 300 μM, respectively) and incubated for 24 h and 48 h. Then, the DCF fluorescence intensity was measured using the GloMax®-Multi Detection System (Promega Corporation, Madison, WI, USA) at the excitation wavelength of 485 nm and the emission wavelength of 535 nm. The intracellular ROS generation in fibroblasts cells was shown as the intensity of fluorescence of the DCF. All the experiments were done in triplicates.

2.13. Intracellular ROS Detection by Flow Cytometry

The level of intracellular reactive oxygen species (ROS) was determined using dichlorodihydrofluorescein diacetate (DCFH-DA), (Sigma, St. Louis, MO, USA). After diffusion through the cell membrane, DCFH-DA is deacetylated by cellular esterases to a non-fluorescent compound, which is later oxidized by intracellular ROS into a fluorescent 2′,7′–dichlorofluorescein (DCF). The cells (2.5×10^5) were seeded in 2 mL of growth medium in 6-well plates. After 24 h, the medium was removed, the cells were stained with 10 μM of DCFH-DA in 2 mL PBS at 37 °C, 5% CO_2 incubator, for 30 min. Next, the dye was removed and replaced with DOX in a concentration of 3 μM, CA in a concentration of 300 μM and with a mixture of DOX and CA (3 μM + 300 μM, respectively) and incubated for 24 h and 48 h. Then, the cells were trypsinized, resuspended in DMEM and then in PBS. The DCF fluorescence intensity was measured according to flow cytometry method, by using FACSCanto II cytometer (Becton Dickinson, Franklin Lakes, NJ, USA). Data were analysed using FACSDiva software (version 6, Becton Dickinson, Franklin Lakes, NJ, USA). The intracellular ROS generation in fibroblasts was depicted as the % of DCF positive cells.

2.14. Fluorescent Microscopy Assay

For apoptotic and necrotic cells nuclear morphology evaluation fluorescent dyes, such as ethidium bromide (10 μM) and acridine orange (10 μM) were used. The MCF-7 cells were seeded on cell imaging dishes with coverglass bottom with DOX in a concentration of 3 μM, CA in a concentration of 300 μM and with a mixture of DOX and CA (3 μM + 300 μM, respectively) and without tested compound as a control, for 24 h and 48 h. After incubation the cells were washed twice with PBS and then stained with dyes solution in the dark in room temperature, for 10 min. After incubation, staining mixture was removed and the cells were washed with PBS in order to analyze under fluorescent microscope (200× magnification). Ethidium bromide stains only cells that have lost their membrane integrity, while acridine orange stains live and dead cells. The cells were analyzed and photographed via using Leica DM IL fluorescent microscope (Leica Microsystems, Wetzlar, Germany). The following criteria were used: living cells—have regularly distributed green chromatin nucleus, early apoptotic cells characterized by bright green nucleus with condensed or often fragmented chromatin, late apoptotic cells—orange nuclei with chromatin condensation or fragmentation, while necrotic cells showed orange-stained cell nuclei. The cells were counted and percentage of apoptotic cells was the sum of early apoptotic and late apoptotic cells percent.

2.15. Statistical Analysis

For parametric data one-way analysis of variance (ANOVA) followed Tukey's test was applied. Results from five independent experiments were expressed as mean ± standard deviation (SD) of mean for parametric data. Significance was considered when $p \leq 0.05$. Statistica 13.0 was used.

3. Results

3.1. Antioxidant (DPPH Assays) and Pro-Oxidant (Trolox Assay) Activity

The anti- and pro-oxidant activity of cichoric acid (CA) was determined and compared with the activity of caffeic acid (CFA), chlorogenic acid (CGA) and quercetin (Q). In Figure 1 the antioxidant properties of selected polyphenolics (determined as antiradical properties against DPPH$^{\bullet}$ radical) are shown. The percent of DPPH$^{\bullet}$ radical inhibition (%I) was the highest for cichoric acid for four out of six studied concentrations and it was equal: 88.44 ± 0.53, 82.37 ± 0.70, 52.52 ± 0.99, 31.81 ± 1.46, 13.60 ± 1.45 and 6.67 ± 0.91%, for the concentrations 8, 5, 3, 2, 1 and 0.5 μM, respectively. Caffeic acid shows slightly lower antioxidant properties than cichoric acid, %I = 85.37 ± 0.41, 80.11 ± 1.67, 42.57 ± 0.48, 9.66 ± 0.76 and 5.45 ± 1.37 for 8, 5, 1 and 0.5 μM, respectively. Quercetin possess similar antioxidant activity as cichoric and caffeic acid, except the 5 and 3 μM concentrations where the %I = 65.96 ± 2.53 and 62.77 ± 0.98, respectively. Chlorogenic acid shows the lowest antioxidant properties among studied compounds, for all studied concentrations (the %I = 49.78 ± 0.14, 36.00 ± 1.98, 26.93 ± 0.38, 21.18 ± 0.59, 5.73 ± 0.63 and 3.01 ± 1.08, respectively; Figure 1). Therefore, taking into account the increasing value of %I as a measure of the antioxidant activity, the studied compounds may be ordered as follows: cichoric acid > caffeic acid~quercetin > chlorogenic acid (for the concentrations 8, 5, 2, 1 and 0.5 μM).

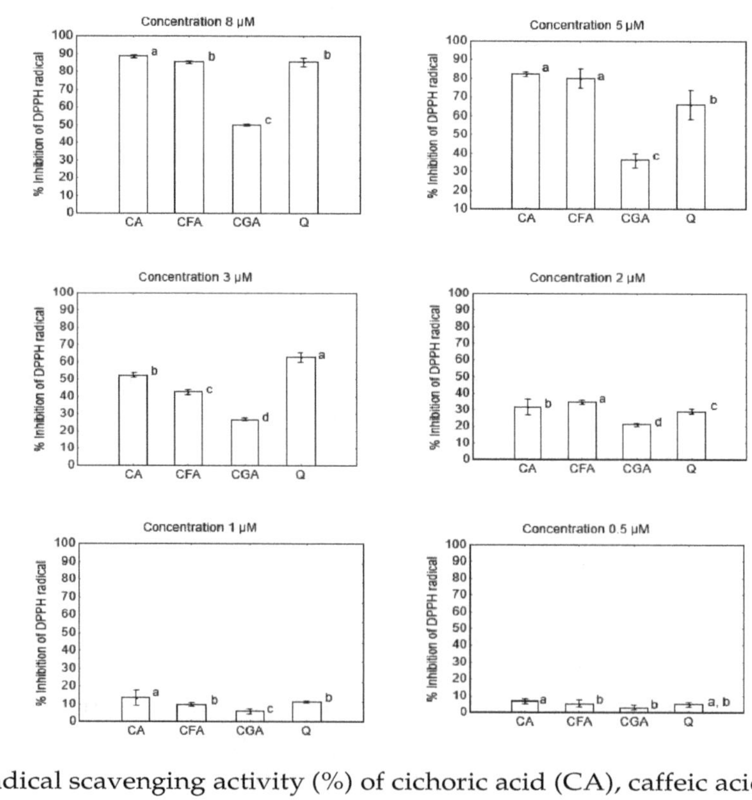

Figure 1. DPPH radical scavenging activity (%) of cichoric acid (CA), caffeic acid (CFA), chlorogenic acid (CGA) and quercetin (Q) for the concentrations 8, 5, 2, 1 and 0.5 μM. The same letter near the means indicate no significant difference (Tukey test, $p < 0.05$).

The pro-oxidant property of phenolic compounds was studied for the concentration 0.25 μM (Figure 2). The rate of oxidation of trolox depends on the type of compounds. For the first 20 min. of measurement chlorogenic acid shows the highest pro-oxidant properties whereas cichoric acid is the lowest (the pro-oxidant activity increases in the series: cichoric acid < quercetin < caffeic acid < chlorogenic acid). For the next 30 min. the pro-oxidant capacity increases as follows: quercetin < cichoric acid < caffeic acid < chlorogenic acid), and after 60 min. all tested compounds reveal similar pro-oxidant properties.

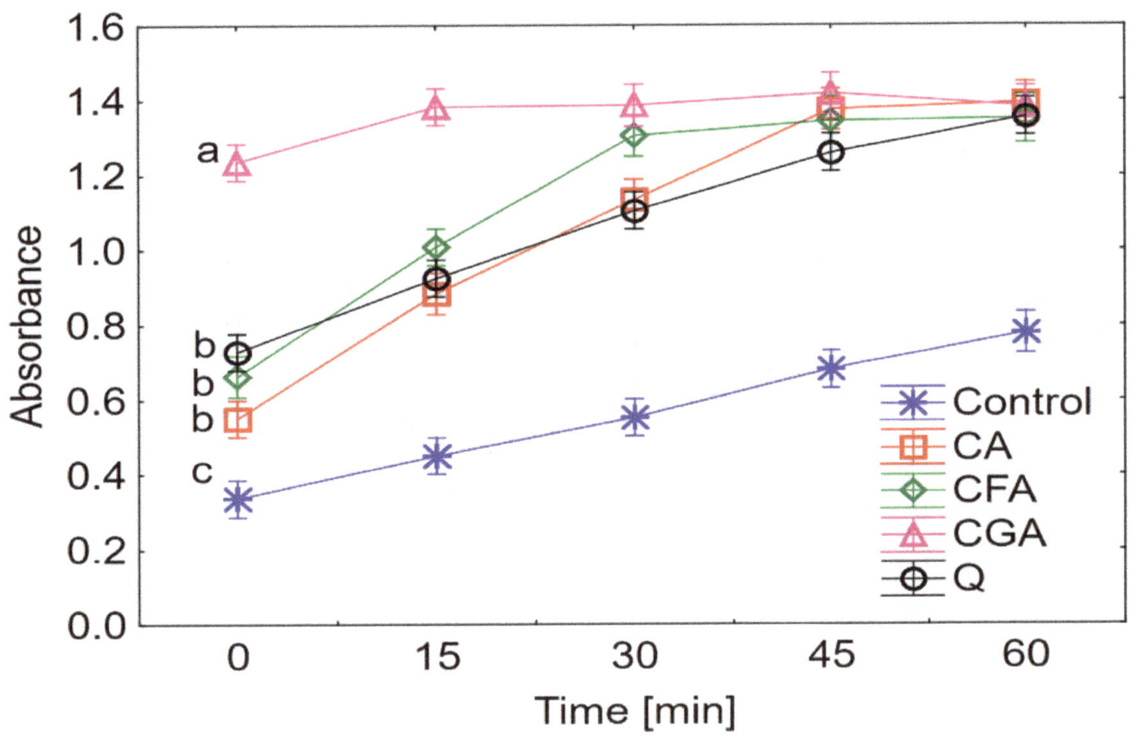

Figure 2. The effect of selected phenolic compounds (0.25 μM) on the oxidation of trolox. CA: cichoric acid, CFA: caffeic acid, CGA: chlorogenic acid, Q: quercetin. The same letters for particular compounds indicate no significant difference (Tukey test, $p < 0.05$).

3.2. CA, DOX and CA-DOX Cytotoxicity

Cell viability was determined using MTT assay. CA significantly increased cell proliferation especially after 24 h of exposure (Figure 3A–C). None of the tested CA concentration resulted in a decrease below the control level. The concentration of 1 μM of CA increased the viability of cells by 46% after 24 h and by about 50% after 48 h treatment. Treatment with 100 μM of CA also increased fibroblast cells proliferation by about 40% in both tested incubation times (Figure 3A). DOX treatment caused decrease in fibroblast viability (Figure 3B). The most significant decrease by about 53% was observed under the influence of 3 μM DOX after 48 h treatment. We didn't observe any increases above the control level in viability of cells under the influence of DOX. Therefore we selected one concentration of DOX, which is 3 μM and combined it with all of the tested concentrations of CA (ranged from 0.5 μM to 300 μM). We observed significant increase in viability of cells after 24 h and 48 h treatment with 200 and 300 μM CA combined with 3 μM DOX (Figure 3C). Simultaneous treatment with 300 μM CA and 3 μM DOX for 48 h increased cell proliferation by about 200% as compared to untreated controls. Based on that experiment we chose one combination of DOX and CA, which was 300 μM of CA and 3 μM of DOX for studying oxidative stress and apoptosis.

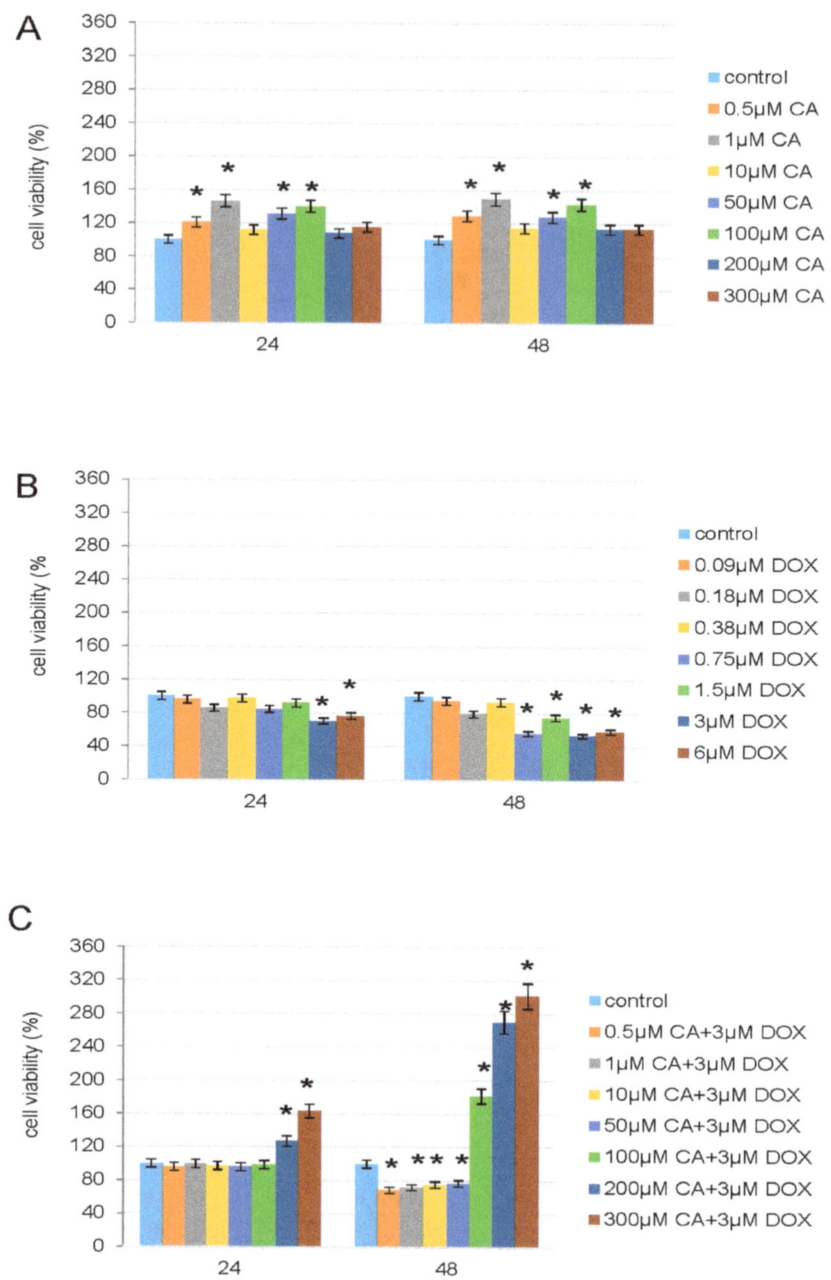

Figure 3. The effect of CA, DOX and CA + DOX on cell viability of fibroblasts. The cells were incubated with 0.5 μM, 1 μM, 10 μM, 50 μM, 100 μM, 200 μM and 300 μM CA for 24 h and 48 h (**A**); 0.09 μM, 0.18 μM, 0.38 μM, 0.75 μM, 1.5 μM, 3 μM and 6 μM DOX for 24 h and 48 h (**B**); mix of CA and DOX in concentrations: 0.5 μM CA + 3 μM DOX, 1 μM CA + 3 μM DOX, 10 μM CA + 3 μM DOX, 50 μM CA + 3 μM DOX, 100 μM CA + 3 μM DOX, 200 μM CA+3 μM DOX and 300 μM CA + 3 μM DOX for 24 h and 48 h (**C**). Mean values from three independent experiments ± SD are shown. Significant alterations are expressed relative to control, untreated cells, and marked with asterisks. Statistical significance was considered if * $p < 0.05$. CA: cichoric acid, DOX: doxorubicin.

3.3. Determination of Caspase 3/7 Activity

Caspase-Glo® 3/7 Assay was used to assess apoptosis level under the influence of the tested substances on fibroblast cell line. The cells were subjected to 3 μM DOX, 300 μM CA and DOX combined with CA in the above-mentioned concentrations for 24 h and 48 h (Figure 4). 300 μM of CA was added to the cell culture 2 h before adding 3 μM DOX. An increased level of apoptosis was observed in the presence of 3 μM DOX and in case of simultaneous treatment with DOX and CA, however when CA was added to the DOX-treated culture the level of apoptosis was decreased as compared to DOX—treated cells. Exposure of fibroblast cells to 300 μM CA significantly decreased caspase 3/7 activity and therefore apoptosis.

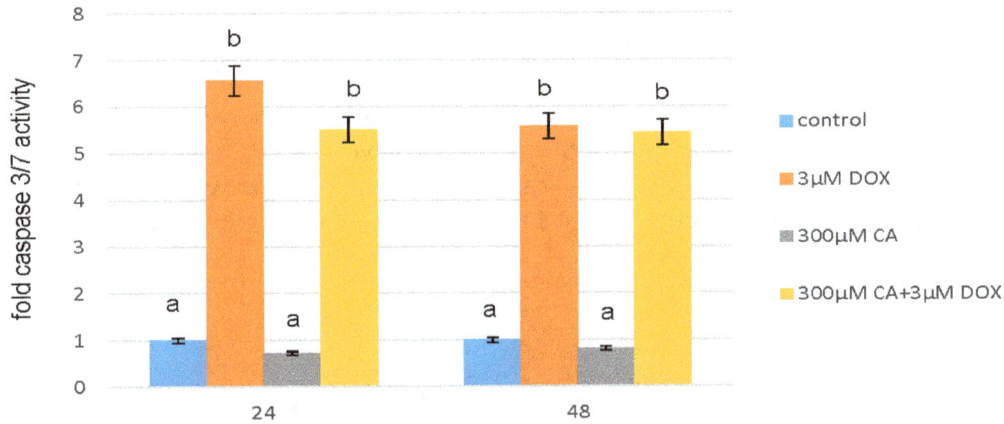

Figure 4. The effect of DOX, CA and CA + DOX on caspase 3/7 activity in fibroblast cells. The cells were incubated with 3 μM DOX, 300 μM CA and DOX (3 μM) combined with CA (300 μM) for 24 h and 48 h Mean values from three independent experiments ± SD are shown. Different letters (a, b) indicate statistical differences ($p \leq 0.05$) between control, 3 μM DOX, 300 μM CA and DOX combined with CA estimated by Tukey's test.

3.4. Determination of Caspase 9 Activity

For the measurement of the caspase 9 activity Caspase-Glo® 9 Assay was applied. Similarly as in case of caspase 3/7 activity results, a significant increase in caspase 9 activity was observed under the influence of 3 μM DOX (Figure 5). CA in 300 μM concentration caused a significant decrease in caspase 9 activity. However, the most interesting and significant result is statistically significant decrease in studied caspase activity under the influence of 300 μM CA combined with 3 μM DOX. The level of apoptosis in this case is even lower than in control, untreated cells, which may mean the CA is effective in counteracting the effect of DOX on healthy cell apoptosis.

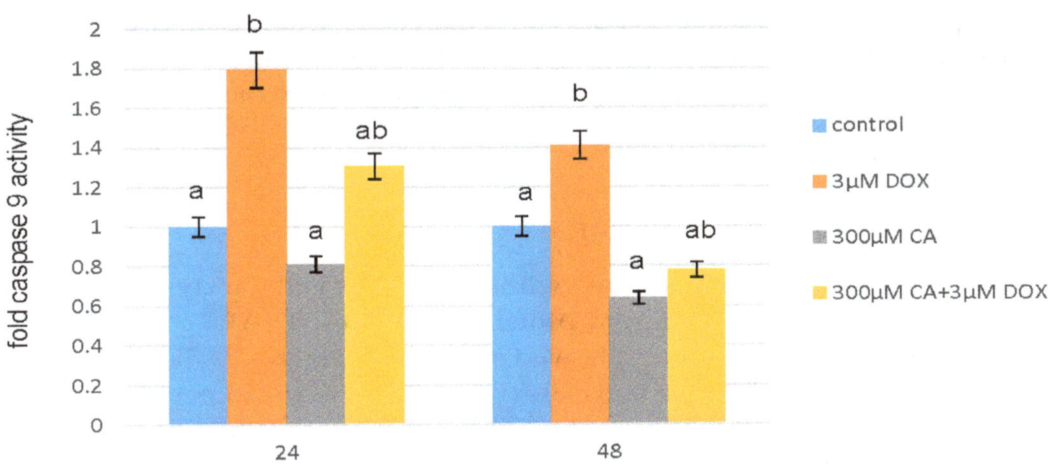

Figure 5. The effect of DOX, CA and CA+DOX on caspase 9 activity in fibroblast cells. The cells were incubated with 3 μM DOX, 300 μM CA and DOX (3 μM) combined with CA (300 μM) for 24 h and 48 h Mean values from three independent experiments ± SD are shown. Different letters (a, b) indicate statistical differences ($p \leq 0.05$) between control, 3 μM DOX, 300 μM CA and DOX combined with CA estimated by Tukey's test.

3.5. Determination of SH Groups

The effect of DOX and CA on SH group content is shown in Figure 6. To determine the oxidation of the SH group, a spectrophotometric assay with Ellman's reagent was used. Thiol group content was evaluated as a marker of protein oxidation. A significant decrease in thiol group content of ~25% compared to the control was observed especially after 48 h of treatment at a concentration of 3 μM DOX. Exposure to CA resulted in ~50% increase in the total cellular content of the thiol groups after 48 h of treatment. Obtained results revealed that 300 μM concentration of CA eliminated pro-oxidative effect of DOX on fibroblasts, because we observed a significant increase in thiol group content under the influence of 3 μM DOX in culture pretreated with 300 μM CA. An observed SH group level after 48 h treatment with DOX combined with CA was even higher than it was in control untreated cells. These data indicate that CA is an effective agent in elimination of the oxidative stress, mainly oxidative damage of proteins, caused by DOX.

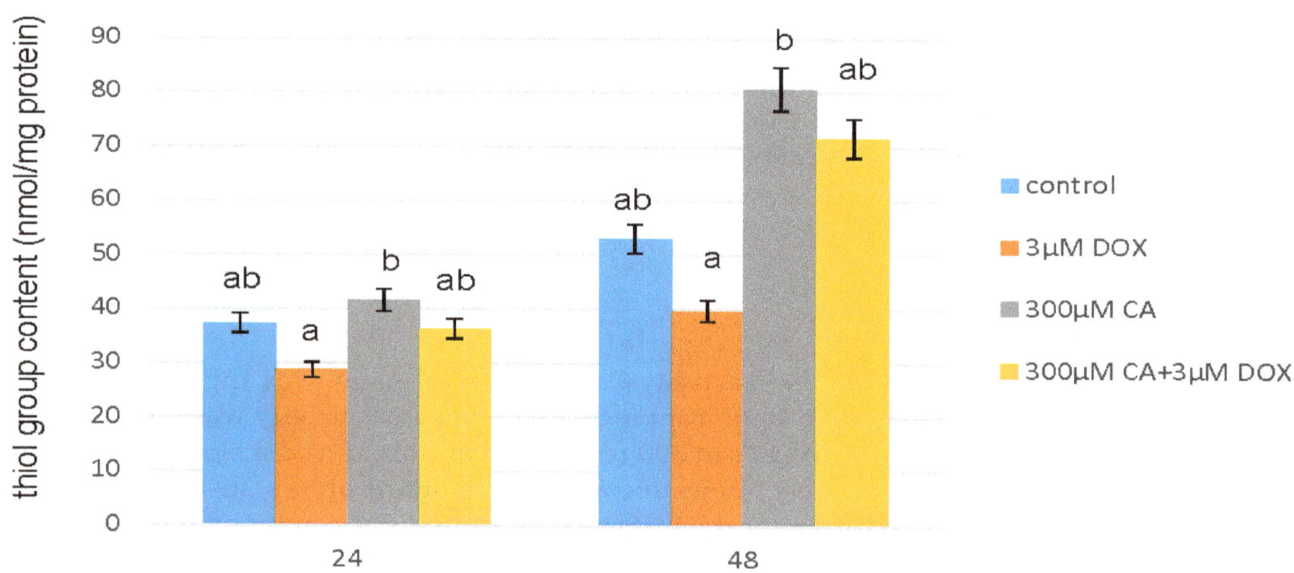

Figure 6. The effect of DOX, CA and CA+DOX on SH group content in fibroblasts. The cells were incubated with 3 μM DOX, 300 μM CA and DOX (3 μM) combined with CA (300 μM) for 24 h and 48 h Mean values from three independent experiments ± SD are shown. Different letters (a, b) indicate statistical differences ($p \leq 0.05$) between control, 3 μM DOX, 300 μM CA and DOX combined with CA estimated by Tukey's test.

3.6. Determination of TBA Reactive Species (TBARS) Levels

Lipid peroxidation is a process connected with a variety of cellular dysfunctions, which result from the inappropriate modifications of lipid-protein complexes. TBARS content was measured as an index of lipid peroxidation. The results showed significant differences between TBARS levels in the control, DOX, CA and DOX-CA—treated cells (Figure 7). The addition of 3 μM DOX to the cells induced a significant increase in TBARS content of ~95% compared to the control after 24 h treatment. CA at a concentration of 300 μM induced a decrease of ~14% compared to the control observed after 24 h of incubation. CA in 300 μM concentration caused a reduction in TBARS content, which was raised because of DOX influence. The obtained results suggest that CA demonstrates protective properties against TBARS production caused by DOX, and as a consequence it decreases membrane phospholipid peroxidation.

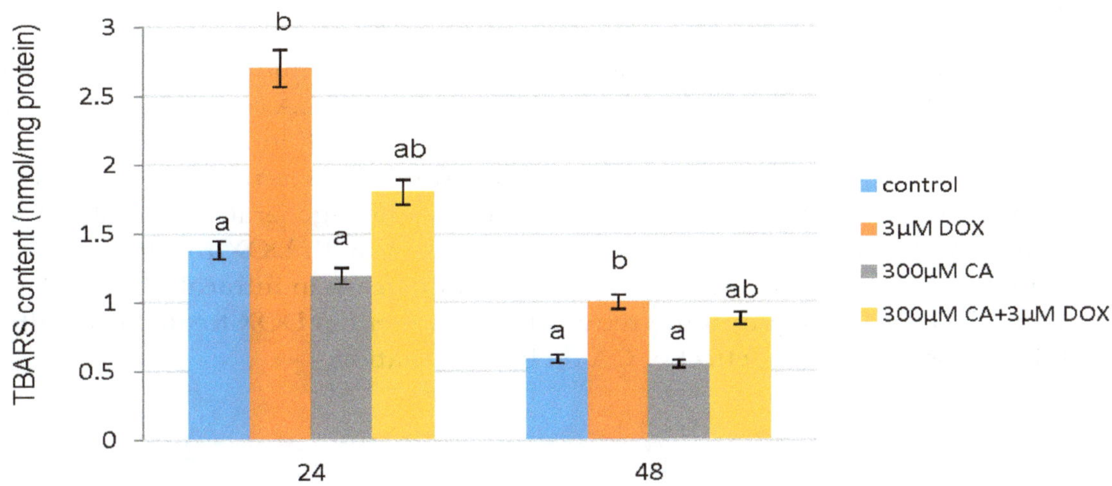

Figure 7. The effect of DOX, CA and CA + DOX on TBARS content in fibroblast cells. The cells were incubated with 3 μM DOX, 300 μM CA and DOX (3 μM) combined with CA (300 μM) for 24 h and 48 h Mean values from three independent experiments ± SD are shown. Different letters (a, b) indicate statistical differences ($p \leq 0.05$) between control, 3 μM DOX, 300 μM CA and DOX combined with CA estimated by Tukey's test.

3.7. Determination of GSH/GSSG

Reduced glutathione is one of the most important low mass antioxidants, therefore the estimation of GSH/GSSG ratio constitute an essential study in oxidative stress parameters research. DOX in 3 μM concentration treatment caused a significant decreases in GSH/GSSG ratio after 24 h and 48 h of incubation, while 300 μM of CA treatment resulted in significant increases in both incubation times as compared to the control, untreated cells. Cell culture pre-treatment with CA in 300 μM concentration resulted in an elevated ration of GSH/GSSG after 24 h and 48 h of incubation even after addition of DOX. After 24 h of incubation with the addition of DOX and CA mixture the level of GSH was elevated even as compared to control untreated cells. The effect of DOX, CA and DOX combined with CA on GSH/GSSG ratio is shown in Figure 8. Obtained results revealed an inhibitory influence of DOX and stimulatory effect of CA on GSH amount in fibroblast cell line.

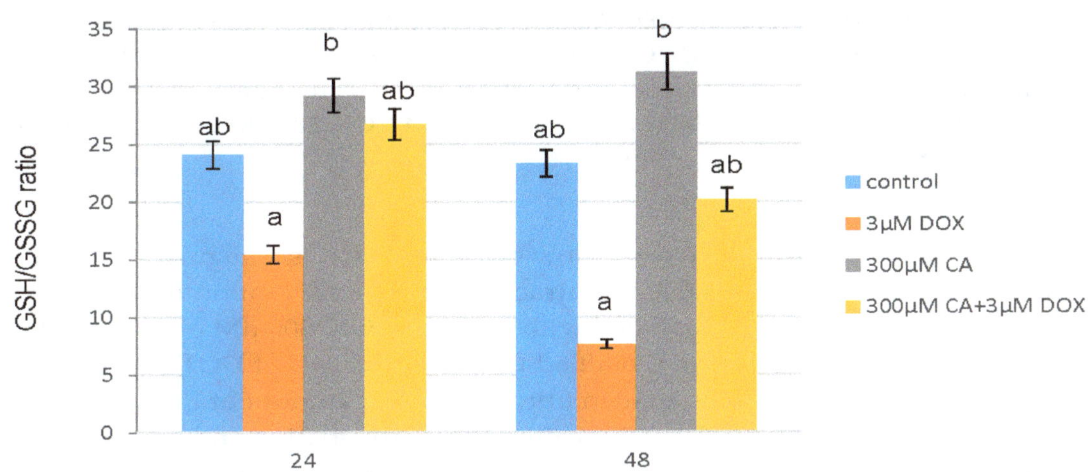

Figure 8. The effect of DOX, CA and CA + DOX on GSH/GSSG ratio in fibroblasts. The cells were incubated with 3 μM DOX, 300 μM CA and DOX (3 μM) combined with CA (300 μM) for 24 h and 48 h Mean values from three independent experiments ± SD are shown. Different letters (a, b) indicate statistical differences ($p \leq 0.05$) between control, 3 μM DOX, 300 μM CA and DOX combined with CA estimated by Tukey's test.

3.8. Intracellular ROS Detection

Figure 9 shows the relative fluorescence intensity of 2′,7′-dichlorofluorescein (DCF) as a percent of control in fibroblast cells incubated with 3 μM of DOX or 300 μM of CA or 3 μM of DOX and 300 μM of CA for 24 and 48 h. An increase in the intracellular ROS production resulted in higher intensity of DCF fluorescence and it was dependent on the concentration of studied compounds. After 24 h incubation of fibroblast cells with 3 μM DOX, the intracellular ROS generation was about 50% higher in comparison to control, untreated cells. The 48 h incubation with DOX resulted in 35% increase in ROS production. CA treatment caused non-significant decrease in intracellular ROS production. Pre-treatment with 300 μM CA significantly reduced ROS content in DOX treated cell culture. These data show inhibitory and protective effect of CA on ROS formation.

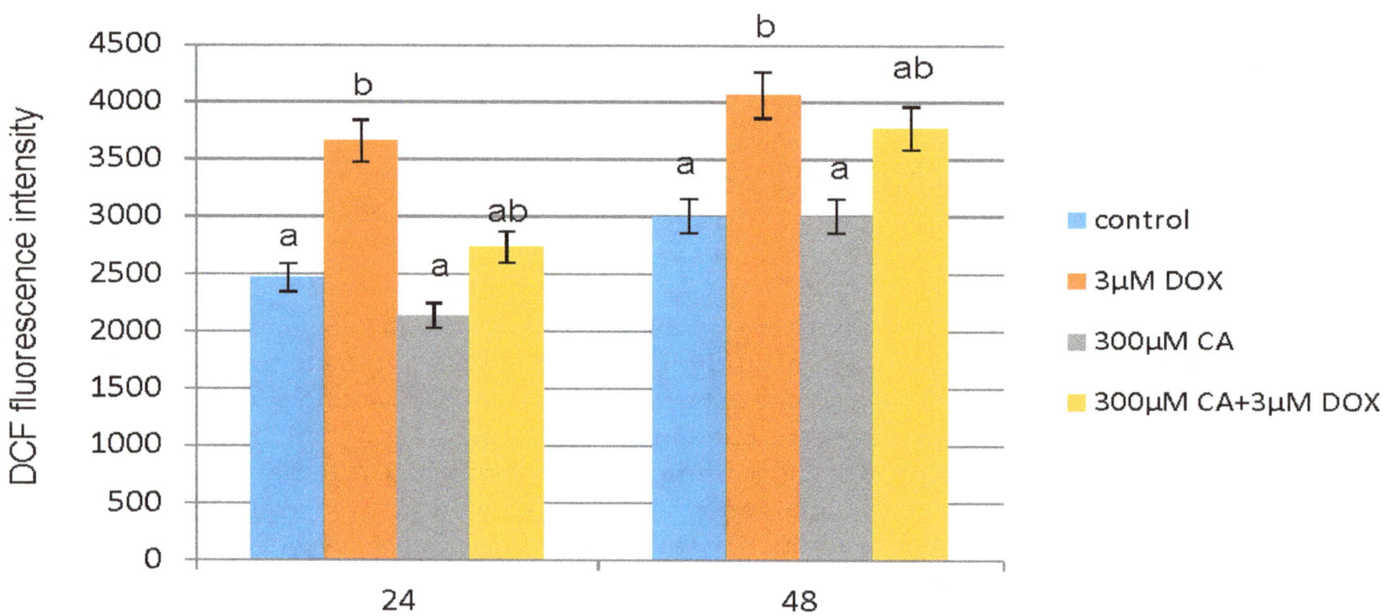

Figure 9. The effect of DOX, CA and CA + DOX on the level of intracellular ROS in fibroblasts. The cells were incubated with 3 μM DOX, 300 μM CA and DOX (3 μM) combined with CA (300 μM) for 24 h and 48 h Mean values from three independent experiments ± SD are shown. Different letters (a, b) indicate statistical differences ($p \leq 0.05$) between control, 3 μM DOX, 300 μM CA and DOX combined with CA estimated by Tukey's test.

Obtained results were confirmed by using flow cytometry analysis. Figure 10 indicates the effect of DOX, CA and DOX combined with CA on intracellular ROS generation in fibroblasts. It shows the % of DCF positive fibroblast cells incubated with 3 μM of DOX, 300 μM of CA and the mixture of two tested compounds for 24 h and 48 h. Obtained results indicate that DOX in 3 μM concentration is efficient in enhancing oxidative stress level in fibroblasts. The amount of ROS under the influence of DOX was significantly elevated by about 20% after 24 h of incubation and by about 45% after 48 h of incubation as compared to control, non-treated cells. Presented results are statistically significant. Pretreatment with 300 μM of CA caused a significant reduction in ROS content in DOX-treated culture. The difference in ROS formation in cultures treated with CA mixed with DOX and cultures treated with DOX only amounted approximately 40% after 48 h of incubation. This results confirmed protective properties of CA against ROS generation in DOX-treated fibroblasts.

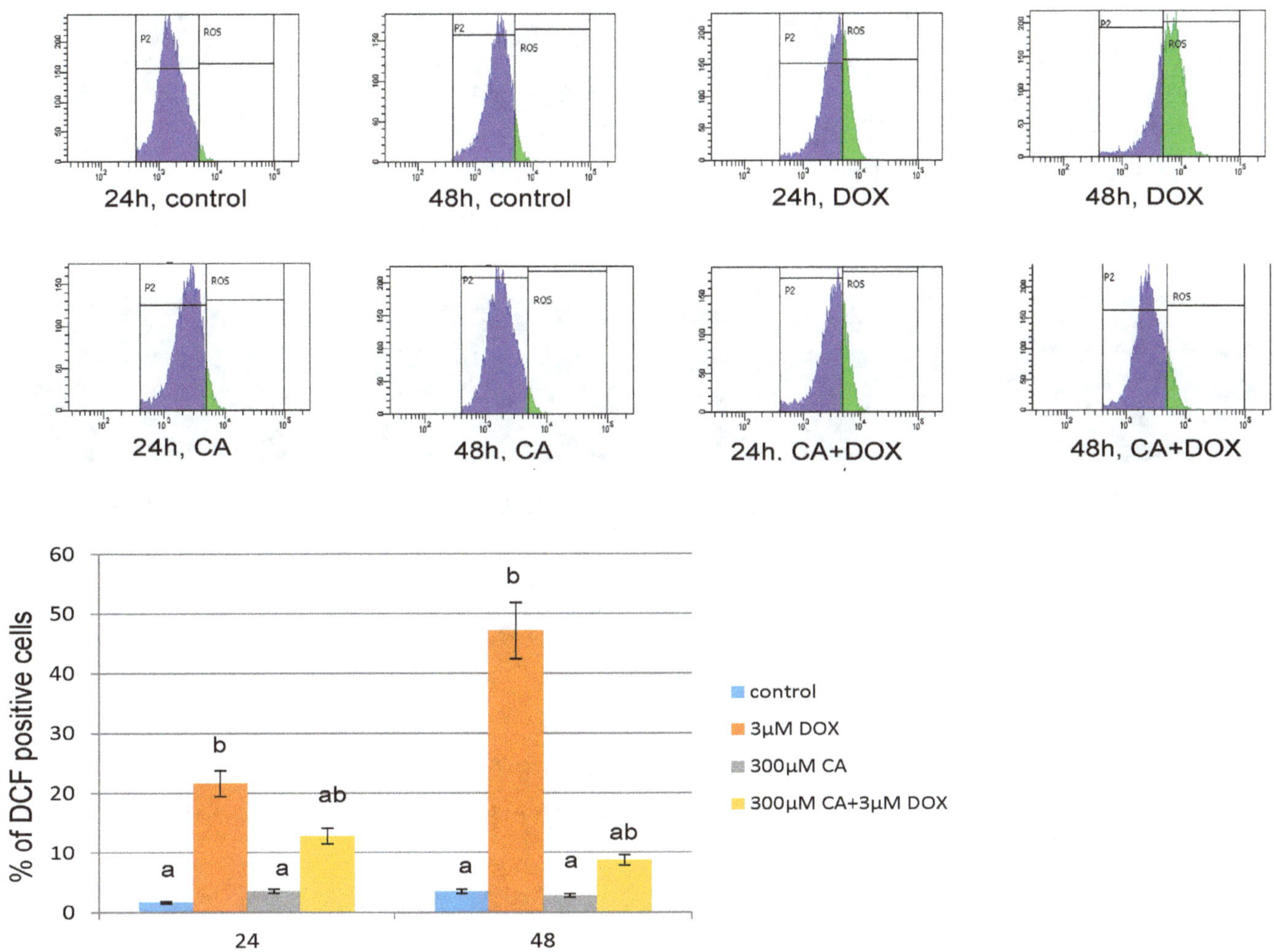

Figure 10. The effect of DOX, CA and CA + DOX on the level of intracellular ROS examined by flow cytometry in fibroblast cells. This Figure shows representative histograms of fibroblasts FACS analysis and the percentage of fibroblast cells generating intracellular ROS. The cells were incubated with 3 μM DOX, 300 μM CA and DOX (3 μM) combined with CA (300 μM) for 24 h and 48 h Mean values from three independent experiments ± SD are shown. Different letters (a, b) indicate statistical differences ($p \leq 0.05$) between control, 3 μM DOX, 300 μM CA and DOX combined with CA estimated by Tukey's test

3.9. Fluorescent Microscopy Assay

In order to evaluate the apoptotic and necrotic cells morphology and for the confirmation of the apoptosis process measured in above described methods, fluorescent staining was used (Figure 11). Similar to luminescence analysis we observed changes between the control, DOX and CA—treated cells. In control cells lack of chromatin condensation and a few to over a dozen of bright green stained nucleoli were observed. At a 3 μM concentration of DOX, numerous of apoptotic cells with visible chromatin condensation and apoptotic bodies especially after 48 h treatment were seen. DOX treatment also caused chromatin marginalization. However, CA treated cells did not reveal any significant apoptotic changes and CA pretreatment in cells before addition of DOX caused a significant reduction in apoptosis level.

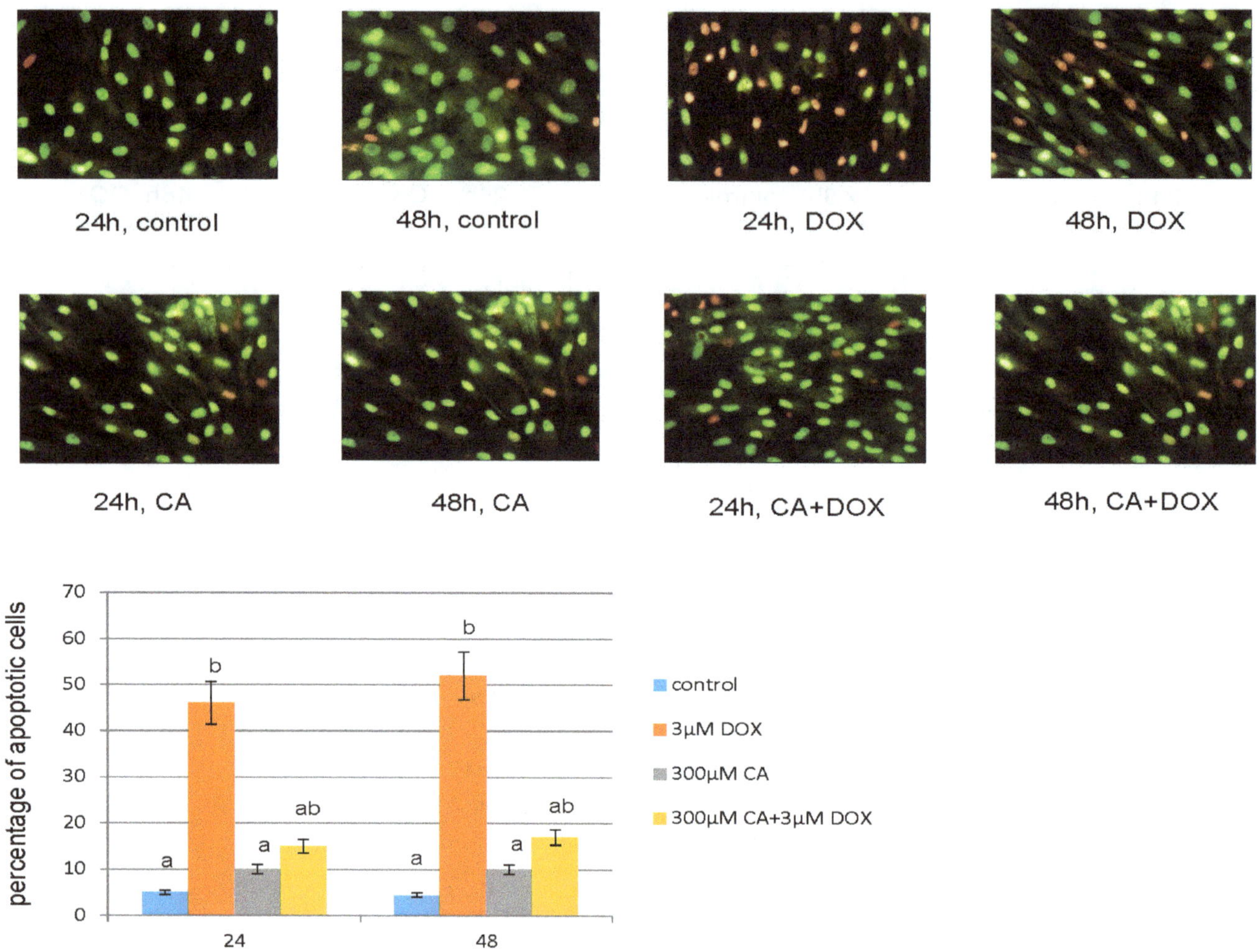

Figure 11. The effect of DOX, CA and CA + DOX on apoptosis and necrosis in the fibroblasts evaluated by fluorescence microscope assay. The cells were incubated in 3 μM DOX, 300 μM CA and DOX (3 μM) combined with CA (300 μM) for 24, and 48 h and stained with acridine orange and ethidium bromide. The cells were photographed under a fluorescence microscope at 200× magnification. We presented representative images from one of three independent experiments and the percentage of apoptotic cells on the graph. Different letters (a, b) indicate statistical differences ($p \leq 0.05$) between control, 3 μM DOX, 300 μM CA and DOX combined with CA estimated by Tukey's test

4. Discussion

The selected natural phenolic compounds are common components of human diet and their antioxidant and as well as anti-inflammatory and anticancer properties are widely described, e.g., CA could be beneficial for preventing dermal injury in the setting of DOX treatment [31–34]. Cichoric acid is a compound with many potentially beneficial properties. It can be obtained from isolated and purified plant and vegetables and it has been described as a one daily nutraceutical which enhances antioxidant activity [35]. The consumption of CA, its derivatives and CA containing plants may significantly influence redox balance in human organism and provide excellent health benefits. CA has been reported as potential anti-diabetic and anti-obesity compound [36]. However, what is important in the context of nutrition in pathological conditions, its oral intake alleviates severe side effects of an excessive alcohol consumption, which was studied in case of acute alcohol-induced hepatic steatosis in mice. Mechanism of CA action in above described study resulted from oxidative stress inhibition and CA anti-inflammation properties [37].

The anti- and pro-oxidant activity of cichoric acid was determined and compared with the activity of caffeic acid, chlorogenic acid and quercetin. Cichoric acid is the derivative of caffeic acid and tartaric acid. The presence of the two caffeic acid moieties in the cichoric acid molecule determines its high antioxidant properties. Therefore the caffeic acid was chosen in this comparative study. Chlorogenic acid is another chosen phenolic compound which is an ester of caffeic and quinic acids. It was selected in this study in order to estimate whether the number of caffeic acid moieties or the present of additional structure (e.g., quinic acid fragment) affect the anti-/pro-oxidant properties of molecules. Quercetin was chosen as one of the most intensively studied antioxidants. Obtained results indicate that according to the increasing antioxidant activity the studied compounds may be ordered as follows: cichoric acid > caffeic acid~quercetin > chlorogenic acid. The selected compounds were studied for their pro-oxidative effect on trolox oxidation. In this assay the radicals of polyphenolics are produced in their reaction with H_2O_2 catalysed by horseradish peroxidase. Then the phenoxyl radicals react with trolox and cause its oxidation to trolox radicals and trolox quinones. In the same time the phenoxyl radicals are transformed to phenolic compounds. The maximum absorption for trolox quinone is 272 nm. This is a general procedure for study the pro-oxidant activity of phenolic compounds [27]. Obtained results showed that the pro-oxidant activity increases in the series: cichoric acid < quercetin < caffeic acid < chlorogenic acid. Cichoric acid was selected for this study because of its high antioxidant properties and relatively lower pro-oxidant activity compared to compounds which display structural similarities.

An increasing interest in the evaluation of clinical effectiveness of natural extracts, dietary supplements, plant origin antioxidants, especially from the polyphenol group of compounds is being observed. The understanding of the molecular mechanisms underlying dietary antioxidants action in diseases prevention and treatment is important to effectively complete these improvements with healthy lifestyle changes. The aim of this actions is mainly to improve human health, prevent diseases and eliminate some severe side effects of the commonly used chemotherapeutics, especially in the cancer treatment. An example of such chemotherapeutic, widely used in the treatment of a variety of cancers, both hematological malignancies and solid tumors is DOX. However, the clinical application of DOX is limited, which results from its high, cumulative dose-dependent toxicity, especially cardiotoxicity, leading to cardiomyopathy. An observed DOX-induced toxicity may be a result of DOX-induced mitochondrial dysfunction and accumulation of oxidative stress products, such as lipid peroxidation products and/or protein oxidation products [17,38].

In order to study possible protective properties of CA on DOX-treated normal human fibroblasts we decided to choose, based on prior experiments, a range of DOX [39] and CA [40] concentrations and estimate the most effective concentrations for both tested compounds. MTT assay revealed that in normal conditions, without any stress factors, CA is efficient in the stimulation of fibroblasts proliferation especially in 0.5 μM, 1 μM, 50 μM and 100 μM concentration. On the other hand, DOX inhibits fibroblasts viability most effectively at the concentration of 3 μM. Therefore, this DOX concentration was chosen for further analysis. The third part of MTT assay showed that pretreatment of fibroblasts with CA (0.5–300 μM) for 2 h before stimulate with DOX was the most effective at 300 μM of CA. Because of that reason, this combination of DOX with CA was applied for the evaluation of the anti-apoptotic and antioxidative effect. Literature data indicate the fact that CA has positive influence on normal cells, e.g., human dermal fibroblasts, where it induces Hepatocyte Growth Factor production on hepatocytes and where it may act as an anti-viral agent [41,42].

Reactive oxygen species (ROS) occurring due to too high level of oxidative stress are chemically reactive molecules that may damage main cellular macromolecules, such as DNA, lipids and proteins, subsequently causing genetic mutations. An excessive exposure to ROS may be seriously deleterious because of oxidative damage to important molecules in cell [43]. To assess the effect of CA on proteins in this work we used one of the most widely studied markers of protein oxidation—protein thiol groups content. We observed the oxidative action of DOX, which conforms that DOX exhibits pro-oxidant properties against proteins and this action is connected with its cytotoxic activity. On the other hand stimulation with CA caused a significant increase in thiol group content, which means that tested compound act as an antioxidant. Especially after 48 h of treatment we can observe that prooxidative activity of DOX was effectively reversed by CA treatment. Study by Tsai KL et al. confirmed that pretreatment with CA may inhibit oxidative stress caused by external factors [44].

Many natural compounds from the polyphenol group, which also include CA, are characterized by high antioxidant capacities and have been considered as a potential protectors against DOX-induced toxicity. This protective effect may be also connected with the reduction of lipid peroxidation process [19]. In support of this report, we observed that CA does not cause oxidative alterations of membrane lipids and protects against DOX-induced TBARS production, which is probably related with antioxidant properties of CA. Already after 24 h we noticed significant increase in TBARS content in DOX-treated cells and a decrease in cells pretreated with 300 μM of CA. CA activity as a compound that prevents lipid peroxidation process was confirmed by several studies [45–47]. Polyphenols exhibit antioxidative properties at several levels, among others they prevent the lipid peroxidation of biological membranes and inhibit the oxidation of lipoproteins and polyunsaturated fatty acids, which is in consistence with our results [48].

Low ROS concentration within the cell is essential for keeping redox balance and for the stimulation of cell proliferation rate. However, an excessive level of accumulated in cell ROS may cause serious damage in protein, lipid and DNA structures through their oxidation and subsequently apoptosis and cell death [49,50]. According to the literature CA, which belongs to the polyphenols group of compounds, may provoke ROS generation in cancer cells and also in preadipocytes, but in normal cells CA was a potent ROS scavenger, reducing ROS accumulation under basal as well as oxidative stress conditions [51]. It is in accordance with our results regarding ROS generation in fibroblast cells. We observed a significant increase in ROS production under the influence of DOX and a decrease in ROS content caused by CA. Pretreatment of fibroblast cells with CA (300 μM) for 2 h before stimulate with DOX significantly inhibited the formation of ROS. Flow cytometry results confirm that intervention with CA mitigated DOX-caused oxidative stress and reduced ROS formation in fibroblasts stimulated with DOX. Therefore we presume that the primary mechanism through which CA alleviates DOX-facilitated cell death of fibroblast cells is its antioxidant function. An observed, DOX-induced significant increase in ROS content was accompanied by a decrease in GSH/GSSG ratio, especially after 48 h of treatment. Similarly as in other tested oxidative stress parameters, GSH/GSSG ratio was significantly reduced after exposure to DOX and these results were effectively reversed by CA treatment. Our results are in accordance with literature data indicating positive influence of selected polyphenols on GSH content. One of the main phenolic compounds of curry spice turmeric is curcumin, the consumption of which brings beneficial effects. It was shown that curcumin plays a protective role against adriamycin-induced toxicity through three main mechanisms: first—it inhibits lipid peroxidation, second – it stabilizes cell membranes and third—it raises glutathione level [52]. Therefore we presume that CA likewise influences GSH level in fibroblast cells. According to Fauser JK et al. a reduced level of the main GSH antioxidant may result in apoptosis and it also may be connected with a reduction of G0/G1 and arrest of the S and M cell cycle phases, together with increased ROS generation [53]. Apoptosis is a programmed cell death that is extremely important for human organism homeostasis maintaining, for tissue development and malignancies treatment. Regulation of this process is main target for anticancer drugs, however chemotherapeutics, such as anthracycline antibiotics, e.g., DOX, may also induce apoptosis in normal, non-cancerous cells. At least two pathways have been described by which an apoptosis occurs: first is an extrinsic death-receptor dependent apoptosis and the second—intrinsic mitochondrial dependent apoptosis. In both pathways selected caspases activation occurs, which means activation of initiator caspases (e.g., caspase-8 and -9) and effector caspases (e.g., caspase-3, -6, and -7) [54,55]. A variety of evidence support also the role of reactive oxygen species in apoptotic cell death. It has been shown that oxygen free radicals are directly involved in the pathogenesis of apoptosis. Caspase 3/7 assay, caspase 9 assay and fluorescent microscopy assay showed that at 3 μM of DOX concentration, numerous apoptotic cells were seen, while pretreatment with 300 μM of CA reduced the number of positive fluorescent cells and decreased the activity of studied caspases significantly. We observed an increase in caspase 3, 7 and 9 activity under the influence of DOX as compared to control non-treated cells, which was accompanied by a decrease in GSH/GSSG ratio and a significant increase in ROS content. Apoptosis is particularly related to the cascade of caspases. Literature data indicated that the release of cytochrome c from the mitochondria into the cytosol, may result in the caspase-9 activation, which subsequently activates effector caspase, such as caspase-3, which causes DNA fragmentation and eventually—cell death [56]. In our study, we found that CA significantly prevented DOX-induced activation of caspase 3 and 7, which is in accordance with literature data that confirms such CA activity. It may thus be hypothesized that this anti-apoptotic effect of CA might be attributed to observed increase in the levels of antioxidant glutathione (reduced GSH) and subsequently to a decrease in oxidative stress level. Tsai KL et al. revealed that CA precluded the activation of caspase 3 and subsequent DNA strand breaks, through the inhibition of the translocation of NF-κB from the cytosol to the nucleus, suppression of Bax and promotion the Bcl-2 expression [44]. In our experiment pretreatment with CA was associated with the inhibition of the downstream apoptotic signaling pathways, finally preventing activation of caspase-3, caspase-7 and caspase -9 induced by DOX. It is suggested that CA is a natural food-derived compound that inhibits apoptosis [57]. Our findings confirm this hypothesis, because under the influence of CA we showed a significant increase in cells proliferation and an decrease in caspase 3/7 and 9 level, which is accompanied by an increase in GSH content and a decrease in ROS content. Anti-apoptotic effect of CA in DOX-treated fibroblasts was confirmed by fluorescence microscopy assay, which indicated that tested compound was efficient both in time and dose-dependent manner.

5. Conclusions

In conclusion, our findings suggest that CA mitigates DOX-induced oxidative stress and inhibits DOX-facilitated ROS formation. Chicoric acid treatment also inhibited DOX-facilitated apoptosis. It is likely that these beneficial effects contribute to the overall antioxidative and anti-apoptotic function of chicoric acid. However, only in vitro investigations were used to test the cytoprotective effects of chicoric acid from DOX-caused fibroblasts dysfunction. Above results may be the first step in explaining important mechanisms underlying the protective effects of CA observed in DOX cytotoxicity. However, additional studies are indispensable to evaluate long-term effect of CA on dermal injuries caused by DOX treatment. Further analysis must also be conducted on the other skin cell types, such as keratinocytes and melanocytes. Further analysis must also be conducted on the molecular level of the anti-oxidative and anti-apoptotic effects of CA, which may be considered as lead compounds for the development of functional food.

Acknowledgments: This work was financially supported by National Science Centre, Poland, under the research project number 2015/17/B/NZ9/03581.

Author Contributions: Agata Jabłońska-Trypuć—corresponding author, wrote the paper, planned experiments; performed experiments; analysed data; Rafał Krętowski—planned flow cytometry experiments; performed flow cytometry experiments; analysed data; Monika Kalinowska—planned chemical experiments, performed chemical experiment, analysed data; Grzegorz Świderski—analyzed the data; Marzanna Cechowska-Pasko—analyzed data; Włodzimierz Lewandowski—analyzed the data.

Compliance with ethical standards: The manuscript does not contain clinical studies or patient data.

References

1. Shroff, A.; Mamalis, A.; Jagdeo, J. Oxidative Stress and Skin Fibrosis. *Curr. Pathobiol. Rep.* **2014**, *2*, 257–267. [CrossRef] [PubMed]
2. Bickers, D.R.; Athar, M. Oxidative stress in the pathogenesis of skin disease. *J. Investig. Dermatol.* **2006**, *126*, 2565–2575. [CrossRef] [PubMed]

3. Ji, H.; Li, X.K. Oxidative Stress in Atopic Dermatitis. *Oxid. Med. Cell. Longev.* **2016**, *2016*, 2721469. [CrossRef] [PubMed]
4. Komuro, T. Re-evaluation of fibroblasts and fibroblast-like cells. *Anat. Embryol.* **1990**, *182*, 103–112. [CrossRef] [PubMed]
5. Atkins, F.M.; Friedman, M.M.; Rao, P.V.S.; Metcalfe, D.D. Interactions between mast cells, fibroblasts and connective tissue components. *Int. Arch. Allergy Appl. Immunol.* **1985**, *77*, 96–102. [CrossRef] [PubMed]
6. Gebicki, J.M.; Bartosz, G. The role of proteins in propagation of damage induced by reactive oxygen species in vivo. *Postepy Biochem.* **2010**, *56*, 115–123. [PubMed]
7. Bartosz, G. Total antioxidant capacity. *Adv. Clin. Chem.* **2003**, *37*, 219–292. [PubMed]
8. Menzel, D.B. The toxicity of air pollution in experimental animals and humans: The role of oxidative stress. *Toxicol. Lett.* **1994**, *72*, 269–277. [CrossRef]
9. Kohen, R.; Gati, I. Skin low molecular weight antioxidants and their role in aging and in oxidative stress. *Toxicology* **2000**, *148*, 149–157. [CrossRef]
10. Jabłońska-Trypuć, A.; Świderski, G.; Krętowski, R.; Lewandowski, W. Newly Synthesized Doxorubicin Complexes with Selected Metals-Synthesis, Structure and Anti-Breast Cancer Activity. *Molecules* **2017**, *22*, 1106. [CrossRef] [PubMed]
11. Coldwell, K.; Cutts, S.M.; Ognibene, T.J.; Henderson, P.T.; Phillips, D.R. Detection of adriamycin-DNA adducts by accelerator mass spectrometry. *Met. Mol. Biol.* **2010**, *613*, 103–118. [CrossRef]
12. Sauter, K.A.; Magun, E.A.; Iordanov, M.S.; Magun, B.E. ZAK is required for doxorubicin, a novel ribotoxic stressor, to induce SAPK activation and apoptosis in HaCaT cells. *Cancer Biol. Ther.* **2010**, *10*, 258–266. [CrossRef] [PubMed]
13. Cao, B.; Li, M.; Zha, W.; Zhao, Q.; Gu, R.; Liu, L.; Shi, J.; Zhou, J.; Zhou, F.; Wu, X.; et al. Metabolomic approach to evaluating adriamycin pharmacodynamics and resistance in breast cancer cells. *Metabolomics* **2013**, *9*, 960–973. [CrossRef] [PubMed]
14. Ta, H.Q.; Thomas, K.S.; Schrecengost, R.S.; Bouton, A.H. A novel association between p130Cas and resistance to the chemotherapeutic drug adriamycin in human breast cancer cells. *Cancer Res.* **2008**, *68*, 8796–8804. [CrossRef] [PubMed]
15. Taskin, E.; Dursun, N. Recovery of adriamycin induced mitochondrial dysfunction in liver by selenium. *Cytotechnology* **2015**, *67*, 977–986. [CrossRef] [PubMed]
16. Yapislar, H.; Taskin, E.; Ozdas, S.; Akin, D.; Sonmez, E. Counteraction of apoptotic and inflammatory effects of adriamycin in the liver cell culture by clinopitolite. *Biol. Trace Elem. Res.* **2016**, *170*, 373–381. [CrossRef] [PubMed]
17. De Beer, E.L.; Bottone, A.E.; Voest, E.E. Doxorubicin and mechanical performance of cardiac trabeculae afteracute and chronic treatment: A review. *Eur. J. Pharmacol.* **2001**, *415*, 1–11. [CrossRef]
18. Singal, P.K.; Li, T.; Kumar, D.; Danelisen, I.; Iliskovic, N. Adriamycin-induced heart-failure: Mechanism and modulation. *Mol. Cell. Biochem.* **2000**, *207*, 77–85. [CrossRef] [PubMed]
19. Quiles, J.L.; Huertas, J.R.; Battino, M.; Mataix, J.; Ramírez-Tortosa, M.C. Antioxidant nutrients and adriamycin toxicity. *Toxicology* **2002**, *180*, 79–95. [CrossRef]
20. Pellati, F.; Benvenuti, S.; Magro, L.; Melegari, M.; Soragni, F. Analysis of phenolic compounds and radical scavenging activity of Echinacea spp. *J. Pharm. Biomed. Anal.* **2004**, *35*, 289–301. [CrossRef]
21. Barnes, J.; Anderson, L.A.; Gibbons, S.; Phillipson, J.D. Echinacea species (*Echinacea angustifolia* (DC.) Hell., *Echinacea pallida* (Nutt.) Nutt., *Echinacea purpurea* (L.) Moench): A review of their chemistry, pharmacology and clinical properties. *J. Pharm. Pharmacol.* **2005**, *57*, 929–954. [CrossRef] [PubMed]
22. Robinson, W.E.; Reinecke, M.G.; Abdel-Malek, S.; Jia, Q.; Chow, S.A. Inhibitors of HIV-1 replication that inhibit HIV integrase. *Proc. Natl. Acad. Sci. USA* **1996**, *93*, 6326–6331. [CrossRef] [PubMed]
23. Kour, K.; Bani, S. Chicoric acid regulates behavioral and biochemical alterations induced by chronic stress in experimental Swiss albino mice. *Pharmacol. Biochem. Behav.* **2011**, *99*, 342–348. [CrossRef] [PubMed]
24. Kour, K.; Bani, S. Augmentation of immune response by chicoric acid through the modulation of CD28/CTLA-4 and Th1 pathway in chronically stressed mice. *Neuropharmacology* **2011**, *60*, 852–860. [CrossRef] [PubMed]
25. Zhu, D.; Wang, Y.; Du, Q.; Liu, Z.; Liu, X. Cichoric Acid Reverses Insulin Resistance and Suppresses Inflammatory Responses in the Glucosamine-Induced HepG2 Cells. *J. Agric. Food Chem.* **2015**, *63*, 10903–10913. [CrossRef] [PubMed]

26. Rice-Evans, C.A.; Diplock, A.T.; Symons, M.C.R. *Techniques in Free Radical Research*; Elsevier: Amsterdam, The Netherlands, 1991.
27. Zeraik, M.L.; Petrono, M.S.; Coelho, D.; Regasini, L.O.; Silva, D.H.S.; da Fonseca, L.M.; Machado, S.A.S.; Bolzani, V.S.; Ximenes, V.F. Improvement of pro-oxidant capacity of protocatechuic acid by esterification. *PLoS ONE* **2014**, *9*, e110277. [CrossRef] [PubMed]
28. Carmichael, J.; DeGraff, W.G.; Gazdar, A.F.; Minna, J.D.; Mitchell, J.B. Evaluation of a tetrazolium-based semiautomated colorimetric assay: Assessment of chemosensitivity testing. *Cancer Res.* **1987**, *47*, 936–942. [PubMed]
29. Jabłońska-Trypuć, A.; Pankiewicz, W.; Czerpak, R. Traumatic acid reduces oxidative stress and enhances collagen biosynthesis in cultured human skin fibroblasts. *Lipids* **2016**, *51*, 1021–1035. [CrossRef] [PubMed]
30. Krętowski, R.; Kusaczuk, M.; Naumowicz, M.; Kotyńska, J.; Szynaka, B.; Cechowska-Pasko, M. The Effects of Silica Nanoparticles on Apoptosis and Autophagy of Glioblastoma Cell Lines. *Nanomaterials* **2017**, *7*, 230. [CrossRef] [PubMed]
31. Kalinowska, M.; Bielawska, A.; Lewandowska-Siwkiewicz, H.; Priebe, W.; Lewandowski, W. Apple: Phenolic compounds, extraction and health benefits—A review. *Plant Phys. Biochem.* **2014**, *84*, 169–188. [CrossRef] [PubMed]
32. Lewandowska, H.; Kalinowska, M.; Lewandowski, W.; Stępkowski, T.M.; Brzóska, K. The role of natural polyphenols in cell signaling and cytoprotection against cancer development. *J. Nutr. Biochem.* **2016**, *32*, 1–19. [CrossRef] [PubMed]
33. Bajko, E.; Kalinowska, M.; Borowski, P.; Siergiejczyk, L.; Lewandowski, W. 5-*O*-Caffeoylquinic acid: A spectroscopic study and biological screening for antimicrobial activity. *LWT Food Sci. Technol.* **2016**, *65*, 471–479. [CrossRef]
34. Facino, R.M.; Carini, M.; Aldini, G.; Saibene, L.; Pietta, P.; Mauri, P. Echinacoside and caffeoyl conjugates protect collagen from free radical-induced degradation: A potential use of Echinacea extracts in the prevention of skin photodamage. *Planta Med.* **1995**, *61*, 510–514. [CrossRef] [PubMed]
35. Azay-Milhau, J.; Ferrare, K.; Leroy, J.; Aubaterre, J.; Tournier, M.; Lajoix, A.D.; Tousch, D. Antihyperglycemic effect of a natural chicoric acid extract of chicory (*Cichorium intybus* L.): A comparative *in vitro* study with the effects of caffeic and ferulic acids. *J. Ethnopharmacol.* **2013**, *150*, 755–760. [CrossRef] [PubMed]
36. Xiao, H.; Wang, J.; Yuan, L.; Xiao, C.; Wang, Y.; Liu, X. Chicoric acid induces apoptosis in 3T3-L1 preadipocytes through ROS-mediated PI3K/Akt and MAPK signaling pathways. *J. Agric. Food Chem.* **2013**, *61*, 1509–1520. [CrossRef] [PubMed]
37. Landmann, M.; Kanuri, G.; Spruss, A.; Stahl, C.; Bergheim, I. Oral intake of chicoric acid reduces acute alcohol-induced hepatic steatosis in mice. *Nutrition* **2014**, *30*, 882–889. [CrossRef] [PubMed]
38. Wouters, K.A.; Kremer, L.C.; Miller, T.L.; Herman, E.H.; Lipshultz, S.E. Protecting against anthracycline-induced myocardial damage: A review of the most promising strategies. *Br. J. Haematol.* **2005**, *131*, 561–578. [CrossRef] [PubMed]
39. Guerriero, E.; Sorice, A.; Capone, F.; Storti, G.; Colonna, G.; Ciliberto, G.; Costantini, S. Combining doxorubicin with a phenolic extract from flaxseed oil: Evaluation of the effect on two breast cancer cell lines. *Int. J. Oncol.* **2017**, *50*, 468–476. [CrossRef] [PubMed]
40. Tsai, Y.L.; Chiu, C.C.; Chen, J.Y.F.; Chan, K.C.; Lin, S.D. Cytotoxic effects of Echinacea purpurea flower extracts and cichoric acid on human colon cancer cells through induction of apoptosis. *J. Ethnopharmacol.* **2012**, *143*, 914–919. [CrossRef] [PubMed]
41. Kurisu, M.; Nakasone, R.; Miyamae, Y.; Matsuura, D.; Kanatani, H.; Yano, S.; Shigemori, H. Induction of hepatocyte growth factor production in human dermal fibroblasts by caffeic acid derivatives. *Biol. Pharm. Bull.* **2013**, *36*, 2018–2021. [CrossRef] [PubMed]
42. Zhang, H.L.; Dai, L.H.; Wu, Y.H.; Yu, X.P.; Zhang, Y.Y.; Guan, R.F.; Liu, T.; Zhao, J. Evaluation of hepatocyteprotective and anti-hepatitis B virus properties of Cichoric acid from Cichorium intybus leaves in cell culture. *Biol. Pharm. Bull.* **2014**, *37*, 1214–1220. [CrossRef]
43. Rucinska, A.; Roszczyk, M.; Gabryelak, T. Cytotoxicity of the isoflavone genistein in NIH 3T3 cells. *Cell Biol. Int.* **2008**, *32*, 1019–1023. [CrossRef] [PubMed]
44. Tsai, K.L.; Kao, C.L.; Hung, C.H.; Cheng, Y.H.; Lin, H.C.; Chu, P.M. Chicoric acid is a potent anti-atherosclerotic ingredient by anti-oxidant action and anti-inflammation capacity. *Oncotarget* **2017**, *8*, 29600–29612. [CrossRef] [PubMed]

45. Dalby-Brown, L.; Barsett, H.; Landbo, A.K.; Meyer, A.S.; Mølgaard, P. Synergistic antioxidative effects of alkamides, caffeic acid derivatives, and polysaccharide fractions from Echinacea purpurea on in vitro oxidation of human low-density lipoproteins. *J. Agric. Food Chem.* **2005**, *53*, 9413–9423. [CrossRef] [PubMed]
46. Sloley, B.D.; Urichuk, L.J.; Tywin, C.; Coutts, R.T.; Pang, P.K.; Shan, J.J. Comparison of chemical components and antioxidants capacity of different Echinacea species. *J. Pharm. Pharmacol.* **2001**, *53*, 849–857. [CrossRef] [PubMed]
47. Ahn, H.R.; Lee, H.J.; Kim, K.A.; Kim, C.Y.; Nho, C.W.; Jang, H.; Pan, C.H.; Lee, C.Y.; Jung, S.H. Hydroxycinnamic acids in Crepidiastrum denticulatum protect oxidative stress-induced retinal damage. *J. Agric. Food Chem.* **2014**, *62*, 1310–1323. [CrossRef] [PubMed]
48. Granados-Principal, S.; Quiles, J.L.; Ramirez-Tortosa, C.L.; Sanchez-Rovira, P.; Ramirez-Tortosa, M.C. New advances in molecular mechanisms and the prevention of adriamycin toxicity by antioxidant nutrients. *Food Chem. Toxicol.* **2010**, *48*, 1425–1438. [CrossRef] [PubMed]
49. Tsai, C.W.; Lin, C.Y.; Lin, H.H.; Chen, J.H. Carnosic acid, a rosemary phenolic compound, induces apoptosis through reactive oxygen species-mediated p38 activation in human neuroblastoma IMR-32 cells. *Neurochem. Res.* **2011**, *36*, 2442–2451. [CrossRef] [PubMed]
50. Lee, Y.S. Role of NADPH oxidase-mediated generation of reactive oxygen species in the mechanism of apoptosis induced by phenolic acids in HepG2 human hepatoma cells. *Arch. Pharm. Res.* **2005**, *28*, 1183–1189. [CrossRef] [PubMed]
51. Schlernitzauer, A.; Oiry, C.; Hamad, R.; Galas, S.; Cortade, F.; Chabi, B.; Casas, F.; Pessemesse, L.; Fouret, G.; Feillet-Coudray, C.; et al. Chicoric acid is an antioxidant molecule that stimulates AMP kinase pathway in L6 myotubes and extends lifespan in Caenorhabditis elegans. *PLoS ONE* **2013**, *8*, e78788. [CrossRef] [PubMed]
52. Quiles, J.L.; Ochoa, J.J.; Huertas, J.R.; López-Frías, M.; Mataix, J. Olive oil and mitochondrial oxidative stress: Studies on adriamycin toxicity, physical exercise and ageing. In *Olive Oil and Health*; Quiles, J.L., Ramirez-Tortosa, M.C., Yaqoob, P., Eds.; CABI Publishing: Oxford, UK, 2006; pp. 119–151.
53. Fauser, J.K.; Matthews, G.M.; Cummins, A.G.; Howarth, G.S. Induction of apoptosis by the medium-chain length fatty acid lauric acid in colon cancer cells due to induction of oxidative stress. *Chemotherapy* **2013**, *59*, 214–224. [CrossRef] [PubMed]
54. Jacobson, M.D.; Weil, M.; Raff, M.C. Programmed cell death in animal development. *Cell* **1997**, *88*, 347–354. [CrossRef]
55. Wong, R.S. Apoptosis in cancer: From pathogenesis to treatment. *J. Exp. Clin. Cancer Res.* **2011**, *30*, 87. [CrossRef] [PubMed]
56. Kumar, D.; Kirshenbaum, L.; Li, T.; Danelisen, I.; Singal, P. Apoptosis in isolated adult cardiomyocytes exposed to adriamycin. *Ann. N. Y. Acad. Sci.* **1999**, *874*, 156–168. [CrossRef] [PubMed]
57. Zhu, D.; Zhang, X.; Niu, Y.; Diao, Z.; Ren, B.; Li, X.; Liu, Z.; Liu, X. Cichoric acid improved hyperglycaemia and restored muscle injury via activating antioxidant response in MLD-STZ-induced diabetic mice. *Food Chem. Toxicol.* **2017**, *107*, 138–149. [CrossRef] [PubMed]

4

Bioactive Dietary VDR Ligands Regulate Genes Encoding Biomarkers of Skin Repair that are Associated with Risk for Psoriasis

Amitis Karrys [1,2,†], Islam Rady [3,4,†], Roxane-Cherille N. Chamcheu [3], Marya S. Sabir [5], Sanchita Mallick [5], Jean Christopher Chamcheu [3,6,*], Peter W. Jurutka [2,5], Mark R. Haussler [2] and G. Kerr Whitfield [2]

1 School of Life Sciences, Arizona State University, Tempe, AZ 85281, USA; tkarrys12@gmail.com
2 Department of Basic Medical Sciences, University of Arizona College of Medicine–Phoenix, Phoenix, AZ 85004, USA; peter.jurutka@asu.edu (P.W.J.); haussler@email.arizona.edu (M.R.H.); gkw@email.arizona.edu (G.K.W.)
3 Department of Dermatology, School of Medicine and Public Health, University of Wisconsin, Madison, WI 53706, USA; irady@dermatology.wisc.edu (I.R.); roxanechamcheu@gmail.com (R.-C.N.C.)
4 Department of Zoology, Faculty of Science, Al-Azhar University, P.O. Box 11884 Nazr City, Cairo, Egypt
5 School of Mathematical and Natural Sciences, Arizona State University, Phoenix, AZ 85306, USA; msabir@asu.edu (M.S.S.); smallic5@asu.edu (S.M.)
6 Department of Basic Pharmaceutical Sciences, School of Pharmacy, College of Health & Pharmaceutical Sciences, University of Louisiana at Monroe, 1800 Bienville Drive, Bienville 362, Monroe, LA 71201, USA
* Correspondence: chamcheu@ulm.edu
† These authors contributed equally to this work.

Abstract: Treatment with 1,25-dihydroxyvitamin D_3 (1,25D) improves psoriasis symptoms, possibly by inducing the expression of late cornified envelope (*LCE*)3 genes involved in skin repair. In psoriasis patients, the majority of whom harbor genomic deletion of *LCE3B* and *LCE3C* (*LCE3C_LCE3B-del*), we propose that certain dietary analogues of 1,25D activate the expression of residual *LCE3A/LCE3D/LCE3E* genes to compensate for the loss of *LCE3B/LCE3C* in the deletant genotype. Herein, human keratinocytes (HEKn) homozygous for *LCE3C_LCE3B-del* were treated with docosahexaenoic acid (DHA) and curcumin, two low-affinity, nutrient ligands for the vitamin D receptor (VDR). DHA and curcumin induce the expression of *LCE3A/LCE3D/LCE3E* mRNAs at concentrations corresponding to their affinity for VDR. Moreover, immunohistochemical quantitation revealed that the treatment of keratinocytes with DHA or curcumin stimulates *LCE3* protein expression, while simultaneously opposing the tumor necrosis factor-alpha (TNFα)-signaled phosphorylation of mitogen activated protein (MAP) kinases, p38 and Jun amino-terminal kinase (JNK), thereby overcoming inflammation biomarkers elicited by TNFα challenge. Finally, DHA and curcumin modulate two transcription factors relevant to psoriatic inflammation, the activator protein-1 factor Jun B and the nuclear receptor NR4A2/NURR1, that is implicated as a mediator of VDR ligand-triggered gene control. These findings provide insights into the mechanism(s) whereby dietary VDR ligands alter inflammatory and barrier functions relevant to skin repair, and may provide a molecular basis for improved treatments for mild/moderate psoriasis.

Keywords: vitamin D receptor; late cornified envelope genes; docosahexaenoic acid; curcumin; epidermis; keratinocytes; psoriasis treatment; nutraceuticals; differentiation; activator protein-1

1. Introduction

Psoriasis is a skin disease of largely unknown etiology with an estimated prevalence of over three percent in the United States [1]. Prominent features include overproliferation and incomplete differentiation of epidermal keratinocytes, as well as epidermal inflammation. Chemical analogs of 1,25 dihydroxyvitamin D_3 (1,25D), the hormonal metabolite of vitamin D, are routinely used as topical agents to treat mild/moderate psoriasis. The success of 1,25D-based agents is presumably related to the reported role of vitamin D in skin biology, in particular its role in regulating keratinocyte proliferation and differentiation, but also its known ability to regulate components of the immune system in skin (reviewed in [2]). In support of the role of vitamin D (or lack thereof) in psoriasis pathogenesis, several studies have associated low vitamin D status with psoriasis (e.g., [3,4]). However, 1,25D analog therapy, even when combined with an anti-inflammatory drug (e.g., betamethasone), is not effective in approximately 40% of patients with mild to moderate psoriasis [5]. Severe cases of psoriasis can be treated effectively with injectable anti-inflammatory agents such as etanercept, adalimumab, infliximab, or secukinumab [6]; however, these agents are not approved for patients with mild/moderate cases [7]. Thus, developing improved topical agents for mild/moderate psoriasis remains an important goal.

The currently accepted paradigm of 1,25D action is that 1,25D, or an analog thereof, binds with high affinity to the nuclear vitamin D receptor (VDR), which then forms a heterodimer with a retinoid X receptor (RXR) isoform on vitamin D-responsive elements (VDREs) in chromosomal DNA, modulating the expression of nearby target genes [8]. Although 1,25D and its analogs are known to improve psoriasis symptoms in many patients, presumably by serving as VDR ligands, the key epidermal genes that are regulated to ameliorate psoriasis are poorly characterized. One approach to enhancing topical therapies for psoriasis is therefore to identify key genes affected by treatment as well as VDR analogs or other ligands that may optimize these effects. Our approach has been to examine those genes for which genetic variations have been shown to confer risk for psoriasis as potential targets for VDR-mediated regulation.

Psoriasis susceptibility loci (*PSORS)* include the *PSORS4* locus, which is contained within the epidermal differentiation complex (EDC), a large assemblage of over 60 genes expressed during the process of epithelial differentiation (Figure 1). Five closely related late cornified envelope genes (*LCE3A–E*) exist in a cluster within the EDC and have been reported to play a role in skin repair [9]. The *PSORS4* risk allele is a deletion of two of these genes, *LCE3C_LCE3B-del*, leading to the hypothesis that the loss of two (of five) *LCE3* genes might reduce the ability of psoriatic lesions to heal [9]. This deletion is very common and studies have indicated that the frequency of *LCE3C_LCE3B-del* is over 50% in many human populations, and is significantly overrepresented in patients with psoriasis, where its frequency increases to 65–75% of the patient population [10].

The endocrine VDR ligand (1,25D), as well as novel VDR ligands delphinidin and cyanidin, have previously been shown to upregulate *LCE3* gene expression to some extent [11,12]. Further, a VDRE has been identified adjacent to the *LCE3A* gene [11] and is not affected by the *LCE3C_LCE3B* deletion (Figure 1). We have proposed that activation by liganded VDR from this VDRE could coordinately upregulate the expression of the *LCE3A/LCE3D/LCE3E* genes to compensate for the *LCE3C_LCE3B* deletion under the assumption that the highly homologous *LCE3* genes have overlapping functions [13]. We have additionally suggested that delphindin and cyanidin represent candidate lead compounds that could be developed into agents to treat mild to moderate psoriasis in a similar manner to how 1,25D was utilized as a lead compound to create therapeutically effective analogs such as calcipotriol [14].

For the current study, we analyzed the ability of two additional bioactive lipids of nutritional origin, namely docosahexaenoic acid (DHA) and curcumin, to upregulate *LCE3* mRNAs as well as proteins. These two compounds were chosen not only for their demonstrated affinity for the vitamin D receptor [15], but also for their reported beneficial effects in skin. Curcumin has been used since ancient times to treat skin inflammation and other ailments, and its anti-inflammatory actions have been studied in the context of various skin conditions, including pruritus, facial photoaging, radiodermatitis, and diabetic microangiopathy (reviewed in [16]). DHA and other omega-3 fatty acids have also been studied for their anti-inflammatory effects, mediated via a variety of mechanisms (reviewed in [17]), including serving as the precursor for the anti-inflammatory molecule resolvin D1 that was recently shown to improve inflammatory symptoms in a mouse imiquimod-induced model of psoriasis [18]. Both DHA [19,20] and curcumin [21,22] have been examined as treatments for psoriasis, but corresponding studies enrolled only a relatively small number of patients and the molecular mechanism(s) accounting for the positive effects observed in a subset of patients were not investigated.

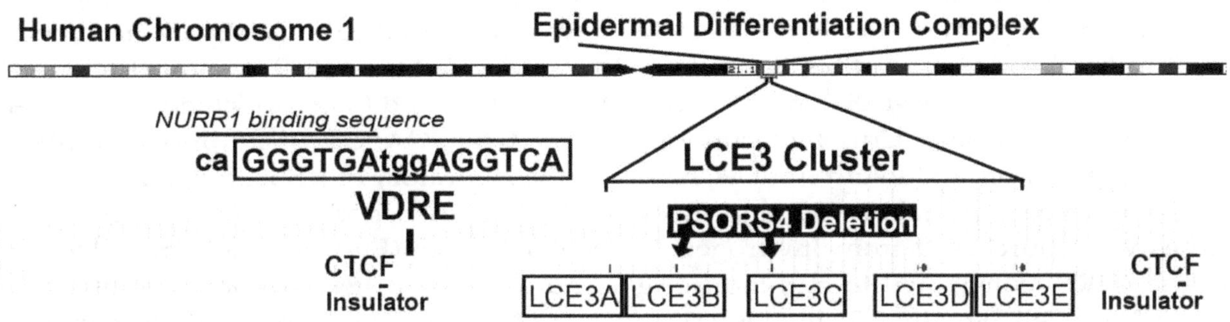

Figure 1. Location of the *LCE3* gene cluster (exact location of each gene indicated by a tiny bars above the boxed LCE3 designation) and the common *PSORS4* gene deletion within the epidermal differentiation complex on human chromosome 1 that also contains other skin genes such as *filaggrin, loricrin, involucrin,* and *S100A* (not shown). The *PSORS4* deletion eliminates two *LCE3* genes (*LCE3C_LCE3B-del*), but leaves *LCE3A/LCE3D/LCE3E* intact. A putative vitamin D-responsive element (VDRE) is located adjacent to the *LCE3A* gene, but within the boundaries established on either side of the *LCE3* gene cluster by sites for the CCCTC-binding factor (CTCF) that may serve to insulate this gene cluster from other nearby genes. This VDRE has been shown to confer responsiveness to both 1,25D and delphinidin in transfection experiments using a heterologous reporter gene construct [11]. Shown above the VDRE sequence is the location of an overlapping recognition sequence for the nuclear receptor subfamily 4 group A member 2 (NR4A2), also known as NURR1 (see text for explanation).

We also examined the ability of 1,25D, curcumin, and DHA to upregulate the expression of two other disease biomarkers, the activator protein-1 factor Jun B and the nuclear receptor NR4A2, to illuminate additional pathways by which 1,25D, curcumin, and/or DHA might improve psoriasis symptoms. Jun B was selected since the *Jun B* gene is localized in psoriasis susceptibility locus 6 (*PSORS6*). Additionally, an inducible epidermal knockout of *Jun B* in adult mice was reported to yield a phenotype possessing the histological and molecular hallmarks of psoriasis [23]. Further, *Jun B* expression, similar to *LCE3* gene expression, is associated with skin repair [24]. NR4A2, also known as NURR1, nuclear receptor of T cells (NOT), or transcriptionally inducible nuclear receptor (TINUR), was selected for study because a putative VDRE located near the *LCE3* gene cluster overlaps with a consensus NR4A2 binding site (Figure 1, caGGGTGA). An additional reason why NR4A2 was of interest is our previously published hypothesis that part of the actions of liganded VDR might be mediated via the upregulation of NR4A2 [25]. Based on the current study, we conclude that both Jun B and NR4A2 may play a role in the action of 1,25D and DHA, and to some extent of curcumin, on skin, but higher doses of ligands are required to demonstrate a statistically significant effect on mRNA levels.

Finally, several literature reports have implied that the effects of DHA in the skin are mediated, not by VDR as we have hypothesized, but rather via peroxisome proliferator-activated receptor (PPAR) isoforms, with PPARδ being the dominant isoform in human skin [26]. To assess whether PPARδ is a major regulator of *LCE* genes, we probed GW501516, a selective ligand for PPARδ, for its ability to upregulate *LCE3* genes in keratinocytes.

2. Materials and Methods

2.1. Source of Ligands and Reagents

Crystalline 1,25D was obtained from Roche Diagnostics (Indianapolis, IN, USA). Docosahexaenoic acid was purchased from Sigma Aldrich Corporation (St. Louis, MO, USA). GW510516 was secured from Santa Cruz Biotechnology (Dallas, TX, USA). GW501516 and 1,25D were dissolved in ethanol at 1000 times the concentrations needed for cell culture experiments (1000×) and stored at −20 °C. Curcumin was obtained from Cayman Chemical Co. (Ann Arbor, MI, USA), dissolved in dimethyl sulfoxide (DMSO) at 1000×, and stored at −20 °C. Figure 2A depicts the structures of these ligands. An antibody against NR4A2/NURR1 (LS-C99204) was purchased from LifeSpan BioSciences, Inc. (LSBio, Seattle, WA, USA). Antibodies to LCE3B–E (clone C-14, sc-138974), Jun B (clone N-17X, sc-46X), p-JNK (clone G-7, sc-6254), p-p38 (clone D-8, sc-7973), and filaggrin (clone AKH1, sc-66192) were purchased from Santa Cruz Biotechnology (Santa Cruz, CA, USA). Additional antibodies to LCE3B–E proteins were a kind gift from M. Narita in the laboratory of J. Shalkwijk [27]. Alexa Fluor 488-conjugated goat anti-rabbit IgG and Texas Red-conjugated goat anti-mouse IgG secondary antibodies were purchased from Invitrogen Molecular Probes (Eugene, OR, USA). Horseradish peroxidase (HRP) conjugated to anti-mouse IgG and anti-rabbit IgG secondary antibodies were purchased from Cell Signaling Technology (Danvers, MA, USA). The Pierce BCA Protein Assay Kit was from Thermo Scientific (Waltham, MA, USA), and Novex precast Tris-Glycine gels were purchased from Invitrogen (Carlsbad, CA, USA) or Bio-Rad Laboratories (Hercules, CA, USA). Recombinant human Tumor Necrosis Factor-alpha (rhTNFα) was purchased from R & D Systems (Minneapolis, MN, USA). ProLong® Gold Anti-fade Reagent containing 4′,6-diamidino-2-phenylindole (DAPI) for nuclear staining was obtained from Invitrogen (Carlsbad, CA, USA) and Life Technologies (Grand Island, NY, USA).

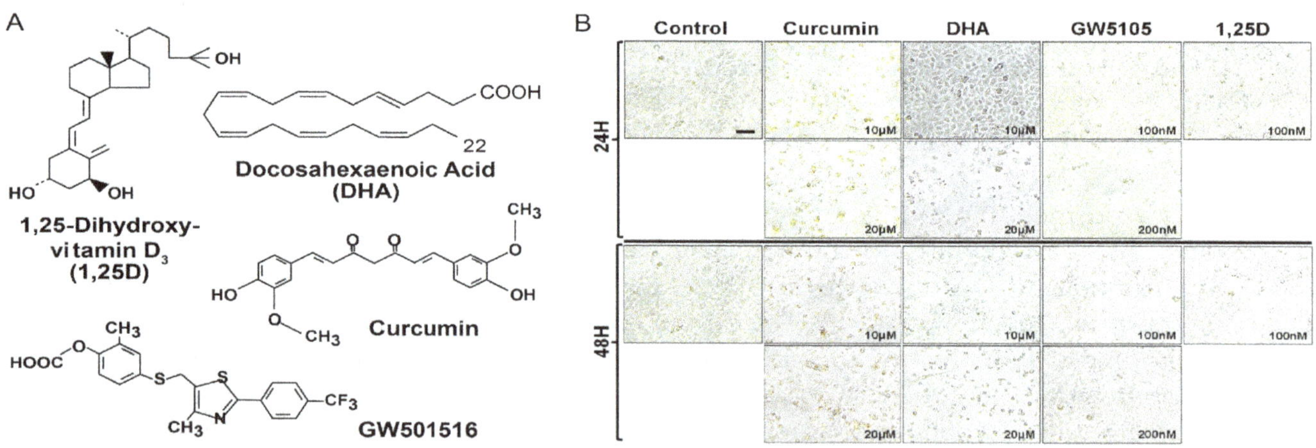

Figure 2. (**A**) Ligands used in the current study. 1,25D is the natural high affinity ligand for vitamin D receptor (VDR). Curcumin and docosahexaenoic acid (DHA) are natural, low-affinity ligands for VDR, and GW501516 is a specific synthetic ligand for peroxisome proliferator-activated receptor (PPAR)δ, with the latter nuclear receptor also having a reported affinity for DHA. (**B**) Morphology of normal human epidermal keratinocytes (NHEKs) treated without ligand (control) or with various ligands at the indicated concentrations and time of incubation. Magnification = 300×.

2.2. Cell Culture and Treatment

Human primary neonatal keratinocytes (HEKn) from single donors were purchased from Invitrogen Corp. (Carlsbad, CA, USA) and cultured in low calcium serum-free EpiLife medium supplemented with the Human Keratinocytes Growth Supplement Kit (HKGS Kit; Cat# S-001-K, Thermo Fisher Scientific, Rockford, IL, USA) along with gentamicin and amphotericin from GIBCO (Carlsbad, CA, USA). Cells were re-fed every 2–4 days and split as necessary. Cells were plated at

550,000 cells per 60-mm dish and treated with 1000× stocks of calcium chloride (dissolved in water) and/or the ligands of interest (Figure 2A). Rat osteosarcoma cells (UMR-106) were obtained from the American Type Culture Collection (Manassas, VA, USA) and maintained in Dulbecco's Modified Eagles Medium (Hyclone, GE Healthcare, Logan, UT, USA) supplemented with gentamicin/amphotericin in a humidified atmosphere at 37 °C and 5% carbon dioxide. For immunofluorescence and Western blot analyses, cells were treated with different concentrations of agents at different time points (24–48 h) prior to harvest and analysis. In some experiments, cells were first pre-incubated or pre-treated for 48 h with respective ligands/agents and then treated with or without TNFα (15 ng/mL) for 30 min prior to harvest.

2.3. Morphology, Immunocytochemistry, and Immunofluorescence Analysis

Keratinocytes were seeded in four-chamber tissue culture glass slides and pre-treated with concentrations of each ligand as follows: curcumin (10–20 μM), 1,25D (0.1 μM), DHA (10–20 μM), and GW501516 (100–200 nM), for 24–48 h and processed as earlier described [28]. Briefly, after treatment with (or without) VDR ligands for 48 h, the cells were stimulated for 30 min before harvest with or without 15 ng/mL TNFα prior to being washed twice with 1× phosphate-buffered saline (PBS) (Ca^{2+}/Mg^{2+}-free). Subsequently, cells were fixed in 2% paraformaldehyde in a 1:1 mix of cold acetone/methanol in PBS for 20 min at room temperature, followed by 15 min at 4 °C, followed by three washes in 1× PBS. Cells were then permeabilized for 5 min at room temperature with Triton stabilization buffer (0.5% Triton X-100, 100 mM piperazine-N,N′-bis(2-ethanesulfonic acid (PIPES) buffer (K^+-free), 4% PEG, and 1 mM ethyleneglycol-bis(aminoethylether)-tetraacetic acid (EGTA)) and washed three times in 1× PBS. Nonspecific epitopes were blocked with blocking solution (10% normal goat serum, 2.5% bovine serum albumin) in PBS for 20 min. Samples were blotted and subsequently incubated overnight at 4 °C with one of the following monoclonal or polyclonal primary antibodies diluted in blocking buffer: NR4A2/NURR1 (1:100 dilution), LCE3B–E (cross-reacts with four of the five LCE3 protein isoforms [27]) (1:100 dilution), Jun B (1:100 dilution), p-JNK (1:40 dilution), p-p38 (1:100 dilution), or filaggrin (1:50 dilution). Hereafter, the cells were washed three times and incubated with goat anti-rabbit IgG Alexa Fluor 488 or goat anti-mouse IgG-Texas Red secondary antibodies conjugated to HRP, all at 1:600 dilution in blocking buffer, for 45 min at 37 °C. Slides were washed twice in PBS for 10 min each followed by washing once in double-distilled water, and the cover slips were mounted on glass slides using ProLong® Gold Anti-fade Reagent containing DAPI from Thermo Fisher Scientific (Cat# P36941, Rockford, IL, USA) for nuclear counter-staining. The mounted slides were allowed to cure overnight in the dark at room temperature. Automated images were acquired using the Nuance Imaging system with a camera equipped on a light microscope as described below.

2.4. Nuance Multispectral Imaging System FX—Software

Automated immunofluorescence images were acquired using an Olympus BX43 light microscope (Olympus America Inc., Center Valley, PA, USA) equipped with a CRI camera on a Nuance™ Imaging FX system version 3.0.2 (Perkin Elmer, Inc., Waltham, MA, USA) using 20×/0.5 or 40×/0.75 objectives connected to a computer and an X-Cite® Series 120 Q Sport light source. Data acquisition and image analysis using Nuance software technology plate-form were conducted as previously described [29,30]. Briefly, a spectral library was created using image cubes to define distinctive spectral curves for each fluorophore, and counterstained to adjust for background effects and to accurately quantify the positive staining of biomarkers using InForm version 1.4.0 software (Perkin Elmer Inc., Waltham, MA, USA), which allows for an objective analysis of biomarkers with increased accuracy. Isotype controls were used for immunostaining (proportion of green/red pixels for antigen staining) with values averaged from at least five fields for each slide sample.

2.5. PSORS4 Genotyping of HEKn Cell Lots

Genomic DNA was isolated from cells using a DNAeasy kit (Qiagen Corp., Valencia, CA, USA) according to the manufacturer's protocol. A triple primer set was utilized to genotype cells: LCE3CF 5′-TCACCCTGGAACTAGACCTCA-3′; LCE3CR 5′-CTCCAACCACTTGTTCTTCTCA-3′; LCE3CR2D 5′-CATCCCAGGGATGCTGCATG-3′ [31]. PCR reactions contained approximately 130 ng/μL of HEKn genomic DNA from a single lot of cells, 0.5 μL of an 18 μM stock of the above three primers (0.9 μM final concentration of each primer), and 5 μL of Fast Start Universal SYBR Green Master Mix from Roche Applied Science (Indianapolis, IN, USA) in a total volume of 10 μL. An Applied Biosystems 2400 machine was programmed for 35 cycles: 94 °C for 30 s, 60 °C for 30 s, and 72 °C for 1 min, followed by a 72 °C step for 10 min. PCR products were resolved on 3% agarose gels. A single band at 199 bp indicates that cells harbor a homozygous *LCE3C_LCE3B* deletion (*LCE3C_LCE3B-del*), a single band at the position 240 bp indicates a homozygous intact locus, and the presence of both bands signifies a heterozygote.

2.6. Transient Transfection and Treatment of UMR-106 Cells

UMR-106 cells were plated at 650,000 cells/well in a 6-well plate. After 24 h of incubation, the cells were transfected with PolyJet reagent (SignaGen Laboratories, Gaithersburg, MD, USA) according to the manufacturer's protocol. Briefly, each well received 20 μL/well PolyJet and 500 ng/well of pSG5-VDR M4, an expression plasmid containing the human VDR cDNA with translation starting at codon 4 (one of the common polymorphic variants of VDR [32]). After 24 h of incubation, the cells were treated with ethanol vehicle or 1, 10, or 100 nM 1,25D. RNA was harvested after 22–24 h of incubation.

2.7. Cell Harvesting and Total RNA Preparation

Cultured cells were harvested by trypsinization using standard techniques and cell pellets were washed with sterile phosphate-buffered saline. RNA isolation was performed using an Aurum Total RNA Mini Kit (Bio-Rad Corp., Hercules, CA, USA) from HEKn cells seeded at 550,000 cells per 60-mm plate and grown to a final confluency of approximately 65–70%. The quantity and purity of prepared RNAs were assessed by UV absorbance at 260 vs. 280 nm. Similar procedures were employed for the UMR-106 cells.

2.8. Primer Design and Testing

The UC Santa Cruz Genome Browser [33] was utilized to determine the coding sequence of the genes to be investigated. Unless otherwise referenced, Primer3Plus [34] was used to design primers that spanned an intro-exon junction. For the detection of human *LCE3* transcripts, the following primers were used: *LCE3A* forward primer 5′-CTGAGTCACCACAGATGCCG-3′ and reverse primer 5′-CTTGCTGACCACTTCCCCTG-3′; *LCE3B* forward primer 5′-CTC CTGCTGTGCTCCAAGAC-3′ and reverse primer 5′-ATCTTGCTGACCACTGCCTC-3′; *LCE3C* forward primer 5′-GGTCTG AGGGTTCTGTGCTC-3′ and reverse primer 5′-ACACTTGGGT GAGGGACAAC-3′; *LCE3D* forward primer 5′-CCCCAAAGAGCCCAGTACAG-3′ and reverse primer 5′-CTGTGGTGGTTCAGGAAGCA-3′; *LCE3E* forward primer 5′-CCCAAGTGTCCCCCAAAGAA-3′ and reverse primer 5′-CTGTGGTGGTTCAGGAAGCA-3′. For the detection of human *Jun B* and *NR4A2* transcripts, the following primers were used: human *Jun B* forward primer 5′-CGGCAGCTACTTTTCTGGTC-3′ and reverse primer 5′-GAAGAGGCGAGCTTGAGAGA-3′; human *NR4A2 (NURR1)* forward primer 5′-CTACGACGTCAAGCCACCTT-3′ and reverse primer 5′-TCATCTCCTCAGACTGGGGG-3′. Human glyceraldehyde 3-phosphate dehydrogenase (*GAPDH*) mRNA was amplified using forward primer 5′-TGACAACTTTGGTATCGTGGAAGG-3′ and reverse primer 5′-AGGGATGATGTTCTGGAGAGCC-3′. For the detection of rat transcripts, the following primers were used: rat *Nr4a2* forward primer 5′-CTACGCTTAGCATACAGGTC-3′ and reverse primer 5′-TTCCTTGAGCCCGTGTCT-3′ [35]. Rat *GAPDH* was amplified using forward primer

5′-AGGTCGGTGTGAACGGATTTG-3′ and reverse primer 5′-CATTCTCAGCCTTGACTGTGC-3′. All primer pairs were prepared as 18 μM stocks and stored at −20 °C.

2.9. Real-Time PCR

First strand cDNA was synthesized using a Bio-Rad iScript kit from total RNA isolated from HEKn cells. Quantitative real-time PCR was performed with Fast Start Universal SYBR Green Master Mix (Roche Applied Science) in an ABI 7500 Fast thermal cycler, or a BioRad CFX96 thermal cycler for data in Figure 7B only. Each GAPDH PCR well contained 0.5 μL of primers, 0.25 μL cDNA, and 5 μL of SYBR Green reagent mixed in a total volume of 10 μL. Wells for the detection of other gene products contained 0.5 μL of primers, 0.75 μL of cDNA, and 5 μL of SYBR Green. The temperature profile included 40 cycles with a melting step of 15 s at 95 °C and an annealing/elongation step of 1 min at 60 °C. Real-time PCR data were analyzed via the comparative C_t method and normalized to GAPDH. Fold effects for ligand treatments were calculated in relation to the samples treated with ethanol or DMSO vehicle.

2.10. Protein Extraction and Immunoblotting

After treatment with different concentrations of ligands at different time points, normal human keratinocyte cells were harvested and whole cell lysates were prepared for Western blot analysis. Briefly, cells were homogenized by sonication in ice-cold 1× RIPA lysis buffer (50 mM Tris-HCl, pH 7.4, 150 mM NaCl, 1 mM EGTA, 1 mM EDTA, 20 mM NaF, 100 mM Na_3VO4, 0.5% NP-40, 1% Triton X-100, 1 mM PMSF) with freshly added protease inhibitor cocktail (Protease Inhibitor Cocktail Set III, Calbiochem, La Jolla, CA, USA). The homogenate was then centrifuged at 14,000× *g* for 25 min at 4 °C, and the supernatant was collected, aliquoted, and stored at −80 °C. For immunoblotting, 10–20 μg of protein was resolved on 8–12% SDS polyacrylamide (SDS-PAGE) gels and transferred onto nitrocellulose membranes. Blots were incubated in blocking buffer (5% non-fat dry milk/1% Tween 20; in 20 mM Tris-buffered saline (TBS), pH 7.6) for 45 min at room temperature, followed by incubation with a primary antibody directed against either LCE3B–E, Jun B, or NR4A2/NURR1 in blocking buffer overnight at 4 °C. Following several washes, membranes were incubated with the appropriate HRP-conjugated secondary antibody and detected by enhanced chemiluminescence (ECL) and autoradiography using a Bio-Rad Gel-Doc System (Bio-Rad Laboratories Inc., Hercules, CA, USA). Densitometric measurements of the bands were performed with image analysis software using the Biorad ChemiDoc MP imaging system (Bio-Rad, Hercules, CA, USA). To ensure equal protein loading, membranes were re-probed with antibodies to appropriate house-keeping proteins (GAPDH or vinculin) and processed as above. GAPDH or vinculin data were then used as normalization factors.

3. Results

To examine the effects of DHA and curcumin on human neonatal epidermal keratinocytes, we initially monitored the morphology of HEKn cells treated with different concentrations of ligands or vehicle control over time using phase contrast microscopy. As depicted in Figure 2B, we observed that these ligands differentially induced changes in cellular morphology reminiscent of keratinocyte differentiation.

We hypothesized that many of the effects of both DHA and curcumin on keratinocytes are mediated via the vitamin D receptor (VDR) acting to upregulate the expression of the *LCE3A/LCE3D/LCE3E* genes. First, we determined if the single-patient sample of HEKn cells harbored the *PSORS4* deletion and, if so, whether the deletion was homozygous or heterozygous, using a PCR protocol that incorporated a triple set of primers (see Methods Section 2.5). This reaction yielded a single PCR product at 199 bp (data not shown), indicative of a homozygous *LCE3C_LCE3B* deletion (*LCE3C_LCE3B-del*). Utilizing a homozygous deletant allowed for a direct test of the hypothesis that DHA and/or curcumin upregulate *LCE3A/LCE3D/LCE3E* mRNA expression without interfering background from PCR primers annealing to the similar *LCE3B* and/or *LCE3C* mRNAs.

The first experiment was performed by treating HEKn cells homozygous for *LCE3C_LCE3B-del* with two concentrations of DHA. The selection of concentrations was based on a previously published competition binding assay [15] which indicated that DHA competes with radioactively labeled 1,25D for VDR binding with an IC_{50} of approximately 10 μM. As shown in Figure 3A, DHA indeed upregulates *LCE3* mRNA expression in a dose-dependent manner, with 20 μM DHA eliciting 11-fold, 5.5-fold, and 7-fold increases in mRNAs for *LCE3A, LCE3D,* and *LCE3E,* respectively. These mRNA effects are superior to the respective 3.6-fold, 4.5-fold, and 4.7-fold increases in mRNAs for *LCE3A, LCE3D,* and *LCE3E* reported previously by our group for HEKn cells treated with 100 nM 1,25D [11], which serves as a published positive control (employing the hormonal VDR ligand) for the present experiments. To confirm this effect of DHA at the protein level, cells were treated in the presence or absence of single doses of DHA (10 μM) with or without activation by recombinant human TNFα. Protein expression of *LCE3* gene products was monitored by double immunofluorescent microscopy as described in the Methods section; the antibody for LCE3 expression recognizes LCE3B, LCE3C, LCE3D, and LCE3E. As shown in Figure 3B, treatment with 10 μM DHA alone for 48 h strongly induced the expression of LCE3 proteins compared to vehicle control cells (see LCE3B–E column, comparing top two panels), with no discernible effect on the levels of phosphorylated p38 MAP kinase (p-p38). Phospho-p38 was included in the study because it is a pro-inflammatory factor that is activated in psoriasis [36]. Because the pro-inflammatory cytokine TNFα is critically involved in the early phase of psoriasis [37], we next examined the effect of TNFα activation on the response to DHA ligands. As shown in Figure 3B, treatment with TNFα did not discernibly modulate LCE3B–E protein expression, whether in the presence or absence of DHA (LCE3B–E column, compare bottom two panels with top two panels), but strongly induced the phosphorylation of p38 (see p-p38 column, second panel from the bottom). Additionally, the pre-treatment of keratinocytes with DHA for 48 h, prior to activation with TNFα for 30 min, appeared to block the effect of TNFα on p38 phosphorylation (Figure 3B; p-p38 column, bottom panel). A subset of these results was further corroborated by Western blot analyses (see last section of Results below).

A second dietary agent, namely curcumin, a turmeric derivative and bioactive polyphenol, was similarly evaluated in cultured keratinocytes. Because curcumin exhibits a comparable VDR competition profile to DHA (an IC_{50} of approximately 5–10 μM [15]), and has been reported to be a bona fide VDR ligand [38] with beneficial effects on skin repair [24], we treated HEKn cells with concentrations of curcumin similar to those used for DHA, namely 6.7 and 10 μM for mRNA studies and 5, 10, and 20 μM for immunocytochemistry. Also, DMSO rather than ethanol was employed as the solvent vehicle for curcumin. The results in Figure 4A reveal that curcumin is capable of upregulating *LCE3A, LCE3D,* and *LCE3E* mRNAs 3- to 4-fold in a dose-dependent manner at concentrations corresponding closely to the concentrations capable of competing with 1,25D for binding to the VDR. This magnitude of induction of *LCE3* genes is quite comparable to that of 3.6- to 4.7-fold achieved by 100 nM 1,25D as previously published [12]. Immunostaining for protein expression in human keratinocytes confirmed that curcumin treatment alone strongly induced the protein expression of LCE3B–E (Figure 4B; LCE3B–E column, compare top two panels). Analogous to the DHA study shown in Figure 3B, a 30-min treatment with TNFα (±curcumin) was also included (lower two rows of Figure 4B), and there is a suggestion that the combination of curcumin and TNFα yields a higher induction of LCE3B–E protein expression than curcumin alone (Figure 3B, LCE3D–E column, compare second and fourth panels). Finally, the phosphorylation of MAPK p38 in response to the various treatments was also included, with curcumin showing effects similar to DHA, namely an ability to block p38 phosphorylation in response to TNFα (Figure 4B, p-p38 column, compare third and fourth panels). A subset of these results was further corroborated by Western blot analyses (see last section of Results).

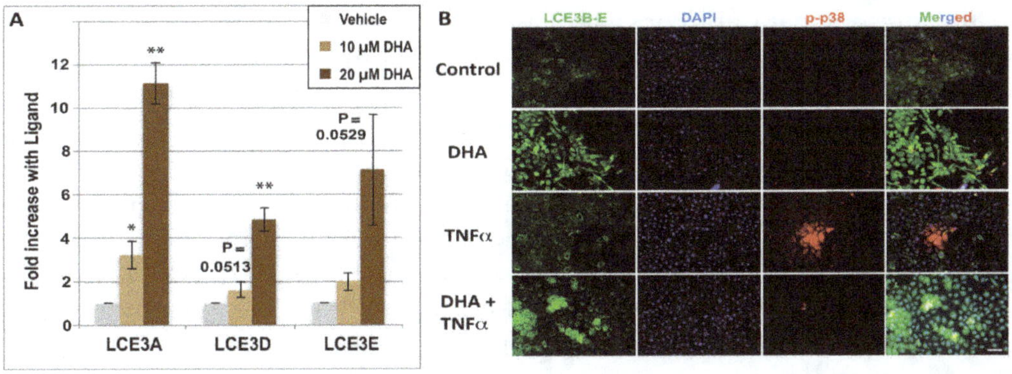

Figure 3. (**A**) Regulation by docosahexaenoic acid (DHA) of the *LCE3A, LCE3D* and *LCE3E* genes spared by the *PSORS4* deletion. Human primary neonatal keratinocytes (HEKn) cells homozygous for the deletion were treated with ethanol vehicle (negative control) or DHA (10 or 20 μM), and total RNA was prepared and analyzed for the expression of mRNA using specific primers for each LCE3 isoform. Bar graphs represent the average of three independent experiments ± STDEV. Asterisks denote results with ligands that are significantly different from ethanol controls as determined by the Student's two-tailed *t*-test: * $p < 0.05$; ** $p < 0.01$. *p*-Values approaching 0.05 are given above the corresponding bar. (**B**) Regulation of LCE3 proteins (and p-p38) by DHA and tumor necrosis factor-alpha (TNFα) as monitored by immunohistochemistry using an antibody that cross-reacts with LCE3B, LCE3C, LCE3D, and LCE3E proteins. Cells were cultured in four chamber tissue culture glass slides and treated for 48 h with (10 μM) or without DHA as indicated. Treatment with TNFα (15 ng/mL) occurred 30 min prior to fixing and binding of permeabilized cells to the indicated antibodies. Image acquisition is described in Methods and representative images are shown. Images in right-hand column represent a merging of all three signals (LCE3B–3E antibody (green), 4′,6-diamidino-2-phenyl (DAPI) (blue), and p-p38 antibody (red)) at a magnification of ×200.

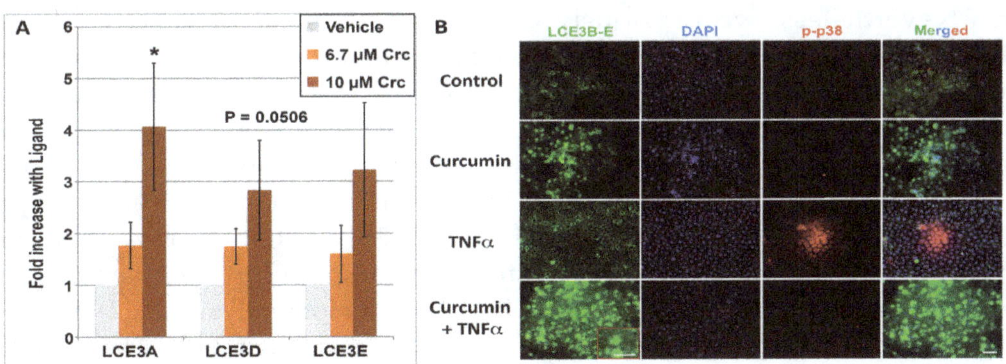

Figure 4. (**A**) Regulation of *LCE3A, LCE3D*, and *LCE3E* mRNA by curcumin (Crc). HEKn cells were treated with ETOH vehicle (negative control) or curcumin (at 6.7 or 10 μM concentration). Bar graphs show real-time PCR results, which are the average of four independent experiments ± STDEV. An asterisk denotes ligand-treated averages that are significantly different from ethanol controls as determined by two-tailed Student's *t*-test, * $p < 0.05$. One of the four replicates of this experiment was performed with HEKn cells heterozygous for the *PSORS4* deletion, which yielded results very similar to the three replicates from homozygous cells. (**B**) Regulation of LCE3 and p-p38 proteins by curcumin and TNFα as monitored by immunohistochemistry. Cells were cultured in four chamber tissue culture glass slides and treated for 48 h with (15 μM) or without curcumin as indicated. Treatment with TNFα (15 ng/mL) occurred 30 min prior to fixing and binding of permeabilized cells to the indicated antibodies. Image acquisition is described in Methods and representative images are shown. Images in right-hand column represent a merging of all three signals (LCE3B-3E (green), DAPI (blue), and p-p38 antibody (red)) at a magnification of ×200. Insets in red boxes indicate a higher power magnification (×400) of the selected section.

Although the present data are consistent with the conclusion that DHA is acting as a VDR ligand, literature reports indicate that DHA effects in skin may be mediated by a peroxisome proliferator-activated receptor (PPAR), presumably PPARδ, which is the predominant isoform expressed in skin [26]. We and others have recently shown that PPARδ is overexpressed in human psoriatic as well as in murine psoriasis-like skin lesions [39], and that treatment with delphinidin, another VDR ligand, normalized the expression in a preclinical mouse model of psoriasis [30]. To determine whether PPARδ is capable of upregulating LCE3 mRNAs in human keratinocytes, a selective ligand for PPARδ (GW501516) was examined at a single 100 nM concentration which, according to published reports, represents a saturating dose for activating PPARδ [40]. The results (data not shown) indicated a nonsignificant trend toward a very slight (<1.5-fold) upregulation of *LCE3A*, *LCE3D*, and *LCE3E* mRNA expression. Moreover, Western blot data from keratinocytes treated for 24 to 48 h with two doses of GW501516 (100 and 200 nM) yielded no significant increase in the expression of LCE3 proteins (see last section of Results). In this same experiment, 10–20 μM DHA or curcumin elicited a statistically significant enhancement in LCE3 protein levels, providing a positive control and indicating that liganded PPARδ is not an inducer of LCE3 protein in HEKn cells. Based on these data, we conclude that liganded PPARδ plays little or no role in *LCE3* gene expression, and this result allows us to distinguish the relative contributions of VDR and PPARδ in mediating the actions of DHA with respect to LCE3 maintenance. The conclusion is that VDR alone executes the function of DHA to induce *LCE3* gene and protein expression. This does not eliminate potential cross-talk between the signaling of the VDR and PPAR systems in skin, at least with regard to the regulation of genes other than those of the LCE3 class. For example, GW501516 is a strong inducer of NR4A2 protein in HEKn cells, as are 1,25D and curcumin (see last part of Results).

We next assessed whether DHA upregulates *Jun B*, for which depressed expression or gene deletion has been noted to be associated with psoriasis. Quantitative real-time PCR results (Figure 5A) indicate that DHA significantly upregulates *Jun B* mRNA expression, but the effect is minimal (2-fold) after 24 h of treatment, and is not evident until DHA is present at the higher 20 μM concentration. Nevertheless, we previously demonstrated *Jun B* induction by 1,25D in KERTr human keratinocytes, utilizing microarray technology to quantitate mRNA [8]. In the present report, utilizing immunofluorescence to determine the effects of 48 h of DHA treatment, we observed an increase in Jun B protein expression (Figure 5B) in both the presence and absence of TNFα treatment. The immunofluorescence experiment also included the monitoring of JNK phosphorylation using a specific phospho-JNK antibody (see p-JNK column in Figure 5B). As expected, JNK is phosphorylated in response to 30 min of treatment with TNFα, an effect that is largely abolished when TNFα-treated cells are pretreated with DHA (Figure 5B, p-JNK column, compare bottom two panels). The upregulation of Jun B by DHA was confirmed by Western blot analysis (see last section of Results), exhibiting a significant, dose-dependent upregulation of Jun B protein at both 24 and 48 h, approaching the dramatic action of 100 nM 1,25D to enhance Jun B protein levels.

The ability of curcumin ± TNFα to upregulate Jun B expression was also investigated, and Figure 6 illustrates the immunofluorescence results using an anti-Jun B antibody. Treatment with curcumin increased levels of Jun B (Figure 6, Jun B column, compare top two panels), an effect that was confirmed with Western blotting (Figure 8B), which demonstrated a significant and dose-dependent increase in Jun B protein after both 24 and 48 h of treatment using doses of 5, 10, and 20 μM. Curcumin also appears to dampen the Jun B-induced phosphorylation of p-JNK by TNFα (Figure 6, p-JNK column, compare bottom two panels). Thus, two low-affinity VDR ligands (DHA and curcumin) evaluated in the present study are able to induce Jun B, as well as to oppose TNFα-induced p-JNK phosphorylation.

Finally, we explored the possibility that VDR ligands, including 1,25D, DHA, and curcumin, regulate the expression of the nuclear receptor NURR1, also known as NR4A2, pursuing a notion previously derived conceptually from the recent demonstration that some VDR actions follow a secondary induction mechanism, whereby liganded VDR first induces NURR1, which in turn activates the expression of the gene(s) of interest [25]. Moreover, as noted above, the LCE3 VDRE shown in

Figure 1 contains within its 5′ half-element a consensus binding sequence for the NR4A2 monomer, caGGGTGA. For these reasons, we examined the level of NURR1 transcripts in DHA-, 1,25D-, and vehicle-treated HEKn cells. The results (Figure 7A) demonstrate that both 1,25D and DHA upregulate *NURR1* mRNA in HEKn cells, although there exists no indication of a classic dose-response relationship for DHA, and the results are variable for treatment with 1,25D and 10 μM DHA. To definitively demonstrate that *NURR1* can be induced in a VDR and ligand dose-dependent fashion, UMR-106 osteoblast-like cells were transfected with human VDR and treated with concentrations of 1,25D from 1 to 100 nM. Data for *NURR1* mRNA levels compared with vehicle controls, as displayed in Figure 7B, exhibit clear 1,25D dose-dependency for a 3- to 4-fold induction of *NURR1* by the hormonal vitamin D. We followed up these mRNA studies by investigating the effect of a single dose of DHA or curcumin treatment using both immunofluorescence as well as Western blotting on the protein expression of NURR1 as well as filaggrin, another biomarker of skin inflammatory disease. Immunofluorescence after 48 h of treatment with ligands reveals a striking ability of both DHA alone and curcumin alone to upregulate both NURR1 and filaggrin (see NURR1 and filaggrin columns in Figure 7C, comparing second and fourth panels to top control panel). These results were confirmed by Western blotting (Figure 8C). Although the DHA effects pictured in Figure 8C are statistically significant only at the higher (20 μM) dose, effects with both DHA and curcumin displayed a dose-response at both time points. Importantly, 1,25D exerts a dramatic positive induction of NURR1 protein in HEKn cells (Figure 8C). Taken together, these results are consistent with the intermediary function of NURR1 as a secondary mediator of at least part of the action of VDR ligands in osteoblasts and skin, with putative occupation of the NURR1 site embedded within the VDRE identified in the LCE gene region being of potential mechanistic significance.

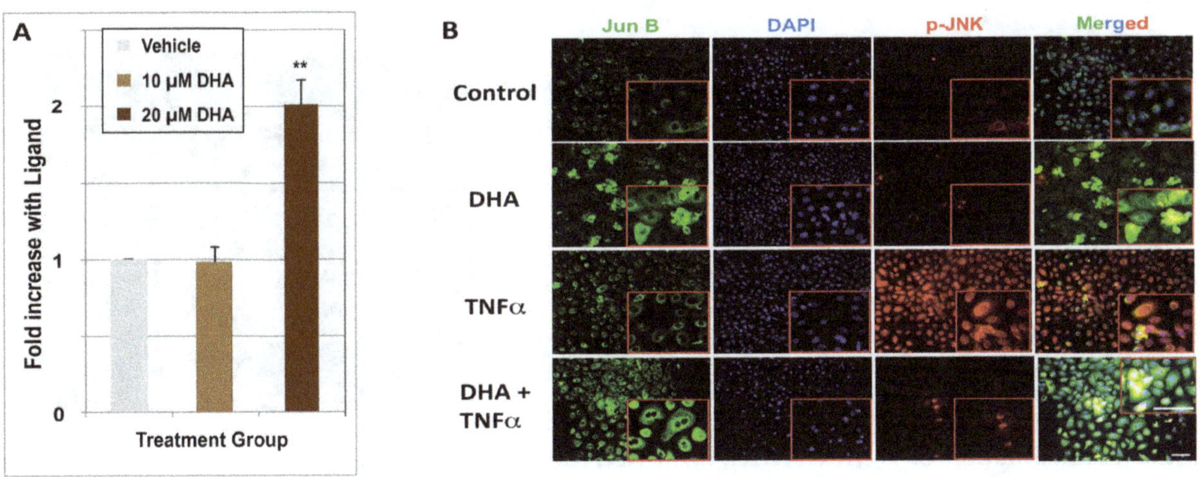

Figure 5. (**A**) Regulation of *Jun B* mRNA by DHA. HEKn cells were treated with ethanol vehicle (control), or with either 10 μM DHA or 20 μM DHA. RNA isolation, synthesis of first strand DNA, and real-time PCR are described in Methods. Results are means from three independent experiments ± STDEV. The double asterisk (**) denotes an average that is statistically significant by Student's *t*-test from the ethanol control, $p < 0.01$. (**B**) Regulation of Jun B and p-JNK proteins by DHA and TNFα as monitored by immunohistochemistry. Cells were cultured in four chamber tissue culture glass slides and treated for 48 h with (10 μM) or without DHA as indicated. Treatment with TNFα (15 ng/mL) occurred 30 min prior to fixing and binding of immobilized proteins to the indicated antibodies. Image acquisition is described in Methods and representative images are shown. Images in the right-hand column represent a merging of all three signals (Jun B antibody, DAPI, and p-JNK antibody), measured using Nuance software as described in Methods. (Magnification ×200). Insets in red boxes indicate a higher power magnification (×400) of the selected section. The yellow color indicates co-localization of both markers.

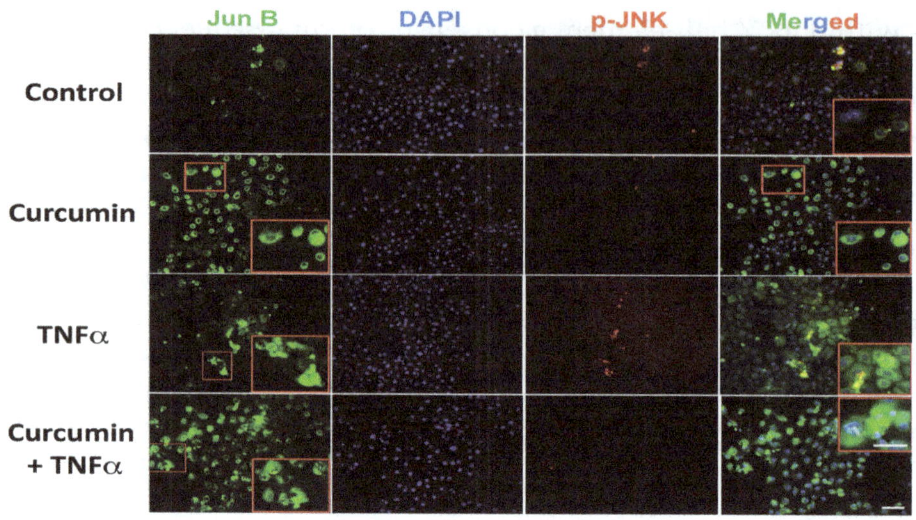

Figure 6. Regulation of Jun B and p-JNK proteins by curcumin and TNFα as monitored by immunohistochemistry. Cells were cultured in four chamber tissue culture glass slides and treated for 48 h with or without curcumin (15 μM) as indicated. Treatment with TNFα (15 ng/mL) occurred 30 min prior to fixing in 2% paraformaldehyde and binding of immobilized proteins to the indicated antibodies. Image acquisition is described in Methods and representative images are shown. Images in right-hand column represent a merging of all three signals (Jun B antibody, DAPI and p-JNK antibody), measured using Nuance software as described in Methods. (Magnification ×200). Insets in red boxes indicate a higher power magnification (×400) of the selected section.

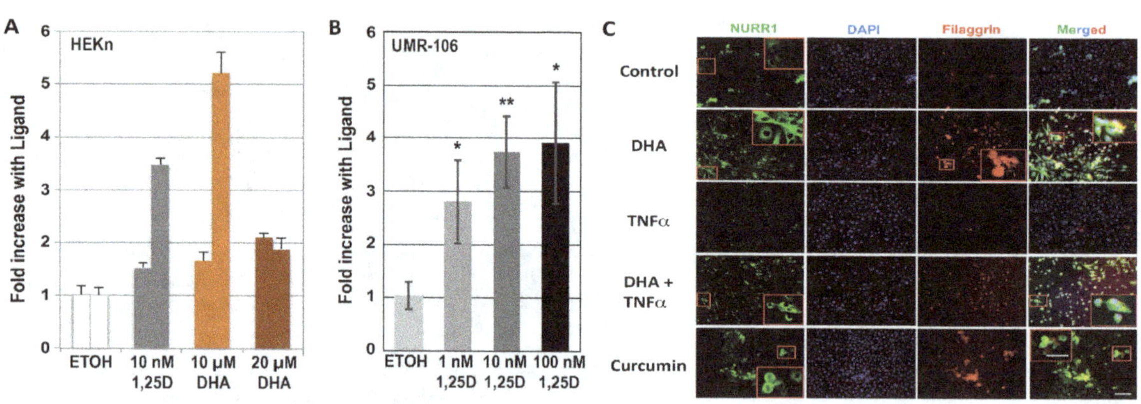

Figure 7. Regulation of *NURR1* (*NR4A2*) mRNA by 1,25D. (**A**) Response of *NURR1* mRNA to 1,25D and DHA in HEKn cells. Cells were plated as described in Methods and dosed with the indicated concentrations of 1,25D or DHA for 22–24 h. Total RNA and first strand cDNA were then prepared, and real-time qPCR was performed using primers to human *NURR1* as described in Methods. Error bars represent STDEV of triplicate real-time PCR wells from each of two independent experiments. (**B**) A similar experiment to (**A**), but performed using increasing doses of 1,25D in rat UMR-106 cultures. Results are means of three independent experiments ± STDEV, * $p < 0.05$, ** $p < 0.01$ compared to control by Student's *t*-test. (**C**) Regulation of NURR1 and filaggrin proteins by DHA and TNFα as monitored by immunohistochemistry. Cells were cultured in tissue culture glass slides and treated for 48 h with (10 μM) or without DHA as indicated. Treatment with TNFα (15 ng/mL) occurred 30 min prior to fixing in 2% paraformaldehyde and binding of immobilized proteins to the indicated antibodies. Image acquisition is described in Methods and representative images are shown. Images in right-hand column represent a merging of all three signals (NURR1 antibody, DAPI and filaggrin antibody), measured using Nuance software as described in Methods. (Magnification ×200). Insets in red boxes indicate a high power magnification (×400) of the highlighted section.

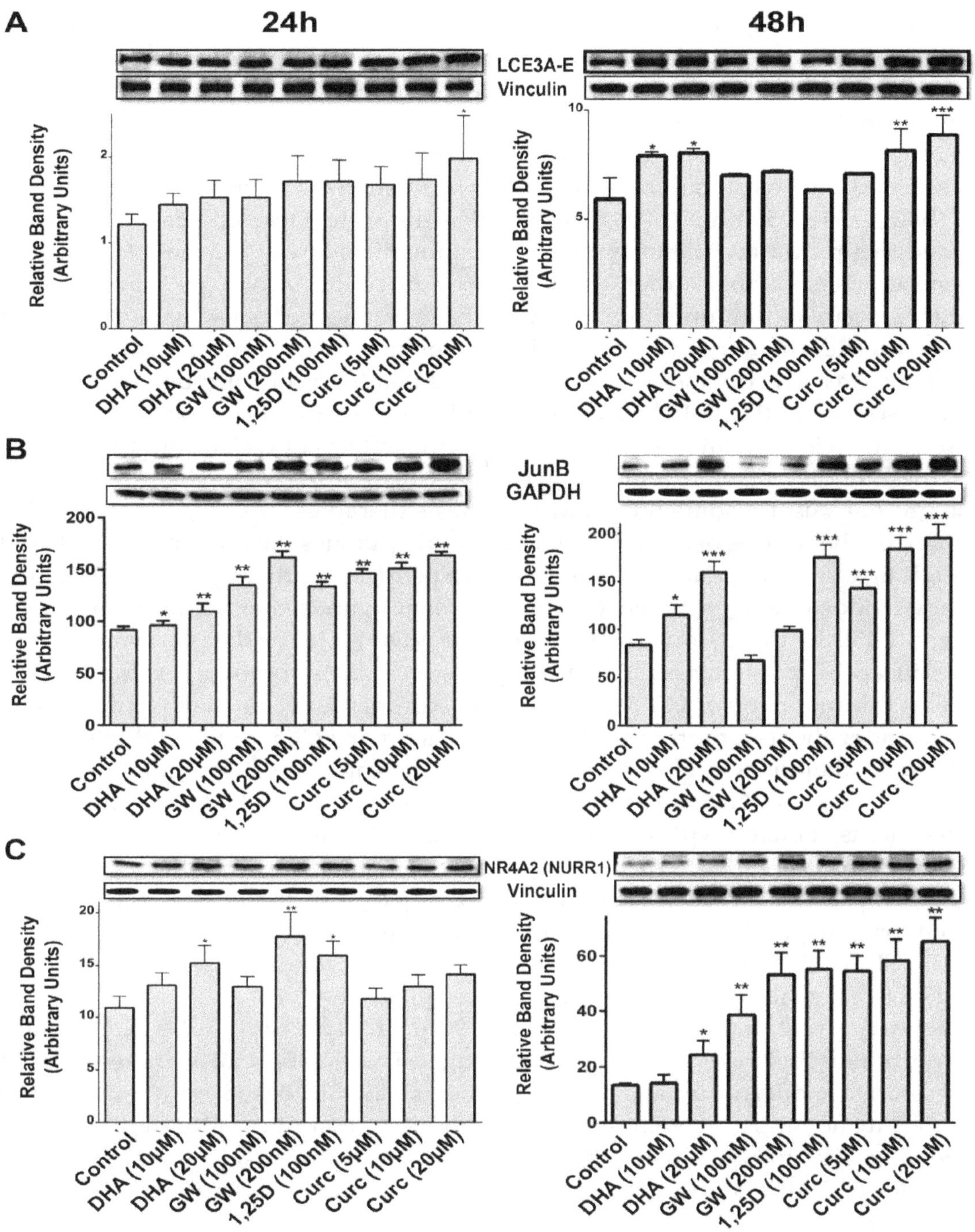

Figure 8. Dose-dependency of protein expression in response to 1,25D, curcumin (Curc) (ligand for the vitamin D receptor), GW501516 (GW; ligand for PPARδ), and DHA (ligand for both receptors). (**A**) Protein expression for LCE3 proteins as monitored by an antibody that recognizes four LCE3 isoforms (LCE3B/LCE3C/LCE3D/LCE3E), using Vinculin expression as an unregulated control to normalize for protein loading. (**B**) Protein expression of Jun B, using GAPDH as an unregulated control. (**C**) Protein expression of NR4A2 (NURR1), using Vinculin as an unregulated control. All bars represent an average of at least five fields for each sample (blots were normalized using Chemidoc quantification analysis software as described in Methods) ±STDEV. * $p < 0.5$, ** $p < 0.01$, *** $p < 0.001$.

4. Discussion and Conclusions

Analogs of 1,25D are used routinely for psoriasis treatment, often in combination with an anti-inflammatory steroid [41]. Previous studies from our laboratory have pursued the hypothesis that 1,25D and other VDR ligands improve symptoms of psoriasis by upregulating skin repair genes, and in two recent publications by our group, we reported that the VDR ligands 1,25D, delphinidin, and cyanidin upregulate *LCE3A/LCE3D/LCE3E* gene expression, potentially to compensate for the common genomic deletion of *LCE3B* and *LCE3C* [11,12].

The dietary lipids DHA (an omega-3 fatty acid) and curcumin (a bioactive component of turmeric spice) were selected for investigation as both have been subjects of clinical trials for the treatment of psoriasis (NCT01351805 and NCT00235625). In addition to these clinical trials, dietary studies have concluded that psoriatic patients typically consume diets low in omega-3 fatty acids, including DHA [42], and conversely, that a diet low in calories but high in omega-3 fatty acids appears to confer a better response to immunomodulatory drugs in a cohort of obese patients with plaque-type psoriasis [43]. Another dietary study found that adherence to a Mediterranean diet was inversely related to psoriasis area severity index (PASI) score, and that high consumption of fish (which contain omega-3 fatty acids including DHA) was independently negatively associated with a high PASI score [44]. Although it is difficult to separate the potential effects of DHA from those of other dietary components, these studies, taken together, suggest that consumption of omega-3 fatty acids, including DHA, may represent a useful adjuvant to other psoriasis therapies.

In addition to other modes of action, the current study pursues the notion that DHA and curcumin may act as VDR ligands to regulate genes involved in psoriasis pathology. Both DHA and curcumin have been shown, like other alternative, low-affinity VDR ligands such as delphinidin and cyanidin, to compete with 1,25D for direct, low-affinity binding to VDR [15]. The data shown in Figure 3 indicate that DHA significantly upregulates *LCE3* gene expression in cells homozygous for *LCE3C_LCE3B-del*. We propose that this induction of *LCE3* gene products compensates for the loss of *LCE3B* and *LCE3C* in skin repair, under the assumption that the highly similar *LCE3* gene products are functionally redundant [27]. Curcumin was also demonstrated to be capable of upregulating *LCE3A*, *LCE3D*, and *LCE3E* genes (Figure 4). Given that the effective concentrations of DHA and curcumin employed in these experiments coincide with those that competitively bind to VDR, we postulate that these ligands upregulate *LCE3* gene expression, at least in part, by binding to, and activating the VDR-RXR heterodimer. Our previous work identified a VDRE adjacent to the *LCE3A* gene (Figure 1) that is capable of conferring regulation onto a heterologous reporter gene by 1,25D, delphinidin, or cyanidin in transfected CCD-1106 KERTr human keratinocyte cells [11], lending further support to the notion that liganded VDR may induce the expression of these genes in vivo.

Recent reports reveal that the presence of *LCE3C_LCE3B-del* within the *LCE3* gene cluster has a lengthy evolutionary history in the hominid lineage. The deletion appears to have arisen in the common ancestor to modern humans and Denisovans [45,46]. Based on an analysis of genomic DNA from ancient hominins as well as modern humans, including a haplotype analysis of the deletion as well as flanking regions in the *LCE3* locus, the authors of these studies conclude that the 32 kb *LCE3C_LCE3B* deletion has been maintained under balancing selection in the human lineage. In considering the potential reasons as to why both LCE3 haplotypes are currently found in all tested human populations, including those from Eurasia, Africa, and the Americas [46,47], these authors quoted Bergboer et al. [48], who hypothesized that *LCE3C_LCE3B-del*, by delaying skin repair, could allow for greater penetration of microbial antigens, which then serve as a natural "vaccine" against future infections (while also posing an increased risk for an autoimmune response). Further, the hypothesis explaining the retention of the intact *LCE3* cluster is that the full complement of five *LCE3* genes confers a superior ability to support skin repair. Whatever the exact explanation, it appears that an interplay between these two sets of advantages/disadvantages has led to the preservation of both alleles in a state of balance over hundreds of thousands of years.

The extent to which DHA upregulates LCE3 mRNA expression exceeds 10-fold in the case of *LCE3A*, which is noticeably greater than the approximate 4-fold achieved by 10^{-8} M 1,25D in prior studies [11,12]. This comparison suggests that, at least for the upregulation of *LCE3* gene expression, DHA may be superior to the currently used therapeutic agent 1,25D (or analogs thereof), taking into account that higher concentrations of DHA are required [19] to achieve this effect due to the lower affinity of DHA for the receptor. This result positions both DHA and the previously tested cyanidin compound [11] as two dietary, non-toxic nutrients that are each capable of upregulating the expression of *LCE3* skin repair genes in a fashion superior to that of 1,25D, the currently used anti-psoriatic agent. Moreover, curcumin is yet another candidate alternative to 1,25D chemical analogs for psoriasis treatment, as its 3- to 4-fold action to induce *LCE3A* mRNA (Figures 4A and 8A) is equivalent in magnitude to the effect of 100 nM 1,25D, but curcumin is less prone than 1,25D to induce toxic hypercalcemia and likely is endowed with beneficial influences not intrinsic to 1,25D.

The results presented herein (Figures 3–5) do not rule out the possibility that DHA, curcumin, or other VDR ligands may act on LCE3 gene transcription via additional mechanisms. Indeed, literature reports have suggested that DHA effects in the skin are mediated, not by VDR, but rather via peroxisome proliferator-activated receptor (PPAR) isoforms such as PPARδ [26]. Furthermore, the doses of DHA that are capable of activating PPARδ are similar to doses necessary for the activation of VDR [49]. By observing that treatment with a saturating concentration of the PPARδ ligand GW501516 only modestly (and not statistically significantly) upregulated *LCE3A*, *LCE3D*, and *LCE3E* mRNAs (data not shown), and did not significantly enhance LCE3 protein expression (Figure 8A), we conclude that the effect of DHA on *LCE3* gene expression is exerted predominantly via the activation of VDR. Thus, DHA appears to function via a mechanism involving the association of liganded VDR with VDREs in target genes. To prove conclusively that liganded VDR docks on the postulated LCE3 gene region VDRE (Figure 1) will require in vivo ChIP-seq experiments in skin, a technical challenge which is beyond the scope of the current investigation, but is warranted for future studies.

The involvement of TNFα in the pathogenesis of psoriasis is well documented [50] and is the target of biological therapies that have proven effectiveness in severe cases [51]. The involvement of the MAP kinase p38 in the pathogenesis of psoriasis and its activation by the TNFα pathway are also well established [52]. We therefore investigated whether the VDR ligands DHA and curcumin could impact p38 phosphorylation in response to TNFα treatment of keratinocytes. Our finding that both ligands inhibit TNFα-induced p38 phosphorylation (Figures 3B and 4B) suggests that these VDR ligands have anti-psoriatic actions besides the induction of skin repair involving *LCE3* gene products. The effects of both ligands on TNFα signaling are similar to those observed in the imiquimod-induced mouse models of psoriasis by curcumin [53], and in other tissues, such as rat endothelial cells, by DHA [54]. In the case of DHA, the involvement of PPAR receptors such as PPARγ in these effects cannot be excluded (see [55]). Similarly, the effect of TNFα on JNK phosphorylation is also relevant to psoriasis [56]. Again, the pretreatment of keratinocytes with either DHA or curcumin inhibited the TNFα-induced phosphorylation of JNK (Figures 5B and 6), another indication that the anti-psoriatic mechanisms of these ligands extend to the TNFα pathway, which is successfully targeted by biologic treatments for moderate to severe psoriasis.

As a concluding experiment in this study, we evaluated whether VDR ligands, including DHA, 1,25D, and curcumin, regulate the expression of the nuclear receptor NURR1, also known as NR4A2, based on recent insight that specific VDR actions appear to involve a secondary mechanism whereby liganded VDR upregulates NURR1 expression, which in turn activates the expression the gene(s) of interest [25]. Moreover, increased expression of *NURR1* mRNA and protein occurs in involved psoriasis skin compared with uninvolved and normal skin [57], which is consistent with another recent report showing that NURR1 expression is crucial for the development of mature, fully functional Th17 cells [58] that have, in turn, been shown to play an important role in psoriasis pathogenesis via the production of IL-17 and IL-23 cytokines [59]. For these reasons, it was of interest to investigate the potential ability of DHA, curcumin, and 1,25D to control NURR1 expression. The results (Figures 7 and 8C) revealed that DHA, curcumin, and 1,25D induce, rather than repress, NURR1 expression, consistent with the hypothesis that NURR1 acts as a secondary mediator of at least part of the function of VDR ligands to induce skin repair genes such as the LCEs. However, because NURR1 is apparently a pro-psoriatic transcription factor in human skin [57], its induction by VDR ligands complicates our understanding of the mechanism whereby vitamin D analogs are effective in suppressing mild to moderate psoriasis symptoms. In other words, by inducing NURR1, VDR ligands could conceivably aggravate inflammation and proliferation as collateral effects to inducing skin repair genes, although one could argue that NURR1 is actually a trigger for normal skin remodeling in place of psoriatic pathology. It is also possible that the relative timing of NURR1 upregulation might be important with respect to its effects on inflammation and/or proliferation versus skin repair, an issue that could be addressed in future studies. In conclusion, identified herein is a secondary induction mechanism whereby VDR ligands increase the expression of NURR1, which in turn may function as the primary inducer of skin repair genes such as the LCE3 ensemble. Again, proof of this concept will require in vivo ChIP-seq experiments in skin, determining whether NURR1 is the transcription factor actually docked on the composite response element for VDR and NURR1 identified in the LCE3 gene region (Figure 1).

Given the lack of understanding of how 1,25D analogs improve symptoms of psoriasis, the effect of these compounds, as well as low-affinity VDR ligands such as DHA, curcumin, cyanidin, delphinidin, and others, could be examined on the expression of genes harbored in different loci. One of many possible examples is secreted mammalian Ly6/urokinase plasminogen activator receptor-related protein (SLURP-2), a gene that is strongly induced in psoriatic skin lesions [60]. Finally, since 14,21-dihydroxy-DHA has been shown to be a dramatic wound healing lipid in murine models [61], it is tempting to speculate that cellular metabolites of DHA, and possibly other low-affinity VDR ligands, could be discovered as high-affinity nuclear receptor ligands. These novel super-bioactive metabolites, if identified, could prove vastly more efficacious than their low-affinity VDR ligand precursors or even than 1,25D itself. In conclusion, the present investigation reveals the ability of nutrient or diet-derived VDR ligands to upregulate specific skin-expressed genes and proteins with relevance for psoriasis, and sets the stage for future studies examining the regulation of psoriasis-related skin-expressed genes by novel metabolites of low-affinity VDR ligands such as DHA and curcumin, potentially leading to drug discovery of new molecular-based treatments for mild/moderate psoriasis. Further studies beyond the scope of the current manuscript are warranted to critically examine these observations and to decipher their detailed molecular mechanisms.

Acknowledgments: This work was supported in part by grants NIH DK033351 to M.R.H., NIH CA140285 to P.W.J., a POHOFI Inc., Pre-College Intern Scholarship Award to R.C.N.C., a American Skin Association (ASA) Carson Research Scholar Award in Psoriasis to J.C.C., a UW-Madison Skin Disease Research Center (SDRC) Pilot and Feasibility Research Award to J.C.C. from NIH/NIAMS grant P30 AR066524, funding from the University of Louisiana at Monroe School of Pharmacy to J.C.C., and a grant from the University of Arizona, Department of Basic Medical Sciences to G.K.W.

Author Contributions: A.K., I.R. and R.C.N.C. performed most of the experimental work, and A.K. wrote the first draft of the manuscript. J.C.C. and G.K.W. designed and supervised the work, and performed most of the data analysis and manuscript editing. M.S.S. and S.M. performed the experiment and data analysis for Figure 7B as well as aided in manuscript editing. P.W.J. and M.R.H. provided laboratory and grant support for the project, as well as key insights into the planning of the project, interpretation of the data, and placing the conclusions into the context of the broader field. All authors read and approved the final submitted version of this manuscript.

References

1. Rachakonda, T.D.; Schupp, C.W.; Armstrong, A.W. Psoriasis prevalence among adults in the United States. *J. Am. Acad. Dermatol.* **2014**, *70*, 512–516. [CrossRef] [PubMed]
2. Barrea, L.; Savanelli, M.C.; Somma, C.D.; Napolitano, M.; Megna, M.; Colao, A.; Savastano, S. Vitamin D and its role in psoriasis: An overview of the dermatologist and nutritionist. *Rev. Endocr. Metab. Disord.* **2017**, *18*, 195–205. [CrossRef] [PubMed]
3. Gisondi, P.; Rossini, M.; Di Cesare, A.; Idolazzi, L.; Farina, S.; Beltrami, G.; Peris, K.; Girolomoni, G. Vitamin D status in patients with chronic plaque psoriasis. *Br. J. Dermatol.* **2012**, *166*, 505–510. [CrossRef] [PubMed]

4. Orgaz-Molina, J.; Buendia-Eisman, A.; Arrabal-Polo, M.A.; Ruiz, J.C.; Arias-Santiago, S. Deficiency of serum concentration of 25-hydroxyvitamin D in psoriatic patients: A case-control study. *J. Am. Acad. Dermatol.* **2012**, *67*, 931–938. [CrossRef] [PubMed]
5. Devaux, S.; Castela, A.; Archier, E.; Gallini, A.; Joly, P.; Misery, L.; Aractingi, S.; Aubin, F.; Bachelez, H.; Cribier, B.; et al. Topical vitamin D analogues alone or in association with topical steroids for psoriasis: A systematic review. *J. Eur. Acad. Dermatol. Venereol.* **2012**, *26*, 52–60. [CrossRef] [PubMed]
6. Kim, I.H.; West, C.E.; Kwatra, S.G.; Feldman, S.R.; O'Neill, J.L. Comparative efficacy of biologics in psoriasis: A review. *Am. J. Clin. Dermatol.* **2012**, *13*, 365–374. [CrossRef] [PubMed]
7. Crow, J.M. Therapeutics: Silencing psoriasis. *Nature* **2012**, *492*, S58–S59. [CrossRef] [PubMed]
8. Haussler, M.R.; Whitfield, G.K.; Kaneko, I.; Haussler, C.A.; Hsieh, D.; Hsieh, J.C.; Jurutka, P.W. Molecular mechanisms of vitamin D action. *Calcif. Tissue Int.* **2013**, *92*, 77–98. [CrossRef] [PubMed]
9. Bergboer, J.G.; Tjabringa, G.S.; Kamsteeg, M.; van Vlijmen-Willems, I.M.; Rodijk-Olthuis, D.; Jansen, P.A.; Thuret, J.Y.; Narita, M.; Ishida-Yamamoto, A.; Zeeuwen, P.L.; et al. Psoriasis risk genes of the late cornified envelope-3 group are distinctly expressed compared with genes of other *LCE* groups. *Am. J. Pathol.* **2011**, *178*, 1470–1477. [CrossRef] [PubMed]
10. Riveira-Munoz, E.; He, S.M.; Escaramis, G.; Stuart, P.E.; Huffmeier, U.; Lee, C.; Kirby, B.; Oka, A.; Giardina, E.; Liao, W.; et al. Meta-analysis confirms the *LCE3C_LCE3B* deletion as a risk factor for psoriasis in several ethnic groups and finds interaction with HLA-CW6. *J. Investig. Dermatol.* **2011**, *131*, 1105–1109. [CrossRef] [PubMed]
11. Austin, H.R.; Hoss, E.; Batie, S.F.; Moffet, E.W.; Jurutka, P.W.; Haussler, M.R.; Whitfield, G.K. Regulation of late cornified envelope genes relevant to psoriasis risk by plant-derived cyanidin. *Biochem. Biophys. Res. Commun.* **2014**, *443*, 1275–1279. [CrossRef] [PubMed]
12. Hoss, E.; Austin, H.R.; Batie, S.F.; Jurutka, P.W.; Haussler, M.R.; Whitfield, G.K. Control of late cornified envelope genes relevant to psoriasis risk: Upregulation by 1,25-dihydroxyvitamin D3 and plant-derived delphinidin. *Arch. Dermatol. Res.* **2013**, *305*, 867–878. [CrossRef] [PubMed]
13. Jackson, B.; Tilli, C.M.; Hardman, M.J.; Avilion, A.A.; MacLeod, M.C.; Ashcroft, G.S.; Byrne, C. Late cornified envelope family in differentiating epithelia-response to calcium and ultraviolet irradiation. *J. Investig. Dermatol.* **2005**, *124*, 1062–1070. [CrossRef] [PubMed]
14. Reichrath, J.; Müller, S.M.; Kerber, A.; Baum, H.P.; Bahmer, F.A. Biologic effects of topical calcipotriol (MC 903) treatment in psoriatic skin. *J. Am. Acad. Dermatol.* **1997**, *36*, 19–28. [CrossRef]
15. Haussler, M.R.; Haussler, C.A.; Bartik, L.; Whitfield, G.K.; Hsieh, J.C.; Slater, S.; Jurutka, P.W. Vitamin D receptor: Molecular signaling and actions of nutritional ligands in disease prevention. *Nutr. Rev.* **2008**, *66*, S98–S112. [CrossRef] [PubMed]
16. Vaughn, A.R.; Branum, A.; Sivamani, R.K. Effects of turmeric (*Curcuma longa*) on skin health: A systematic review of the clinical evidence. *Phytother. Res.* **2016**, *30*, 1243–1264. [CrossRef] [PubMed]
17. Calder, P.C. Omega-3 fatty acids and inflammatory processes: From molecules to man. *Biochem. Soc. Trans.* **2017**, *45*, 1105–1115. [CrossRef] [PubMed]
18. Xu, J.; Duan, X.; Hu, F.; Poorun, D.; Liu, X.; Wang, X.; Zhang, S.; Gan, L.; He, M.; Zhu, K.; et al. Resolvin D1 attenuates imiquimod-induced mice psoriasiform dermatitis through mapks and nf-kappab pathways. *J. Dermatol. Sci.* **2017**. [CrossRef]
19. Mayser, P.; Mrowietz, U.; Arenberger, P.; Bartak, P.; Buchvald, J.; Christophers, E.; Jablonska, S.; Salmhofer, W.; Schill, W.B.; Kramer, H.J.; et al. Omega-3 fatty acid-based lipid infusion in patients with chronic plaque psoriasis: Results of a double-blind, randomized, placebo-controlled, multicenter trial. *J. Am. Acad. Dermatol.* **1998**, *38*, 539–547. [CrossRef]
20. Rahman, M.; Beg, S.; Ahmad, M.Z.; Kazmi, I.; Akhter, S.; Ahmed, A. Omega-3 fatty acids as pharmacotherapeutics in psoriasis: Current status and future of nanomedicine in its effective delivery. *Curr. Drug Targets* **2013**, *14*, 708–722. [CrossRef] [PubMed]
21. Thangapazham, R.L.; Sharma, A.; Maheshwari, R.K. Beneficial role of curcumin in skin diseases. *Adv. Exp. Med. Biol.* **2007**, *595*, 343–357. [PubMed]
22. Kurd, S.K.; Smith, N.; VanVoorhees, A.; Troxel, A.B.; Badmaev, V.; Seykora, J.T.; Gelfand, J.M. Oral curcumin in the treatment of moderate to severe psoriasis vulgaris: A prospective clinical trial. *J. Am. Acad. Dermatol.* **2008**, *58*, 625–631. [CrossRef] [PubMed]

23. Zenz, R.; Eferl, R.; Kenner, L.; Florin, L.; Hummerich, L.; Mehic, D.; Scheuch, H.; Angel, P.; Tschachler, E.; Wagner, E.F. Psoriasis-like skin disease and arthritis caused by inducible epidermal deletion of Jun proteins. *Nature* **2005**, *437*, 369–375. [CrossRef] [PubMed]
24. Florin, L.; Knebel, J.; Zigrino, P.; Vonderstrass, B.; Mauch, C.; Schorpp-Kistner, M.; Szabowski, A.; Angel, P. Delayed wound healing and epidermal hyperproliferation in mice lacking JunB in the skin. *J. Investig. Dermatol.* **2006**, *126*, 902–911. [CrossRef] [PubMed]
25. Kaneko, I.; Saini, R.K.; Griffin, K.P.; Whitfield, G.K.; Haussler, M.R.; Jurutka, P.W. *FGF23* gene regulation by 1,25-dihydroxyvitamin D: Opposing effects in adipocytes and osteocytes. *J. Endocrinol.* **2015**, *226*, 155–166. [CrossRef] [PubMed]
26. Kuenzli, S.; Saurat, J.H. Peroxisome proliferator-activated receptors in cutaneous biology. *Br. J. Dermatol.* **2003**, *149*, 229–236. [CrossRef] [PubMed]
27. Niehues, H.; van Vlijmen-Willems, I.M.; Bergboer, J.G.; Kersten, F.F.; Narita, M.; Hendriks, W.J.; van den Bogaard, E.H.; Zeeuwen, P.L.; Schalkwijk, J. Late cornified envelope (*LCE*) proteins: Distinct expression patterns of LCE2 and LCE3 members suggest nonredundant roles in human epidermis and other epithelia. *Br. J. Dermatol.* **2016**, *174*, 795–802. [CrossRef] [PubMed]
28. Syed, D.N.; Lall, R.K.; Chamcheu, J.C.; Haidar, O.H.M. Involvement of ER stress and activation of apoptotic pathways in fisetin induced cytotoxicity in human melanoma. *Arch. Biochem. Biophys.* **2014**, *563*, 108–117. [CrossRef] [PubMed]
29. Huang, W.; Hennrick, K.; Drew, S. A colorful future of quantitative pathology: Validation of Vectra technology using chromogenic multiplexed immunohistochemistry and prostate tissue microarrays. *Hum. Pathol.* **2013**, *44*, 29–38. [CrossRef] [PubMed]
30. Chamcheu, J.C.; Adhami, V.M.; Esnault, S.; Sechi, M.; Siddiqui, I.A.; Satyshur, K.A.; Syed, D.N.; Dodwad, S.M.; Chaves-Rodriquez, M.I.; Longley, B.J.; et al. Dual inhibition of PI3K/AKT and mTOR by the dietary antioxidant, delphinidin, ameliorates psoriatic features in vitro and in an imiquimod-induced psoriasis-like disease in mice. *Antioxid. Redox Signal* **2017**, *26*, 49–69. [CrossRef] [PubMed]
31. De Cid, R.; Riveira-Munoz, E.; Zeeuwen, P.L.; Robarge, J.; Liao, W.; Dannhauser, E.N.; Giardina, E.; Stuart, P.E.; Nair, R.; Helms, C.; et al. Deletion of the late cornified envelope LCE3B and LCE3C genes as a susceptibility factor for psoriasis. *Nat. Genet.* **2009**, *41*, 211–215. [CrossRef] [PubMed]
32. Jurutka, P.W.; Remus, L.S.; Whitfield, G.K.; Thompson, P.D.; Hsieh, J.C.; Zitzer, H.; Tavakkoli, P.; Galligan, M.A.; Dang, H.T.; Haussler, C.A.; et al. The polymorphic N terminus in human vitamin D receptor isoforms influences transcriptional activity by modulating interaction with transcription factor IIB. *Mol. Endocrinol.* **2000**, *14*, 401–420. [CrossRef] [PubMed]
33. Speir, M.L.; Zweig, A.S.; Rosenbloom, K.R.; Raney, B.J.; Paten, B.; Nejad, P.; Lee, B.T.; Learned, K.; Karolchik, D.; Hinrichs, A.S.; et al. The UCSC genome browser database: 2016 update. *Nucleic Acids Res.* **2016**, *44*, D717–D725. [CrossRef] [PubMed]
34. Untergasser, A.; Nijveen, H.; Rao, X.; Bisseling, T.; Geurts, R.; Leunissen, J.A. Primer3plus, an enhanced web interface to primer3. *Nucleic Acids Res.* **2007**, *35*, W71–W74. [CrossRef] [PubMed]
35. Misund, K.; Selvik, L.K.; Rao, S.; Norsett, K.; Bakke, I.; Sandvik, A.K.; Laegreid, A.; Bruland, T.; Prestvik, W.S.; Thommesen, L. Nr4a2 is regulated by gastrin and influences cellular responses of gastric adenocarcinoma cells. *PLoS ONE* **2013**, *8*, e76234. [CrossRef] [PubMed]
36. Johansen, C.; Kragballe, K.; Westergaard, M.; Henningsen, J.; Kristiansen, K.; Iversen, L. The mitogen-activated protein kinases P38 and ERK1/2 are increased in lesional psoriatic skin. *Br. J. Dermatol.* **2005**, *152*, 37–42. [CrossRef] [PubMed]
37. Ettehadi, P.; Greaves, M.W.; Wallach, D.; Aderka, D.; Camp, R.D. Elevated tumour necrosis factor-alpha (TNF-α) biological activity in psoriatic skin lesions. *Clin. Exp. Immunol.* **1994**, *96*, 146–151. [CrossRef] [PubMed]
38. Bartik, L.; Whitfield, G.K.; Kaczmarska, M.; Lowmiller, C.L.; Moffet, E.W.; Furmick, J.K.; Hernandez, Z.; Haussler, C.A.; Haussler, M.R.; Jurutka, P.W. Curcumin: A novel nutritionally derived ligand of the vitamin D receptor with implications for colon cancer chemoprevention. *J. Nutr. Biochem.* **2010**, *21*, 1153–1161. [CrossRef] [PubMed]

39. Chamcheu, J.C.; Chaves-Rodriquez, M.I.; Adhami, V.M.; Siddiqui, I.A.; Wood, G.S.; Longley, B.J.; Mukhtar, H. Upregulation of PI3K/AKT/MTOR, FABP5 and PPARBETA/DELTA in human psoriasis and imiquimod-induced murine psoriasiform dermatitis model. *Acta Derm. Venereol.* **2016**, *96*, 854–856. [PubMed]
40. Ham, S.A.; Hwang, J.S.; Yoo, T.; Lee, H.; Kang, E.S.; Park, C.; Oh, J.W.; Lee, H.T.; Min, G.; Kim, J.H.; et al. Ligand-activated PPARδ inhibits UVB-induced senescence of human keratinocytes via PTEN-mediated inhibition of superoxide production. *Biochem. J.* **2012**, *444*, 27–38. [CrossRef] [PubMed]
41. Van de Kerkhof, P.C. An update on topical therapies for mild-moderate psoriasis. *Derm. Clin.* **2015**, *33*, 73–77. [CrossRef] [PubMed]
42. Barrea, L.; Macchia, P.E.; Tarantino, G.; Di Somma, C.; Pane, E.; Balato, N.; Napolitano, M.; Colao, A.; Savastano, S. Nutrition: A key environmental dietary factor in clinical severity and cardio-metabolic risk in psoriatic male patients evaluated by 7-day food-frequency questionnaire. *J. Transl. Med.* **2015**, *13*, 303. [CrossRef] [PubMed]
43. Guida, B.; Napoleone, A.; Trio, R.; Nastasi, A.; Balato, N.; Laccetti, R.; Cataldi, M. Energy-restricted, *n*-3 polyunsaturated fatty acids-rich diet improves the clinical response to immuno-modulating drugs in obese patients with plaque-type psoriasis: A randomized control clinical trial. *Clin. Nutr.* **2014**, *33*, 399–405. [CrossRef] [PubMed]
44. Barrea, L.; Balato, N.; Di Somma, C.; Macchia, P.E.; Napolitano, M.; Savanelli, M.C.; Esposito, K.; Colao, A.; Savastano, S. Nutrition and psoriasis: Is there any association between the severity of the disease and adherence to the Mediterranean diet? *J. Transl. Med.* **2015**, *13*, 18. [CrossRef] [PubMed]
45. Lin, Y.L.; Pavlidis, P.; Karakoc, E.; Ajay, J.; Gokcumen, O. The evolution and functional impact of human deletion variants shared with archaic hominin genomes. *Mol. Biol. Evol.* **2015**, *32*, 1008–1019. [CrossRef] [PubMed]
46. Pajic, P.; Lin, Y.L.; Xu, D.; Gokcumen, O. The psoriasis-associated deletion of late cornified envelope genes *LCE3B* and *LCE3C* has been maintained under balancing selection since human denisovan divergence. *BMC Evol. Biol.* **2016**, *16*, 265. [CrossRef] [PubMed]
47. Bassaganyas, L.; Riveira-Munoz, E.; Garcia-Aragones, M.; Gonzalez, J.R.; Caceres, M.; Armengol, L.; Estivill, X. Worldwide population distribution of the common *LCE3C-LCE3B* deletion associated with psoriasis and other autoimmune disorders. *BMC Genom.* **2013**, *14*, 261. [CrossRef] [PubMed]
48. Bergboer, J.G.; Zeeuwen, P.L.; Schalkwijk, J. Genetics of psoriasis: Evidence for epistatic interaction between skin barrier abnormalities and immune deviation. *J. Investig. Dermatol.* **2012**, *132*, 2320–2331. [CrossRef] [PubMed]
49. Nakanishi, A.; Tsukamoto, I. *n*-3 polyunsaturated fatty acids stimulate osteoclastogenesis through PPARγ-mediated enhancement of c-Fos expression, and suppress osteoclastogenesis through PPARγ-dependent inhibition of NFKB activation. *J. Nutr. Biochem.* **2015**, *26*, 1317–1327. [CrossRef] [PubMed]
50. Victor, F.C.; Gottlieb, A.B. TNF-alpha and apoptosis: Implications for the pathogenesis and treatment of psoriasis. *J. Drugs Dermatol.* **2002**, *1*, 264–275. [PubMed]
51. Menter, A.; Gordon, K.B.; Leonardi, C.L.; Gu, Y.; Goldblum, O.M. Efficacy and safety of adalimumab across subgroups of patients with moderate to severe psoriasis. *J. Am. Acad. Dermatol.* **2010**, *63*, 448–456. [CrossRef] [PubMed]
52. Arthur, J.S.; Darragh, J. Signaling downstream of p38 in psoriasis. *J. Investig. Dermatol.* **2006**, *126*, 1689–1691. [CrossRef] [PubMed]
53. Varma, S.R.; Sivaprakasam, T.O.; Mishra, A.; Prabhu, S.M.R.P.R. Imiquimod-induced psoriasis-like inflammation in differentiated human keratinocytes: Its evaluation using curcumin. *Eur. J. Pharmacol.* **2017**, *813*, 33–41. [CrossRef] [PubMed]
54. Yamagata, K.; Suzuki, S.; Tagami, M. Docosahexaenoic acid prevented tumor necrosis factor alpha-induced endothelial dysfunction and senescence. *Prostaglandin. Leukot Essent Fatty Acids* **2016**, *104*, 11–18. [CrossRef] [PubMed]
55. Bernardo, A.; Giammarco, M.L.; De Nuccio, C.; Ajmone-Cat, M.A.; Visentin, S.; De Simone, R.; Minghetti, L. Docosahexaenoic acid promotes oligodendrocyte differentiation via PPAR-γ signalling and prevents tumor necrosis factor-alpha-dependent maturational arrest. *Biochim. Biophys. Acta* **2017**, *1862*, 1013–1023. [CrossRef] [PubMed]

56. Kim, B.E.; Howell, M.D.; Guttman-Yassky, E.; Gilleaudeau, P.M.; Cardinale, I.R.; Boguniewicz, M.; Krueger, J.G.; Leung, D.Y. TNF-α downregulates filaggrin and loricrin through c-Jun N-terminal kinase: Role for TNF-α antagonists to improve skin barrier. *J. Investig. Dermatol.* **2011**, *131*, 1272–1279. [CrossRef] [PubMed]
57. O'Kane, M.; Markham, T.; McEvoy, A.N.; Fearon, U.; Veale, D.J.; FitzGerald, O.; Kirby, B.; Murphy, E.P. Increased expression of the orphan nuclear receptor NURR1 in psoriasis and modulation following TNF-α inhibition. *J. Investig. Dermatol.* **2008**, *128*, 300–310. [CrossRef] [PubMed]
58. Raveney, B.J.; Oki, S.; Yamamura, T. Nuclear receptor NR4A2 orchestrates Th17 cell-mediated autoimmune inflammation via IL-21 signalling. *PLoS ONE* **2013**, *8*, e56595. [CrossRef] [PubMed]
59. Deng, Y.; Chang, C.; Lu, Q. The inflammatory response in psoriasis: A comprehensive review. *Clin. Rev. Allergy Immunol.* **2016**, *50*, 377–389. [CrossRef] [PubMed]
60. Moriwaki, Y.; Takada, K.; Tsuji, S.; Kawashima, K.; Misawa, H. Transcriptional regulation of SLURP2, a psoriasis-associated gene, is under control of IL-22 in the skin: A special reference to the nested gene LYNX1. *Int. Immunopharmacol.* **2015**, *29*, 71–75. [CrossRef] [PubMed]
61. Lu, Y.; Tian, H.; Hong, S. Novel 14,21-dihydroxy-docosahexaenoic acids: Structures, formation pathways, and enhancement of wound healing. *J. Lipid Res.* **2010**, *51*, 923–932. [CrossRef] [PubMed]

5

Elucidating the Skin Delivery of Aglycone and Glycoside Flavonoids: How the Structures Affect Cutaneous Absorption

Shih-Yi Chuang [1,†], Yin-Ku Lin [2,3,†], Chwan-Fwu Lin [1,4], Pei-Wen Wang [5], En-Li Chen [6] and Jia-You Fang [1,6,7,8,*]

1 Research Center for Food and Cosmetic Safety and Research Center for Chinese Herbal Medicine, Chang Gung University of Science and Technology, Kweishan, Taoyuan 333, Taiwan; clemencechuang@gmail.com (S.-Y.C.); cflin@mail.cgust.edu.tw (C.-F.L.)
2 Department of Traditional Chinese Medicine, Chang Gung Memorial Hospital, Keelung 204, Taiwan; lin1266@cgmh.org.tw
3 School of Traditional Chinese Medicine, Chang Gung University, Kweishan, Taoyuan 333, Taiwan
4 Department of Cosmetic Science, Chang Gung University of Science and Technology, Kweishan, Taoyuan 333, Taiwan
5 Department of Medical Research, China Medical University Hospital, China Medical University, Taichung 404, Taiwan; pwwang@hotmail.com
6 Pharmaceutics Laboratory, Graduate Institute of Natural Products, Chang Gung University, Kweishan, Taoyuan 333, Taiwan; fajy5521@gmail.com
7 Chinese Herbal Medicine Research Team, Healthy Aging Research Center, Chang Gung University, Kweishan, Taoyuan 333, Taiwan
8 Department of Anesthesiology, Chang Gung Memorial Hospital, Kweishan, Taoyuan 333, Taiwan
* Correspondence: fajy@mail.cgu.edu.tw
† These authors contributed equally to this work.

Abstract: Flavonoids are bioactive phytochemicals that exhibit protective potential against cutaneous inflammation and photoaging. We selected eight flavonoid aglycones or glycosides to elucidate the chemistry behind their skin absorption capability through experimental and computational approaches. The skin delivery was conducted using nude mouse and pig skins mounted on an in vitro Franz cell assembly. The anti-inflammatory activity was examined using the $O_2^{\bullet-}$ and elastase inhibition in activated human neutrophils. In the equivalent dose (6 mM) application on nude mouse skin, the skin deposition of naringenin and kaempferol was 0.37 and 0.11 nM/mg, respectively, which was higher than that of the other flavonoids. Both penetrants were beneficial for targeted cutaneous therapy due to their minimal diffusion across the skin. The absorption was generally greater for topically applied aglycones than glycosides. Although naringenin could be classified as a hydrophilic flavonoid, the flexibility of the chiral center in the C ring of this flavanone could lead to better skin transport than the flavonols and flavones with a planar structure. An optimized hydrophilic and lipophilic balance of the flavonoid structure was important for governing the cutaneous delivery. The hydrogen bond acceptor and stratum corneum lipid docking estimated by molecular modeling showed some relationships with the skin deposition. The interaction with cholesteryl sulfate could be a factor for predicting the cutaneous absorption of aglycone flavonoids (correlation coefficient = 0.97). Baicalin (3 μM) showed the highest activity against oxidative burst with an $O_2^{\bullet-}$ inhibition percentage of 77%. Although naringenin displayed an inhibition efficiency of only 20%, this compound still demonstrated an impressive therapeutic index because of the high absorption. Our data are advantageous to providing the information on the structure–permeation relationship for topically applied flavonoids.

Keywords: flavonoid; cutaneous absorption; structure–permeation relationship; anti-inflammation; molecular modeling

1. Introduction

Strong evidence links oxidative stress with several pathologies [1]. The skin, the largest organ in the body, is a main target of oxidative stress because of its size [2]. Reactive oxygen species (ROS) play a key role in some cutaneous diseases, including photoaging, psoriasis, dermatitis, acne, rosacea, alopecia, and skin cancer [3]. Flavonoids are antioxidants ubiquitously found in vegetables and fruits. The structure of flavonoids is associated with the derivatives of chalcone. They can prevent or treat cutaneous inflammation and malignancy by maintaining the skin's homeostasis [4]. Some flavonoids, such as naringenin and quercetin, have been reported to exhibit anti-aging activity that slows down the skin's natural senescence [5]. Flavonoids have been largely used in dermatology and cosmeceuticals in the form of crude extracts.

Topical application provides an efficient method for facilitating the local action of drugs on the skin [6]. For an active ingredient to exhibit bioactivity, its delivery into the targeted skin must be successful. It is evidenced that the absorption rate and scavenging activity of some flavonoids depend on their chemical structure [7]. The exploration of the structure–permeation relationship (SPR) offers insights into the understanding of how the physicochemical properties of chemicals influence cutaneous absorption or targeting. The establishment of SPR is useful for predicting the skin delivery of the compounds and for facilitating the development of new topically applied actives. In addition to the aglycone form, flavonoids are present in the form of glycoside in nature. Some aglycones and glycosides, such as quercetin/rutin and baicalein/baicalin, are paired. Glycosides also show potent bioactivity in many cases. For example, baicalin is proven to protect the skin from UV radiation, burning, and aging [8]. Although many reports have dealt with the biological effect of glycoside flavonoids, investigation of how the sugar moiety affects cutaneous absorption is still lacking. In a continuing attempt to elucidate SPR, the objective of this study was to evaluate the physicochemical characteristics and the skin absorption of a series of aglycone flavonoids and their corresponding glycosides. These included myricetin, naringenin, quercetin, baicalein, kaempferol, naringin, rutin, and baicalin (Figure 1).

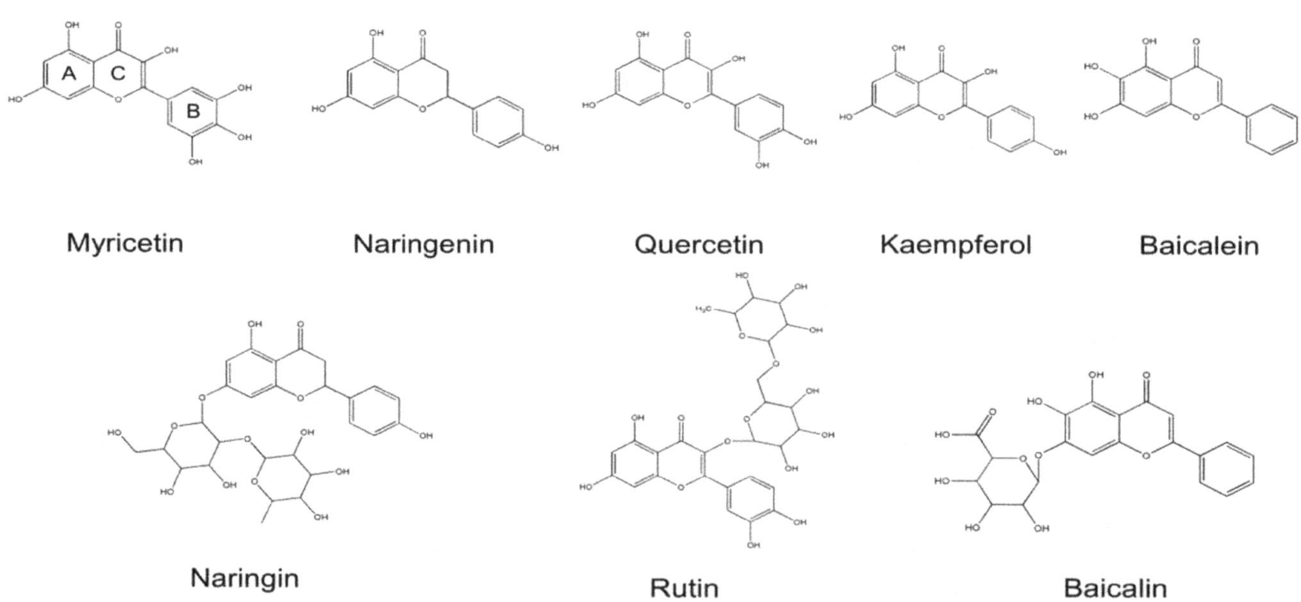

Figure 1. The chemical structures of flavonoids tested in this study.

In the present study, the in vitro Franz cell model was utilized to assess the skin absorption of flavonoids. Both nude mouse skin and baby pig skin were employed as the permeation barriers. In inspecting the permeation behavior of a penetrant, it is important to identify the possible transport pathways [9]. We examined flavonoid permeation via the skin after removal of the stratum corneum (SC), lipid, sebum, and protein in order to understand the delivery routes. Data collected for the capacity factor (log *K'*), the partition coefficient (log *P*), and the aqueous solubility allowed us to distinguish the relative contribution to cutaneous absorption. The anti-inflammatory activity of these compounds was determined by the capacity of inhibiting superoxide anion ($O_2^{\bullet -}$) and elastase of formyl-methionyl-leucyl phenylalanine (fMLF)-activated human neutrophils. A wealth of information on the hydrogen bond acceptor, the hydrogen bond donor, the total polarity surface, and the molecular volume was obtained by the computation of molecular modeling. We also investigated the predicted interaction between flavonoids and SC lipid components to explain the skin permeation trend. The present study sheds light on the effect of the flavonoid structure on skin absorption and targeting, broadening the comprehension of SPR in natural antioxidants.

2. Materials and Methods

2.1. Materials

All flavonoids tested in this study were purchased from Sigma-Aldrich (St. Louis, MO, USA). All other chemicals and solvents were of reagent grade without further purification.

2.2. Capacity Factor (Log K')

The HPLC setup for the calculation of log *K'* was an HPLC system (7-series, Hitachi, Tokyo, Japan) with a LiChrospher® C18 column (200 × 4.6 mm, Merck, Darmstadt, Germany). The mobile phase consisted of a mixture of methanol and pH 2 phosphate buffer solution (1:1). The flow rate and wavelength for determination were 1 mL/min (L-7110 pump) and 256 nm (L-7455 diode array detector), respectively. The retention times of flavonoids were detected, and the log *K'* was computed as $\log [(t_r - t_0)/t_0]$, where t_r and t_0 were the retention time of the flavonoid and the nonretained solvent peak, respectively.

2.3. Partition Coefficient (Log P)

Flavonoids in methanol (0.5 mg/mL) were pipetted into a tube at a volume of 1 mL. Methanol was then evaporated under vacuum. In the amount of 1 mL of each, *n*-Octanol and water were incorporated into the tube. After being shaken for 24 h at 37 °C, the tube was centrifugated at 10,000× *g* for 10 min. The flavonoid content in both phases was analyzed by HPLC. The log *P* was calculated as log (flavonoid content in *n*-octanol/flavonoid content in water).

2.4. Saturated Solubility in 20% PEG400 Aqueous Solution

The saturated solubility of flavonoids in 20% PEG400/pH 7.4 buffer was measured by loading 20 mM compounds in the vehicle and shaking them at 37 °C for 2 h. The suspension was then centrifuged at 10,000× *g* for 10 min. The supernatant was filtered across the polyvinylidene fluoride membrane with a pore size of 0.45 μm. The resulting supernatant was analyzed by HPLC to record the solubility (mM).

2.5. Animals

Eight-week-old female nude mice were provided by the National Laboratory Animal Center (Taipei, Taiwan). One-week-old specific-pathogen-free pigs were obtained from the Animal Technology Institute Taiwan (Miaoli, Taiwan). All animals were treated in strict accordance with the recommendations set forth in the Guidelines for the Institutional Animal Care and Use Committee of Chang Gung University (CGU15-083).

2.6. Preparation of SC-Disrupted Skin

The full-thickness dorsal skin of the nude mouse was excised after sacrifice. The SC-stripped skin was obtained by stripping the skin surface 20 times with adhesive tape (Scotch®, 3M, Maplewood, MN, USA). The delipidized skin was achieved by incubating the skin surface onto a chloroform/methanol solution (2:1) for 2 h [10]. To prepare the desebumed skin, the SC side of the skin was washed with cold hexane (4 °C) five times, based on the procedure of the previous study [11]. The skin's surface was then treated with a 40% ethanol/water solution for 2 h, a process that successfully denatured the skin's proteins.

2.7. In Vitro Franz Cell Assembly

The cutaneous absorption of flavonoids was assessed using a Franz diffusion cell system. The excised animal skin or cellulose membrane was mounted between the donor and receptor compartments with the SC facing up toward the donor. The receptor was filled with 30% ethanol/pH 7.4 buffer and placed on a magnetic stirring plate. The effective permeation area of the cell was 0.785 cm^2. The stirring rate and temperature of the receptor were 600 rpm and 37 °C, respectively. Saturated solution or a 6 mM flavonoid suspension was prepared in 20% PEG400/pH 7.4 buffer to be loaded into the donor compartment. A 300-μL aliquot in the receptor was collected at determined durations, followed by an immediate replacement with fresh receptor medium. The amount of flavonoid in the receptor was determined by HPLC. The skin was removed from the cell after a 24-h application. After being washed with water, the skin sample was weighed and positioned in a vial with 1 mL methanol. MagNA Lyser (Roche) was used to homogenize the skin. The homogenate was centrifuged at 10,000× *g* for 10 min. The supernatant was analyzed by HPLC to quantify the flavonoid deposition in the skin reservoir.

2.8. Inhibition of Neutrophilic Inflammation by Flavonoids

The protocol was approved by the Institutional Review Board at Chang Gung Memorial Hospital, and written informed consent was obtained from all volunteers (201600500B0C101). Whole blood was withdrawn from healthy volunteers between 20 and 30 years of age. Human neutrophils were isolated using a typical method of dextran sedimentation prior to centrifugation in a Ficoll-Hypaque gradient and hypotonic lysis of erythrocytes [12]. The granulocyte layer was harvested and suspended in calcium-free HBSS at pH 7.4, which was maintained at 4 °C until use.

The reduction of ferricytochrome *c* was utilized for measuring the superoxide anion ($O_2^{\bullet -}$) release from the neutrophils [13]. The human neutrophils (6×10^5 cells/mL) were incubated with 0.5 mg/mL ferricytochrome *c* and 1 mM $CaCl_2$ at 37 °C, and were then treated with flavonoids (3 μM) in DMSO for 10 min. Neutrophils were stimulated by adding 0.1 μM fMLF with cytochalasin B (1 μg/mL). The reduction of ferricytochrome *c* was monitored by the absorbance at 550 nm using a U3010 ultraviolet/visible spectrophotometer (Hitachi, Tokyo, Japan). The human neutrophils were equilibrated with an elastase substrate (MeO-Suc-Ala-Ala-Pro-Val-*p*-nitroanilide, 100 μM) at 37 °C for 2 min. Flavonoids at a concentration of 3 μM were added into the neutrophil suspension for 10 min. The cells were activated by fMLF and cytochalasin B for a further 10 min. Elastase release was detected by measuring the change of absorbance at 405 nm.

2.9. Molecular Modeling

The structures of the flavonoids were sketched using Discovery Studio® version 4.1 workstation (Accelrys, San Diego, CA, USA). The hydrogen bond acceptor or donor number, total polarity surface, and molecular volume of the flavonoids were estimated. The superimposition of flavonoids with ceramides, palmitic acid, cholesteryl sulfate, and cholesterol was computed to observe the conformation and ligand-binding activity. The negative CDOCKER energy was calculated after conducting the molecular docking simulation of the flavonoids with these SC lipids.

2.10. *In Vivo Cutaneous Tolerance of Flavonoids*

The 20% PEG400/pH 7.4 buffer loaded with flavonoids at 6 mM was topically applied daily (0.6 mL) on the nude mouse back for 7 days. The flavonoid-containing vehicle was replaced with a new one each day. After removal of the vehicle, the treated skin region was evaluated by Tewameter TM300 (Courage and Khazaka, Köln, Germany) to determine the transepidermal water loss (TEWL). Stained by hematoxylin and eosin (H&E), the treated skin was excised for histological examination after a 7-day flavonoid application.

2.11. *Data Analysis*

In the cutaneous absorption experiment, flavonoid deposition in the skin was estimated as the molar amount per mg of skin (nM/mg). In the case of the skin deposition from the saturated solution, the calibrated skin deposition (CSD) was measured as flavonoid deposition divided by the applied dose (saturated solubility). The flux ($nM/cm^2/h$) was estimated by the slope of the penetrated amount–time curve. The permeability coefficient (PC) was calculated from the flux divided by the saturated solubility of the flavonoids. The dermal/transdermal selectivity index (S value) was calculated using an equation of skin deposition/flux (for equivalent dose application) or CSD/PC (for saturated dose application).

The data in the present study were presented as mean and standard deviation (S.D.). The statistical difference in the data of different experimental groups was evaluated using the Kruskal–Wallis test. The post hoc test for checking individual differences was Dunn's test. A 0.05 level of probability was taken as the statistical significance. The software used for statistical comparison was WINKS (Texasoft, Cedar Hill, TX, USA).

3. Results

3.1. *Physicochemical Properties of Flavonoids*

To understand the relationship between skin permeation and physicochemical properties, the molecular weight (MW), lipophilicity ($\log K'$ and $\log P$), and aqueous solubility of flavonoids were considered as presented in Table 1. Figure 1 demonstrates that the aglycone flavonoids tested in this study have different hydroxyl groups from 3 to 6, with myricetin showing the most abundant hydroxyl moieties and the highest MW. The structures of most aglycones belong to flavonols, with the exception of the flavanone naringenin and flavone baicalein. Naringin, rutin, and baicalin are the glycosides with sugar residue in the structures of naringenin, quercetin, and baicalein, respectively. The glycosides had a higher MW than their corresponding aglycones. Both $\log K'$ and $\log P$ are the indicators of lipophilicity. The capacity factor was increased following the decrease of hydroxyl moieties for flavonols and flavones. The trend of $\log P$ correlated well with that of $\log K'$. Although kaempferol exhibited a higher partition coefficient compared to baicalein (3.71 versus 3.59), no statistically significant difference was found ($p > 0.05$). Naringenin, a flavanone, revealed a lower lipophilicity than baicalein, though both compounds possessed the same hydroxyl group number (3). The lipophilicity of glycosides was less than that of aglycones because of the presence of sugar. As expected, the compounds with lower lipophilicity displayed higher solubility in PEG400/pH 7.4 buffer solution. The flavanone showed much higher solubility compared to the flavonols and flavones. Naringenin was 470-fold more soluble than baicalein. The same result was achieved with naringin, which showed an aqueous solubility of >20 mM.

Table 1. Physicochemical properties of aglycone and glycoside flavonoids.

Category	Compound	MW (Da)	log K'	log P	Solubility in 20% PEG400 (mM)
Aglycone	Myricetin	318.24	0.34	3.18 ± 0.07	0.53 ± 0.01
	Naringenin	272.25	0.51	3.21 ± 0.04	3.62 ± 0.28
	Quercetin	302.24	0.51	3.32 ± 0.09	0.38 ± 0.0025
	Kaempferol	286.24	0.65	3.71 ± 0.57	0.19 ± 0.0047
	Baicalein	270.24	0.73	3.59 ± 0.08	0.0077 ± 0.0019
Glycoside	Naringin	580.54	0.19	0.15 ± 0.04	>20
	Rutin	610.52	0.24	0.76 ± 0.22	1.84 ± 0.04
	Baicalin	446.36	0.42	0.89 ± 0.02	5.32 ± 0.15

MW, molecular weight; log P, partition coefficient measured by n-octanol/water partitioning; log K', logarithm of $(t_r - t_0)/t_0$, t_r is the retention time of compound peak, t_0 is the retention time of solvent peak. Each value represents the mean and S.D (n = 4).

3.2. Cutaneous Absorption of Flavonoids

The cutaneous absorption of the penetrants was compared using a Franz cell assembly. Nude mouse and baby pig dorsal skins were used in this experiment due to their close similarity to human skin. The donor dose was first set at an equivalent concentration (6 mM). This dose surpassed the saturated solubility. This led to a condition of suspension in the donor except for naringin, which showed a solution type because of the extremely high solubility in the aqueous vehicle. Both flavonoid deposition within the skin and the flux across the skin were examined in this study. Dermal delivery should be addressed in the skin deposition that is carried out with the aim of cutaneous targeting with minimizing systemic absorption. Flux is a factor to use in predicting how well the penetrant will reach the systemic circulation. Figure 2A,B depicts the skin permeation profiles of flavonoids via nude mouse skin and pig skin, respectively. Both animal skins demonstrated similar trends of cutaneous absorption. Among the aglycones tested, naringenin and kaempferol showed the greatest skin deposition. Our results showed that myricetin, which had the lowest lipophilicity among the flavonoids examined, was the aglycone with the least deposition. The glycosides may be susceptible to enzymatic hydrolysis in skin tissue with aglycone release. After HPLC analysis, we found no aglycone in the skin deposition and receptor after topical application of glycosides. This indicated that the glycosides were not metabolized in this case. The skin deposition of the glycosides was minor compared to that of the corresponding aglycones.

Naringenin revealed a high cutaneous delivery not only in skin deposition but also in flux. The highest flux of aglycones was observed with naringenin, followed by baicalein. Myricetin and quercetin levels in the receptor were negligible or even below the HPLC detection limit, giving a flux of near zero. Contrary to the result with skin deposition, glycosylation generally increased the flux, except in the case of naringin diffusion across nude mouse skin. The flux of naringin and baicalin was comparable and significantly higher than that of rutin. Cutaneous targeting is a strategy for local skin prevention or therapy with reduced systemic effects. As shown in Figure 2, we calculated S value as an index of selectivity between cutaneous targeting and transdermal delivery. Kaempferol demonstrated the highest S value (2.7 and 1.5 for nude mouse skin and pig skin); Myricetin and quercetin were absorbed into the skin reservoir without reaching the receptor, leading to the infinity of S value (∞). Rutin was the compound with the highest S value (1.3 and 0.4 for nude mouse skin and pig skin, respectively) among the glycosides.

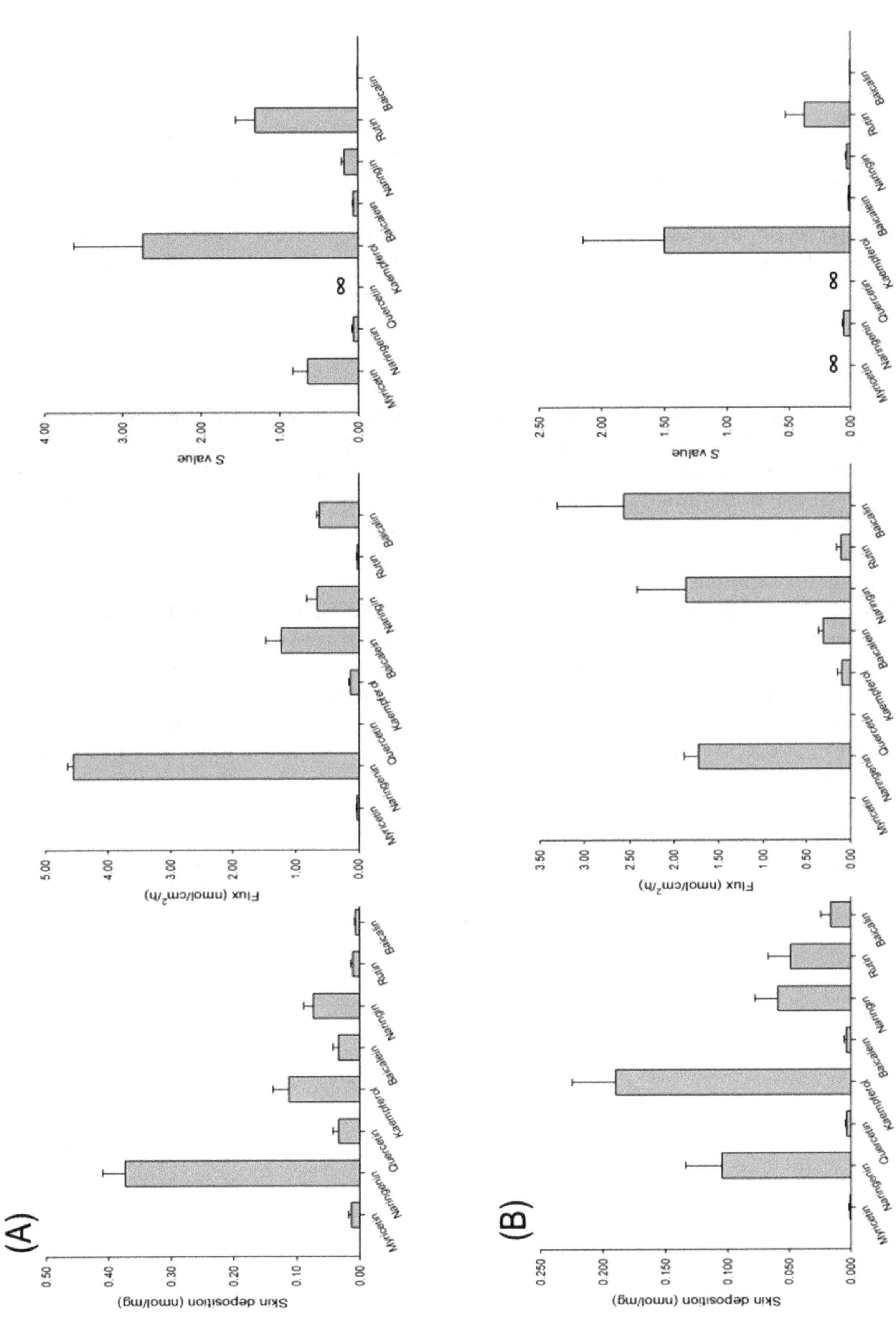

Figure 2. Skin deposition, flux, and *S* value of flavonoids at a dose of 6 mM after topical treatment on nude mouse and pig skins: **(A)** nude mouse skin; and **(B)** pig skin. The donor vehicle is 20% PEG400 in pH 7.4 buffer. All data are presented as the mean of four experiments ± S.D.

The flavonoids in the donor were also dosed with saturated solubility to achieve the maximum thermodynamic equivalents for all penetrants. Naringin was excluded in this experiment because we could not determine the saturated solubility of this compound (>20 mM). The extremely high solubility would lead to skin damage, complicating the discussion of SPR. The trend of the cutaneous absorption profiles was similar for nude mouse skin and pig skin after topical application of saturated solution, as shown in Figure 3A,B, respectively. Equivalent doses of naringenin and kaempferol showed the highest skin deposition in saturated solubility. The CSD of baicalein was below the quantification limit, which may have been due to the negligible solubility (0.0077 mM). Among the topically applied aglycones, only naringenin and baicalein could penetrate across the skin to the receptor. The neglected PC of myricetin, quercetin, and kaempferol led to the infinity of S value. The S value of baicalein was 0. The S value of baicalin was greater than that of rutin. This result was opposite to the S value of glycosides vehiculated at the equivalent dose.

3.3. *Flavonoid Permeation via SC-Disrupted Skin*

The SC is the outermost layer of the skin, consisting of the main barrier of most penetrants. Effective permeation through the SC is necessary to obtain successful skin targeting. The SC-disrupted skin was prepared to explore the possible permeation pathways of flavonoids. These included SC-stripped, delipidized, desebumed, and deproteinized nude mouse skins. The penetrants at the equimolar dose (6 mM) were used as the donor in this experiment. Figure 4A demonstrates the released percentage of flavonoids that penetrated the cellulose membrane at 24 h. The release rate was related to the penetrant escape from the vehicle. The release was a delivery stage before penetrant entrance into the SC. The glycosides showed a higher release percentage compared to the aglycones. Naringenin and kaempferol were the two penetrants with greater release than the other aglycones. Figure 4B–I summarizes the cutaneous deposition of eight flavonoids in different SC-disrupted skins. The deposition in SC-stripped skin and delipidized skin was comparable for all flavonoids tested, indicating that intercellular lipid bilayers are an important route for flavonoid transport. The removal of the SC could evoke skin deposition of myricetin and quercetin by >30 fold compared to the intact skin. Myricetin deposition in desebumed skin was 140-fold higher than that in untreated skin. The other flavonoids showed a 2–6-fold increase in skin deposition after sebum removal. The enhancement of skin deposition by protein denaturation was lower than that by lipid removal. The deproteinization process even failed to change the skin deposition of quercetin and its corresponding glycoside. The result of protein removal suggests the minor role of the intracellular route compared to the intercellular route for flavonoid diffusion across the SC.

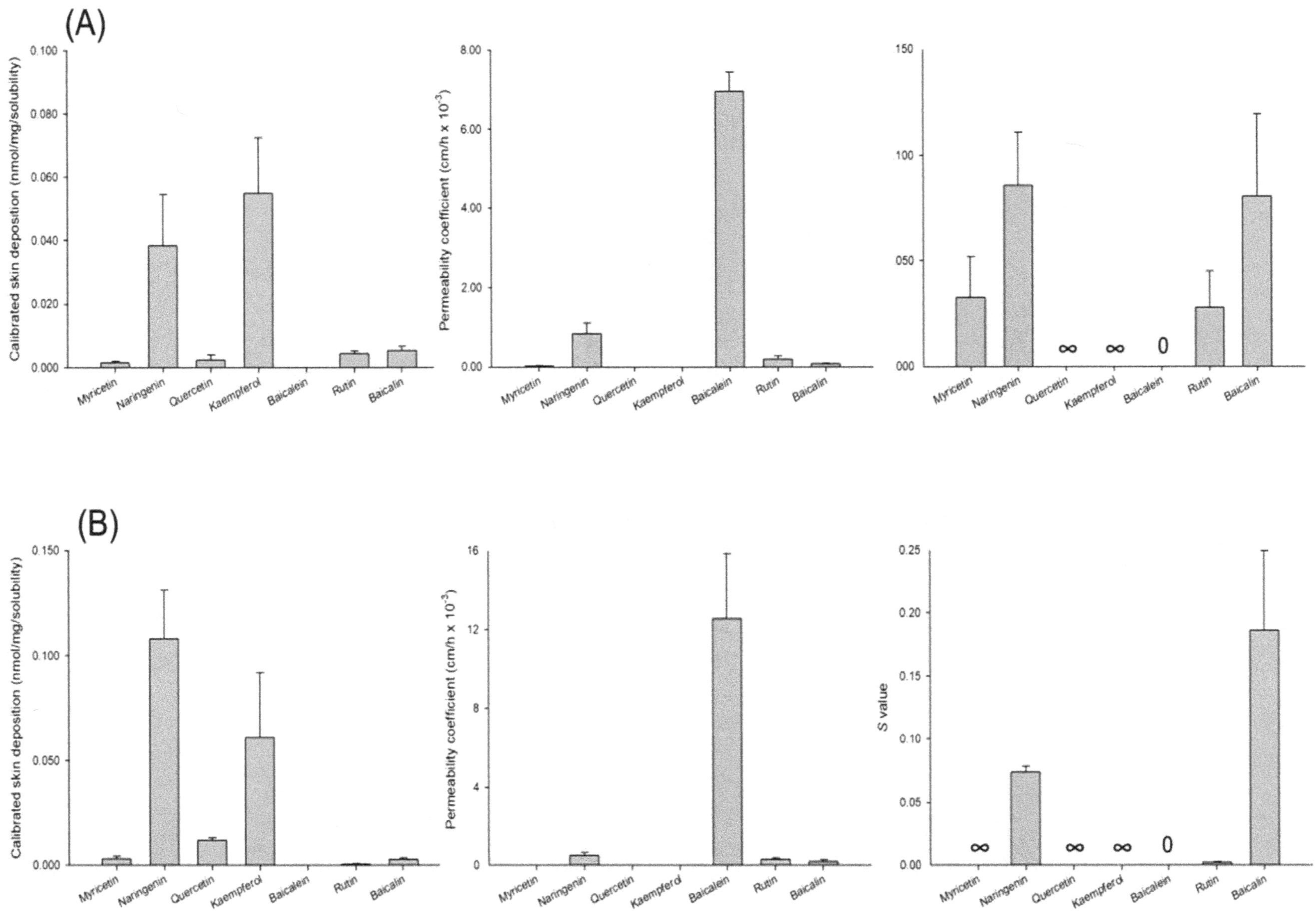

Figure 3. Calibrated skin deposition, permeability coefficient, and *S* value of flavonoids at a dose of saturated solubility after topical treatment on nude mouse and pig skins: (**A**) nude mouse skin; and (**B**) pig skin. The donor vehicle is 20% PEG400 in pH 7.4 buffer. All data are presented as the mean of four experiments ± S.D.

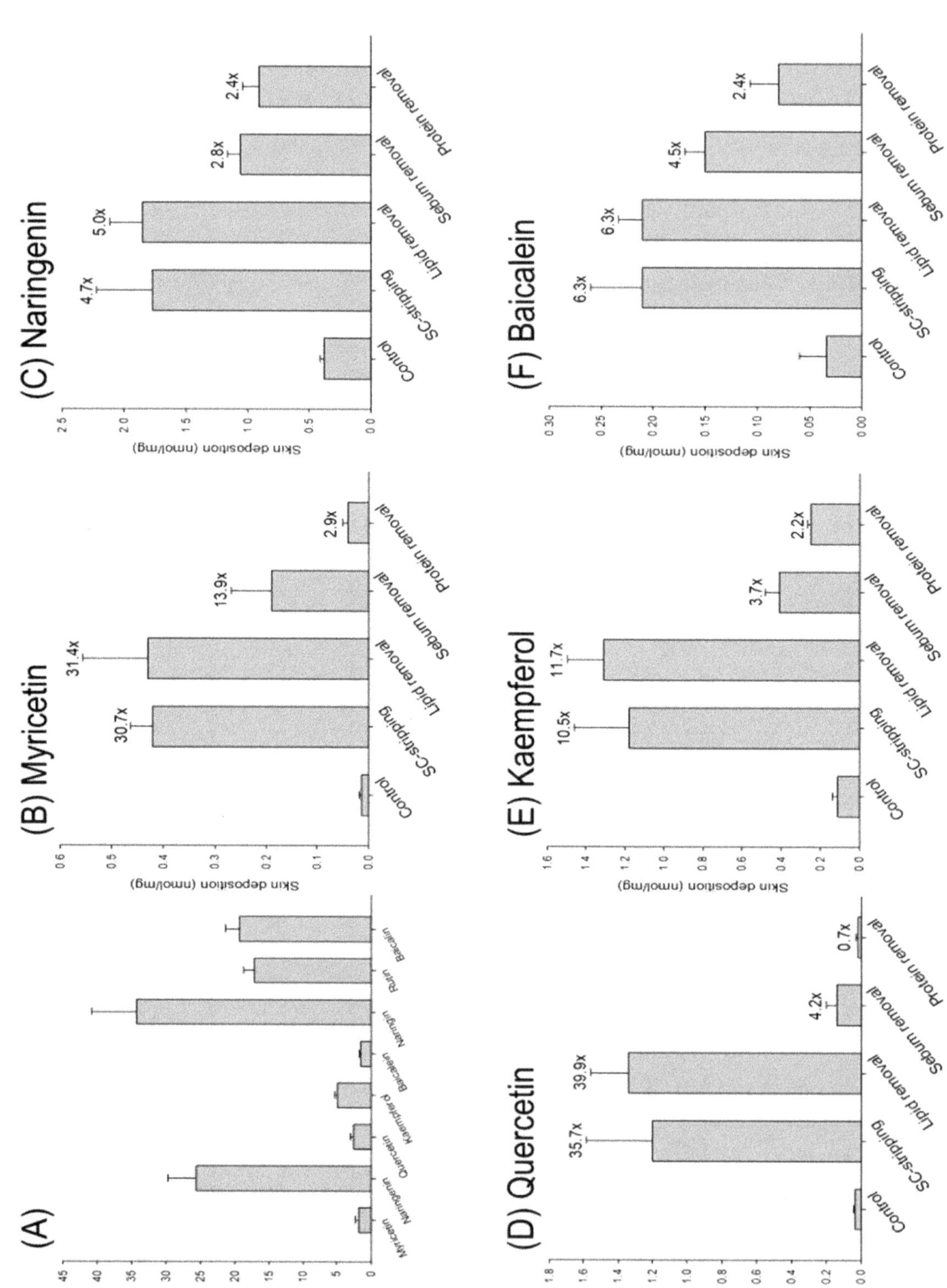

Figure 4. *Cont.*

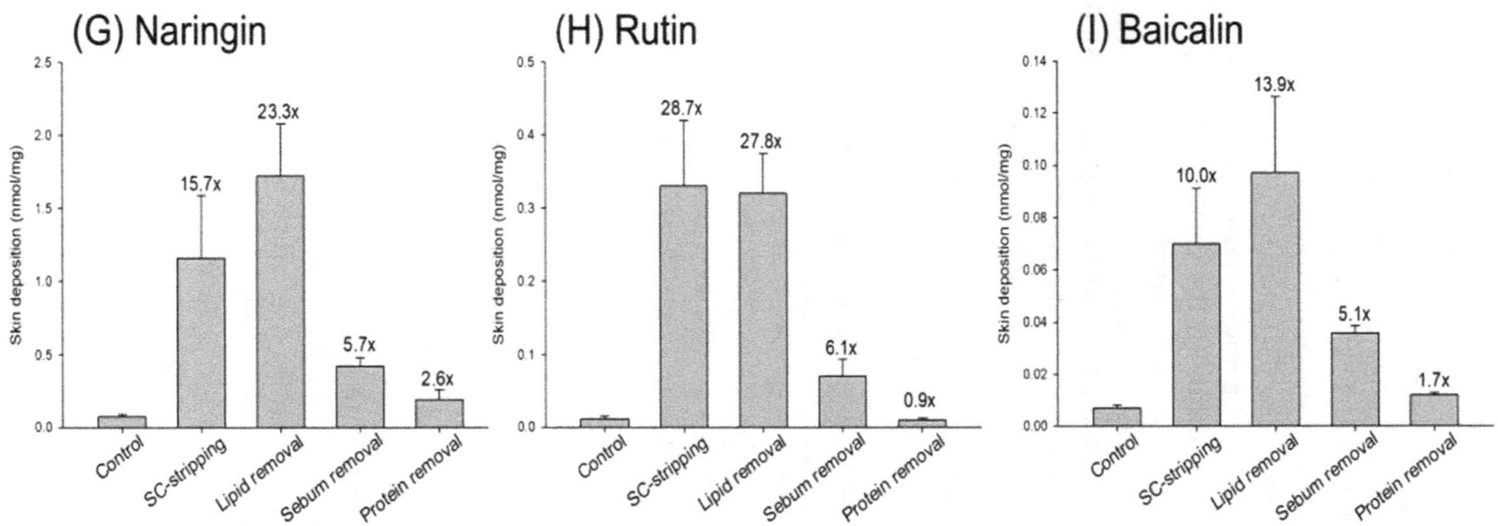

Figure 4. The released percentage and skin deposition of flavonoids (6 mM) via cellulose membrane, stratum corneum (SC)-stripped skin, delipid skin, desebum skin, and deprotein skin: (**A**) released percentage of flavonoids across cellulose membrane; (**B**) skin deposition of myricetin in SC-disrupted skins; (**C**) skin deposition of naringenin in SC-disrupted skins; (**D**) skin deposition of quercetin in SC-disrupted skins; (**E**) skin deposition of kaempferol in SC-disrupted skins; (**F**) skin deposition of baicalein in SC-disrupted skins; (**G**) skin deposition of naringin in SC-disrupted skins; (**H**) skin deposition of rutin in SC-disrupted skins; and (**I**) skin deposition of baicalin in SC-disrupted skins. All data are presented as the mean of four experiments ± S.D.

3.4. Inhibition of Neutrophil Inflammation by Flavonoids

The $O_2^{\bullet-}$ production and elastase release in stimulated neutrophils are indicators reflecting a massive neutrophil infiltration into the inflamed skin. The flavonoids were rated for the inhibition percentage of $O_2^{\bullet-}$ and elastase in response to fMLF, as shown in Table 2. Incubation of fMLF-activated neutrophils in the presence of flavonoids resulted in an inhibition on superoxide anion, with baicalein and baicalin exhibiting the greatest activity (77% and 76%). The $O_2^{\bullet-}$ inhibition effect was comparable for the aglycones and the corresponding glycosides. The flavonoids generated less inhibition on elastase than superoxide. Quercetin was among the most potent flavonoids to repress elastase (29%). The elastase inhibition ranged between 10% and 20% for most of the flavonoids. The glycosides had a lower effect on elastase inhibition than the corresponding aglycones. Baicalin did not change the elastase release of fMLF-stimulated neutrophils. To estimate the possible bioactivity after topical delivery, we calculated TI based on multiplying the nude mouse skin deposition and the inflammatory inhibition percentage as shown in Table 2. Although the $O_2^{\bullet-}$ inhibition of naringenin was weak, this flavanone showed the highest TI because of the preferred delivery into the skin reservoir. The potent activity of baicalein on $O_2^{\bullet-}$ inhibition had led to a TI of 2.60, which approximated the TI level of kaempferol. The compound with the highest TI for elastase inhibition was also found to be naringenin, followed by kaempferol. Naringin was the penetrant with a higher TI than the other glycosides. Naringin demonstrated less TI value compared to naringenin.

Table 2. The inhibition percentage (%) of superoxide anion ($O_2^{\bullet-}$) and elastase and the therapeutic index (TI) of aglycone and glycoside flavonoids at 3 μM.

Category	Compound	$O_2^{\bullet-}$ Inhibition	$TI_{superoxide}$	Elastase Inhibition	$TI_{elastase}$
Aglycone	Myricetin	42.07 ± 6.22	0.58	16.81 ± 4.76	0.23
	Naringenin	19.72 ± 8.23	7.36	17.97 ± 6.62	6.71
	Quercetin	26.44 ± 8.07	0.89	28.67 ± 8.51	0.96
	Kaempferol	26.49 ± 8.41	2.97	18.11 ± 9.01	2.03
	Baicalein	77.48 ± 5.27	2.60	12.25 ± 2.15	0.41
Glycoside	Naringin	21.51 ± 2.53	1.59	13.89 ± 9.67	1.02
	Rutin	33.87 ± 8.67	0.39	13.16 ± 3.39	0.15
	Baicalin	75.73 ± 6.21	0.53	0	0

TI is calculated by the multiplication of inhibition percentage at 3 μM and nude mouse skin deposition at equivalent dose (6 mM). Each value represents the mean and S.D (n = 3).

3.5. Molecular Modeling

The informative explanation of the effect of molecular structure on cutaneous delivery is based on the hydrogen bond number, the total polarity surface, and the molecular volume. The parameters for flavonoids are computed by Discovery Studio® 4.1 as presented in Table 3. The number of hydrogen bond acceptors and donors increased following the increase of hydroxyl groups in the structure. The hydrogen bond number of glycosides was much higher than that of aglycones due to the presence of hydroxyl moieties in the sugar. Rutin exhibited the highest hydrogen bond numbers among all flavonoids examined. The total polarity surface correlated well with the hydrogen bond number, with the glycosides showing a greater polarity surface than aglycones. This indicates more polar interactions of the glycosides in aqueous medium. The molecular volume is a reflection of MW. We found a high positive correlation between molecular volume and MW (correlation coefficient = 0.9979).

To study the cutaneous transport characteristics of the flavonoids in greater detail, we applied computational molecular docking to analyze the possible interaction of the penetrants to SC lipids. The three-dimensional lipid model was generated for their posterior use as the target structure in the in silico calculation. Table 4 summarizes the best docking score (negative CDOCKER) of the flavonoids interacting with SC lipids, including ceramides II, III, and VI, palmitic acid, cholesteryl sulfate, and cholesterol. The flavonoids were docked into conformationally minimized SC lipids. The cooperativity of the interaction included van der Waals, hydrogen bonding, and lipophilic and electrostatic forces. The greater negative energy dictated a stronger binding interaction. The glycosides revealed greater interaction to ceramides than aglycones, with rutin showing the highest interaction. The discrepancy of the negative CDOCKER between ceramides and different aglycones was not large (−24 to −18).

Table 3. The hydrogen bond number, total polarity surface and molecular volume of aglycone and glycoside flavonoids determined by molecular modeling.

Category	Compound	Hydrogen Bond Acceptor Number	Hydrogen Bond Donor Number	Total Polarity Surface	Molecular Volume
Aglycone	Myricetin	8	6	147.68	225.35
	Naringenin	5	3	86.99	204.42
	Quercetin	7	5	127.45	217.11
	Kaempferol	6	4	107.22	203.74
	Baicalein	5	3	86.99	195.85
Glycoside	Naringin	14	8	225.05	437.66
	Rutin	16	10	265.52	444.18
	Baicalin	11	6	183.21	316.93

Table 4. The negative CDOCKER energy of aglycone and glycoside flavonoids to interact with the stratum corneum components determined by molecular modeling.

Compound	Ceramide II	Ceramide III	Ceramide VI	Palmitic Acid	Cholesteryl Sulfate	Cholesterol
Myricetin	−19.454	−25.852	−22.285	−19.048	−117.792	-
Naringenin	−19.143	−25.670	−24.231	−18.155	−121.188	-
Quercetin	−18.928	−21.850	−22.063	−18.032	−118.533	-
Kaempferol	−21.053	−20.831	−19.639	−17.399	−119.485	-
Baicalein	−18.841	−20.637	−20.427	−18.073	−118.632	-
Naringin	−27.144	−28.937	−37.266	−17.326	−109.196	-
Rutin	−33.007	−35.341	−38.940	−23.502	−109.365	−47.1637
Baicalin	−24.573	−30.721	−28.555	−19.751	−112.425	−53.8485

- Means no interaction.

Rutin showed the highest negative CDOCKER level with palmitic acid among the flavonoids detected. A relatively higher negative CDOCKER energy was found for cholesteryl sulfate than for the other lipids. It appears that the flavonoids preferentially interacted with cholesteryl sulfate. In the case of cholesteryl sulfate, the negative CDOCKER of aglycones was higher compared to the corresponding glycosides. Naringenin (−121) and kaempferol (−119) exhibited a more potent interaction with cholesteryl sulfate than the other penetrants. No interaction was detected between cholesterol and the compounds except with rutin and baicalin. Figure 5 illustrates the best docking poses of the flavonoids interacting with cholesteryl sulfate. The flavonoids displayed the ligand binding activity to cholesteryl sulfate but in different conformations.

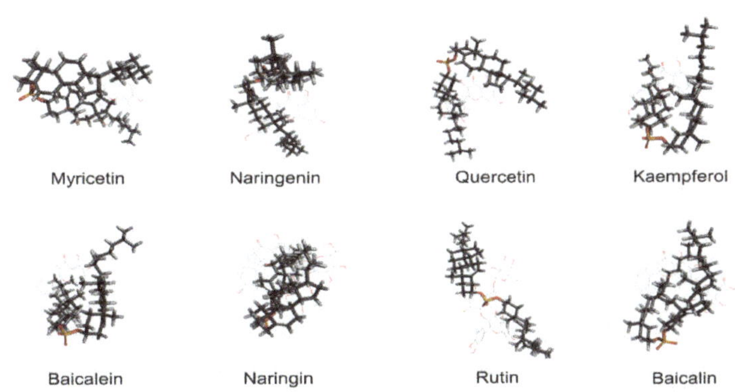

Figure 5. Superimposition of the computed poses for flavonoids with cholesteryl sulfate.

3.6. *In Vivo Cutaneous Tolerance of Flavonoids*

The tolerance at the equivalent dose to the skin was determined by in vivo topical exposure for seven days. We examined ΔTEWL, as shown in Figure 6A. ΔTEWL was calculated by the TEWL value of the treated skin area minus the value of the aqueous vehicle control. Most of the flavonoids exhibited a near-zero point ΔTEWL profile. This suggests that these compounds did not induce a barrier defect of SC. Naringenin and kaempferol even reduced TEWL as compared to the vehicle control. This may imply a protective capability of both compounds on barrier function. Figure 6B–K reveals the histology of flavonoid-treated skin after a seven-day administration. We could see a decrease in the SC layers of the vehicle control compared to the sham group (Figure 6B versus Figure 6C), indicating an interruption of barrier position. The SC layers could be recovered through the application of naringenin, kaempferol, and naringin. The flavonoid treatment did not alter the viable skin morphology, expressing a negligible irritation.

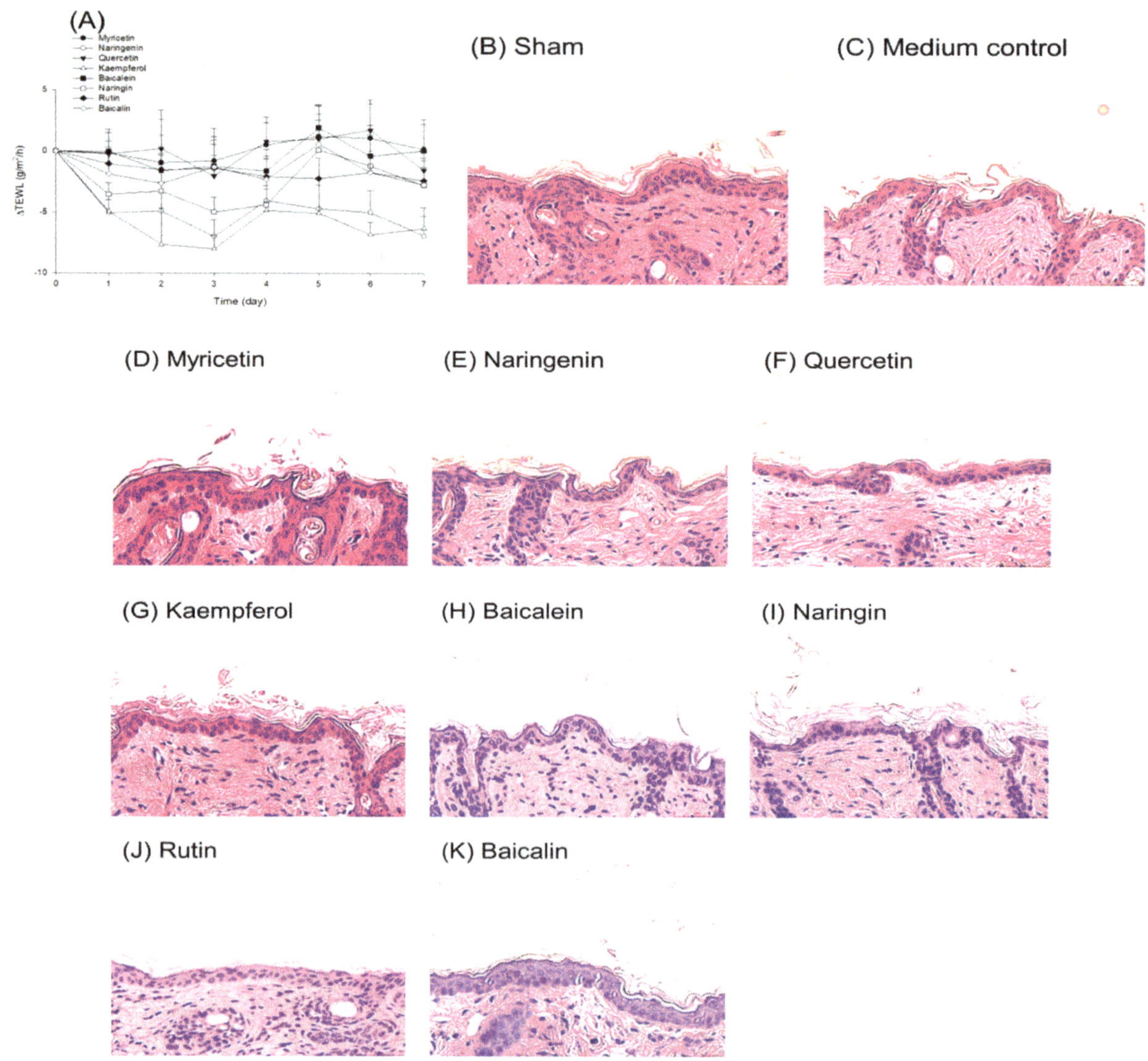

Figure 6. The in vivo safety of topically applied flavonoids on skin after a 7-day exposure: (**A**) ΔTEWL-time curves; (**B**) the histology of sham control skin; (**C**) the histology of aqueous medium-treated skin; (**D**) the histology of myricetin-treated skin; (**E**) the histology of naringenin-treated skin; (**F**) the histology of quercetin-treated skin; (**G**) the histology of kaempferol-treated skin; (**H**) the histology of baicalein-treated skin; (**I**) the histology of naringin-treated skin; (**J**) the histology of rutin-treated skin; and (**K**) the histology of baicalin-treated skin. The TEWL data are presented as the mean of six experiments ± S.D.

4. Discussion

Sustained inflammation contributes to the pathogenesis of some skin disorders, including photoaging, psoriasis, and atopic dermatitis. Flavonoids exert potent anti-inflammatory effects on the skin. Nevertheless, whether the cutaneous absorption of flavonoids is sufficient to trigger the bioactivity is questionable. An ideal topical administration has a much higher absorption accomplished in the cutaneous reservoir compared to that in the systemic circulation to achieve efficient targeting and escape systemic toxicity [14]. We examined the skin delivery and anti-inflammatory activity of aglycone and glycoside flavonoids to select the potential candidates for topical application with the aim of prevention or therapy. The aqueous vehicle was used as the flavonoid donor since most attempts for modeling SPR had been based on the data of aqueous solution application [15]. Naringenin and kaempferol were efficacious for topical application with respect to targeting into the skin and possible treatment capability based on the data of *S* value and TI, respectively. The cutaneous permeation of flavonoids exhibited a similar trend either at an equivalent dose or at the saturated solubility. Both aglycones also produced a protective effect on skin-barrier function. The glycosides generally showed lower absorption than the corresponding aglycones. Previous study [16] also suggests a low skin bioavailability of flavonoid glycosides such as baicalin.

The physicochemical properties of flavonoids from the experimental data and molecular modeling prediction were beneficial to discussing the SPR. The aglycone lipophilicity was decreased following the increase of the hydroxyl group number. An exception was naringenin, which had only 3 hydroxyl groups but low lipophilicity. Different from the flavonols and flavones, naringenin is a flavanone with fewer double bonds in the C ring. The flavonols were more lipophilic and assumed a planar structure [17]. The flexibility of the chiral center in the C ring of naringenin could fold to form a three-dimensional structure. The approximation of the B ring to the A and C rings increased the possibility of the production of intramolecular hydrogen bonds, leading to the decrease of lipophilicity and enhancement of aqueous solubility. This effect did not occur with flavonols and flavones due to the rigidity of the structure.

Some physicochemical factors of penetrants can influence the skin permeation. These include lipophilicity, solubility, release rate, MW, and hydrogen bonding. The penetrants with higher lipophilicity can increase the skin-absorption capacity due to the facile partitioning and entrance into the SC lipids [18]. Both log K' and log P are the parameters of lipophilicity. Another parameter for anticipating the skin absorption is the total polarity surface, which correlates inversely with lipophilicity and biomembrane absorption [19]. The correlation coefficient between log P and the total polarity surface for the flavonoids was 0.9003. The polar surface area is defined as the total sum of the surface of the polar atoms [20]. The highest total polarity surface of myricetin could explain the low skin absorption of this compound. However, the lipophilicity could not explain the high skin deposition of naringenin and kaempferol. There was no correlation between lipophilicity and skin absorption of the flavonoids. The penetrants should first partition into the SC before diffusion across the SC. The sebum spread on the SC surface contributes to a capacity-governing penetrant partitioning from the vehicle to the SC [21]. Theoretically, this partitioning is highly dependent on the lipophilicity [22]. Our results showed that the skin deposition enhancement after sebum removal was less for naringenin and kaempferol than for the other flavonoids. This suggests an ease in the partitioning of naringenin and kaempferol to the SC layer, and sebum was a barrier for the permeation of the other flavonoids. From these data, it can be concluded that the cutaneous absorption of flavonoids cannot be solely ascribed to their lipophilicity. The skin more facilely absorbed the flavonoids with moderate hydrophilicity and aqueous solubility.

Although a lipophilic nature is required for transport across the SC, a hydrophilic property is also needed for entry into the viable skin [23]. The penetrants with the log $P > 3$ show a decrease of viable-skin diffusion following the increase of lipophilicity [24]. Both the SC and the viable epidermis/dermis are the permeation barriers. The role of viable skin in flavonoid absorption could be understood by the permeation via SC-stripped skin. Myricetin and quercetin were the flavonoids with low skin absorption. The SC removal largely promoted the deposition of both flavonoids by >30 fold. This indicates a significant barrier function of the SC for the two penetrants. The skin deposition of myricetin and quercetin was 0.4 and 1.2 nM/mg after the SC's removal, respectively. This value was still lower than the naringenin deposition after stripping. Baicalein was a lipophilic flavonoid with facile entrance into the SC because of the limited enhancement of skin deposition after stripping. However, the baicalein deposition in the stripped skin was only 0.2 nM/mg. These results demonstrate that the viable skin could be a barrier to the flavonoid permeation. The cellulose membrane is like viable skin due to its hydrophilic property. We found that the released percentage across the cellulose membrane was lower for myricetin, quercetin, and baicalein than for naringenin and kaempferol, confirming the diffusion barrier of viable skin. Naringenin and kaempferol could conquer the viable-skin barrier, resulting in the effortless absorption. The much higher aqueous solubility of naringenin compared to the other penetrants was the reason for the easy diffusion into the viable skin. Although kaempferol exerted a comparable lipophilicity to baicalein, the considerable solubility of kaempferol had led to greater absorption than with baicalein. Because of the existence of sugar moiety, the glycoside flavonoids had good solubility in the aqueous vehicle. Although the glycosides might easily permeate into viable skin according to the high percentage of release, the absorption of glycosides was less compared to that of the aglycones. The SC was the main barrier to retard glycoside delivery since SC removal could greatly enhance their deposition.

The SC layer contains lipids and corneocytes cross-linked by keratin. The SC lipids and keratin contribute to the nonpolar and polar pathways for permeation. Similar absorption should be observed for the permeation into SC-stripped skin and delipidized skin if the penetrants predominantly transport via the nonpolar route [25]. Our data supported the lipid pathway being the main diffusion mechanism for the flavonoids. Although proteins occupy 80% of the SC constituents, the polar pathway is not the major route for flavonoids because of the limited skin deposition enhancement after protein denaturation. A high affinity of the penetrants to the SC lipids can generate a reservoir in the skin for plentiful absorption [26]. To obtain detailed information on the absorption of flavonoids, we established the possible flavonoid-lipid interaction employing molecular docking. The lipid content of the SC basically comprises ceramides, fatty acids, cholesteryl sulfate, and cholesterol [27]. There are nine classes of ceramide identified in the SC [28]. We chose ceramides II, III, and VI for docking because of their abundance in human SC [29]. Palmitic acid was used as the model fatty acid. Cholesteryl sulfate presented much stronger interaction with the flavonoids than the other SC lipids. Naringenin and kaempferol showed the highest negative CDOCKER for interacting with cholesteryl sulfate. This result coincided with the highest skin deposition of both compounds. The correlation coefficient between nude mouse skin deposition and CDOCKER of aglycones was 0.9673. The negative CDOCKER of glycosides was inferior to that of aglycones with respect to interacting with cholesteryl sulfate. A contrary result was detected for the other lipids. The aglycones even showed no interaction with cholesterol. Thus, cholesteryl sulfate could offer the most suitable flavonoid-lipid interaction for predicting flavonoid absorption. The CDOCKER of other lipids such as ceramides are infeasible to be the indicator of flavonoid absorption because of the low correlation between the energy and skin deposition. For example, rutin had the highest negative CDOCKER with ceramides and fatty acid but a low skin delivery capability.

The hydrogen bond acceptor is another factor that inversely correlates with cutaneous absorption. Since the SC is the hydrogen bond acceptor [30], an increase in the number of hydrogen bonds reduces the permeation across the SC [31]. Myricetin is the compound with a higher hydrogen bond acceptor number than the other aglycones. The hydrogen bond acceptor number of glycosides was much higher than that of aglycones. Myricetin and glycosides were inferred to have less interaction with the SC according to hydrogen bonding and cholesteryl sulfate docking. Molecular size rather than lipophilicity would impact skin absorption if less interaction was detected between the penetrants and the SC components [32]. The skin diffusion is size-dependent, with the larger penetrants demonstrating lower skin delivery. Both MW and molecular volume illustrated a larger size of myricetin and glycoside structures. The consequence was the low absorption of these compounds. The molecules partially associated with the solvent cage when they traversed the skin from the aqueous vehicle. The permeation rate involved not only the molecule itself but also the entire solvated complex [33]. Myricetin and the glycosides with a higher hydrogen bond number might attract more water molecules to produce a large solvation complex, causing a detrimental effect on skin transport. Although the MW and molecular volume of naringenin were not the lowest, the folding character of this flavanone might generate a smaller size than the flavonols and flavones with a planar structure. The small molecular size after bending favored the diffusion into the skin reservoir.

The aim of topically applied flavonoids was to offer better targeting to the skin with minimal systemic absorption. The *S* value is a parameter for judging the skin-targeting efficacy. With respect to aglycones, naringenin and kaempferol showed efficient targeting to the skin tissue. The high *S* value of myricetin and quercetin was due to there being no or negligible flux. The low cutaneous deposition of myricetin and quercetin might not elicit significant bioactivity on the skin. Rutin presented a high *S* value in the case of the equivalent dose, which could favor the cutaneous efficacy. In the case of a saturated dose, baicalin had the highest *S* value among the glycosides. As with myricetin, the low deposition has limited the topical application of glycosides for therapeutic use.

Neutrophils act as the predominant phagocytic cells for the first line of defense. Although the activation of neutrophils enhances immunity to retard xenobiotic invasion, the overwhelming stimulation contributes to inflammatory disorders and adaptive immune responses [34]. Chronic inflammatory skin diseases such as psoriasis and photoaging can be characterized by neutrophil infiltration [35]. The activated neutrophils damage the skin by the production of reactive oxygen species (ROS). A respiratory burst of neutrophils is an oxygen-dependent process leading to the formation of ROS. The protective effect of flavonoids on the skin is directly linked to the antiradical potency [7]. Our results revealed a flavonoid-driven mitigation of $O_2^{\bullet-}$ in fMLF-stimulated neutrophils. The $O_2^{\bullet-}$ inhibition was the highest for baicalein. Although baicalein reduced $O_2^{\bullet-}$ more effectively, it only exerted moderate TI due to the low efficiency of cutaneous absorption. The lowest superoxide inhibition was found for naringenin. However, this flavanone still exhibited the highest TI because of the efficacious skin targeting. The intramolecular hydrogen bond can suppress antioxidant activity [36]. This is the reason for the low $O_2^{\bullet-}$ inhibition by the flavanone.

The number of hydroxyl groups in the structure of the antioxidants is a factor influencing the antiradical effect, with the presence of more hydroxyl groups resulting in stronger activity [37]. This was not the case in our study since no correlation was observed between the hydroxyl moiety number and the scavenging capacity. The $O_2^{\bullet-}$ inhibition of glycosides was similar to their corresponding aglycones. The lower skin deposition of glycosides had resulted in the lower TI of $O_2^{\bullet-}$ compared to the aglycones. Both neutrophil trafficking and elastase release are elevated in skin photoaging. Elastase plays a role in wrinkling after photoaging [38]. The experimental data provided evidence that the flavonoids showed less inhibition on elastase than $O_2^{\bullet-}$. The glycosylation decreased the inhibitory activity on elastase. The same as $O_2^{\bullet-}$, the greatest TI of elastase proved to be topically applied naringenin.

The ΔTEWL data demonstrated that the flavonoids did not damage the skin barrier as compared to the aqueous vehicle control. No SC disruption was observed for naringenin and kaempferol, though the skin deposition was very high. It is surprising that naringenin and kaempferol even alleviated ΔTEWL. Water contact with the SC in high content can disturb the barrier's nature [39]. The aqueous vehicle used in this study could increase TEWL. The skin histology demonstrated fewer SC layers of the aqueous medium control than the sham group. Naringenin and kaempferol with high cutaneous absorption might protect the skin to reduce the impairment generated by the water. Further work is needed to elucidate the protection mechanism. Naringenin, extensively contained in lemons, oranges, and grapes, is reported to be a potent active of attenuating skin inflammation and oncogenesis [4,40]. Kaempferol has been demonstrated to restrain photoaging and UV-induced carcinogenesis [41]. The synthetic drugs such as indomethacin and celecoxib provide protection against photoaging and skin cancers but have severe adverse effects. Topically applied naringenin and kaempferol can be promising candidates as alternatives for skin-inflammation treatment.

5. Conclusions

This study examined the cutaneous absorption and anti-inflammatory activity of flavonoids with the goal of choosing the optimal candidates for topical delivery. The results revealed that the glycosides showed less absorption and targeting than the aglycones. The low lipophilicity and large molecular size of glycosides contributed to the unsatisfied absorption. Naringenin and kaempferol were the compounds with the greatest deposition in the skin. They also protected the skin from the barrier disruption induced by the aqueous medium. Both flavonoids are potential candidates for topical application to treat skin inflammation. Both the SC and viable skin were the permeation barriers for flavonoid transport. The SPR demonstrated the importance of the hydrophilic and lipophilic balance of the flavonoid structure in order to achieve feasible skin delivery. The hydrogen bond acceptor and docking calculated from molecular modeling described the cutaneous absorption trend. We had utilized the aqueous vehicle as the flavonoid formulation. It is expected that the different compositions of vehicle may largely affect the skin permeation of the penetrants. The flavonoids may exhibit different permeation trend in other vehicles such as oil and nanoparticles. Further study is needed to elucidate the impact of different vehicles on flavonoid absorption. Our results offer essential information for the development of a topically applied flavonoid formulation. The experimental profiles in this study also provide the direction to design or synthesize new compounds for facilitating skin delivery.

Acknowledgments: The authors are grateful to the financial support by Ministry of Science and Technology of Taiwan (MOST-105-2320-B-182-010-MY3) and Chang Gung Memorial Hospital (CMRPG2F0491-3).

Author Contributions: S.-Y.C. and J.-Y.F. conceived the topic. S.-Y.C., Y.-K.L. and E.-L.C. performed the experimental works. Y.-K.L. outlined the paper and mainly wrote it. P.-W.W. and J.-Y.F. contributed to the drafting of the manuscript.

References

1. Petrou, A.L.; Terzidaki, A. A meta-analysis and review examining a possible role for oxidative stress and singlet oxygen in diverse diseases. *Biochem. J.* **2017**, *474*, 2713–2731. [CrossRef] [PubMed]
2. Rinnerthaler, M.; Bischof, J.; Streubel, M.K.; Trost, A.; Richter, K. Oxidative stress in aging human skin. *Biomolecules* **2015**, *5*, 545–589. [CrossRef] [PubMed]
3. Ascenso, A.; Ribeiro, H.M.; Marques, H.C.; Simões, S. Topical delivery of antioxidants. *Curr. Drug Deliv.* **2011**, *8*, 640–660. [CrossRef] [PubMed]
4. George, V.C.; Vijesh, V.V.; Amararathna, D.I.M.; Lakshmi, C.A.; Anbarasu, K.; Kumar, D.R.N.; Ethiraj, K.R.; Kumar, R.A.; Rupasinghe, H.P.V. Mechanism of action of flavonoids in prevention of inflammation-associated skin cancer. *Curr. Med. Chem.* **2016**, *23*, 1–20.
5. Shen, C.Y.; Jiang, J.G.; Yang, L.; Wang, D.W.; Zhu, W. Anti-ageing active ingredients from herbs and nutraceuticals used in traditional Chinese medicine: Pharmacological mechanisms and implications for drug discovery. *Br. J. Pharmacol.* **2017**, *174*, 1395–1425. [CrossRef] [PubMed]
6. Abd, E.; Roberts, M.S.; Grice, J.E. A comparison of the penetration and permeation of caffeine into and through human epidermis after application in various vesicle formulations. *Skin Pharmacol. Physiol.* **2016**, *29*, 24–30. [CrossRef] [PubMed]
7. Arct, J.; Pytkowska, K. Flavonoids as components of biologically active cosmeceuticals. *Clin. Dermatol.* **2008**, *26*, 347–357. [CrossRef] [PubMed]
8. Zhou, B.R.; Liu, W.L.; Luo, D. Protective effect of baicalin against multiple ultraviolet b exposure-mediated injuries in C57BL/6 mouse skin. *Arch. Pharm. Res.* **2011**, *34*, 261–268. [CrossRef] [PubMed]
9. Dayan, N. Pathways for skin penetration. *Cosmet. Toilet.* **2005**, *120*, 67–76.

10. Liu, K.S.; Chen, Y.W.; Aljuffali, I.A.; Chang, C.W.; Wang, J.J.; Fang, J.Y. Topically applied mesoridazine exhibits the strongest cutaneous analgesia and minimized skin disruption among tricyclic antidepressants: The skin absorption assessment. *Eur. J. Pharm. Biopharm.* **2016**, *105*, 59–68. [CrossRef] [PubMed]
11. Campbell, C.S.J.; Contreras-Rojas, L.R.; Delgado-Charro, M.B.; Guy, R.H. Objective assessment of nanoparticle disposition in mammalian skin after topical exposure. *J. Control. Release* **2012**, *162*, 201–207. [CrossRef] [PubMed]
12. Boyum, A.; Lovhaug, D.; Tresland, L.; Nordlie, E.M. Separation of leucocytes: Improved cell purity by fine adjustments of gradient medium density and osmolality. *Scand. J. Immunol.* **1991**, *34*, 697–712. [CrossRef] [PubMed]
13. Yang, S.C.; Chung, P.J.; Ho, C.M.; Kuo, C.Y.; Hung, M.F.; Huang, Y.T.; Chang, W.Y.; Chang, Y.W.; Chan, K.H.; Hwang, T.L.; et al. Propofol inhibits superoxide production, elastase release, and chemotaxis in formyl peptide-activated human neutrophils by blocking formyl peptide receptor 1. *J. Immunol.* **2013**, *190*, 6511–6519. [CrossRef] [PubMed]
14. Sawamura, R.; Sakurai, H.; Wada, N.; Nishiya, Y.; Honda, T.; Kazui, M.; Kurihara, A.; Shinagawa, A.; Izumi, T. Bioactivation of loxoprofen to a pharmacologically active metabolite and its disposition kinetics in human skin. *Biopharm. Drug Dispos.* **2015**, *36*, 352–363. [CrossRef] [PubMed]
15. Riviere, J.E.; Brooks, J.D. Predicting skin permeability from complex chemical mixtures: Dependency of quantitative structure permeation relationships on biology of skin model used. *Toxicol. Sci.* **2011**, *119*, 224–232. [CrossRef] [PubMed]
16. Mir-Palomo, S.; Nácher, A.; Díez-Sales, O.; Busó, O.V.; Caddeo, C.; Manca, M.L.; Manconi, M.; Fadda, A.M.; Saurí, A.R. Inhibition of skin inflammation by baicalin ultradeformable vesicles. *Int. J. Pharm.* **2016**, *511*, 23–29. [CrossRef] [PubMed]
17. Lin, C.F.; Leu, Y.L.; Al-Suwayeh, S.A.; Ku, M.C.; Hwang, T.L.; Fang, J.Y. Anti-inflammatory activity and percutaneous absorption of quercetin and its polymethoxylated compound and glycosides: The relationships to chemical structures. *Eur. J. Pharm. Sci.* **2012**, *47*, 857–864. [CrossRef] [PubMed]
18. Lin, C.F.; Hung, C.F.; Aljuffali, I.A.; Huang, Y.L.; Liao, W.C.; Fang, J.Y. Methylation and esterification of magnolol for ameliorating cutaneous targeting and therapeutic index by topical application. *Pharm. Res.* **2016**, *33*, 2152–2167. [CrossRef] [PubMed]
19. Schaftenaar, G.; De Vlieg, J. Quantum mechanical polar surface area. *J. Comput. Aided Mol. Des.* **2012**, *26*, 311–318. [CrossRef] [PubMed]
20. Ertl, P.; Rohde, B.; Selzer, P. Fast calculation of molecular polar surface area as a sum of fragment-based contributions and its application to the prediction of drug transport properties. *J. Med. Chem.* **2000**, *43*, 3714–3717. [CrossRef] [PubMed]
21. Liu, K.S.; Hsieh, P.W.; Aljuffali, I.A.; Lin, Y.K.; Chang, S.H.; Wang, J.J.; Fang, J.Y. Impact of ester promoieties on transdermal delivery of ketorolac. *J. Pharm. Sci.* **2014**, *103*, 974–986. [CrossRef] [PubMed]
22. Liu, X.; Testa, B.; Fahr, A. Lipophilicity and its relationship with passive drug permeation. *Pharm. Res.* **2011**, *28*, 962–977. [CrossRef] [PubMed]
23. Song, K.; An, S.M.; Kim, M.; Koh, J.S.; Boo, Y.C. Comparison of the antimelanogenic effects of *p*-coumaric acid and its methyl ester and their skin permeabilities. *J. Dermatol. Sci.* **2011**, *63*, 17–22. [CrossRef] [PubMed]
24. Schneider, M.; Stracke, F.; Hansen, S.; Schaefer, U.F. Nanoparticles and their interactions with the dermal barrier. *Dermatoendocrinology* **2009**, *1*, 197–206. [CrossRef]
25. Yan, Y.D.; Sung, J.H.; Lee, D.W.; Kim, J.S.; Jeon, E.M.; Kim, D.D.; Kin, D.W.; Kim, J.O.; Piao, M.G.; Li, D.X.; et al. Evaluation of physicochemical properties, skin permeation and accumulation profiles of salicylic acid amide prodrugs as sunscreen agent. *Int. J. Pharm.* **2011**, *419*, 154–160. [CrossRef] [PubMed]
26. Pierre, M.B.R.; Lopez, R.F.V.; Bentley, M.V.L.B. Influence of ceramide 2 on in vitro skin permeation and retention of 5-ALA and its ester derivatives, for photodynamic therapy. *Braz. J. Pharm. Sci.* **2009**, *45*, 109–116. [CrossRef]
27. Mojumdar, E.H.; Gooris, G.S.; Barlow, D.J.; Lawrence, M.J.; Deme, B.; Bouwstra, J.A. Skin lipids: Localization of ceramide and fatty acid in the unit cell of the long periodicity phase. *Biophys. J.* **2015**, *108*, 2670–2679. [CrossRef] [PubMed]
28. Kessner, D.; Ruettinger, A.; Kiselev, M.A.; Wartewig, S.; Neubert, R.H.H. Properties of ceramides and their impact on the stratum corneum structure: A review. *Skin Pharmacol. Physiol.* **2008**, *21*, 58–74. [CrossRef] [PubMed]

29. Paige, D.G.; Morse-Fisher, N.; Harper, J.I. Quantification of stratum corneum ceramides and lipid envelope ceramides in the hereditary ichthyoses. *Br. J. Dermatol.* **1994**, *131*, 23–27. [CrossRef] [PubMed]
30. N'Da, D.D. Prodrug strategies for enhancing the percutaneous absorption of drugs. *Molecules* **2014**, *19*, 20780–20787. [CrossRef] [PubMed]
31. Alikhan, A.; Farahmand, S.; Maibach, H.I. Correlating percutaneous absorption with physicochemical parameters in vivo in man: Agricultural, steroid, and other organic compounds. *J. Appl. Toxicol.* **2009**, *29*, 590–596. [CrossRef] [PubMed]
32. Yamaguchi, K.; Mitsui, T.; Aso, Y.; Sugibayashi, K. Structure–permeability relationship analysis of the permeation barrier properties of the stratum corneum and viable epidermis/dermis of rat skin. *J. Pharm. Sci.* **2008**, *97*, 4391–4403. [CrossRef] [PubMed]
33. Mohammed, D.; Matts, P.J.; Hadgraft, J.; Lane, M.E. In vitro–in vivo correlation in skin permeation. *Pharm. Res.* **2014**, *31*, 394–400. [CrossRef] [PubMed]
34. Nauseef, W.M.; Borregaard, N. Neutrophils at work. *Nat. Immunol.* **2014**, *15*, 602–611. [CrossRef] [PubMed]
35. Kim, J.; Krueger, J.G. The immunopathogenesis of psoriasis. *Dermatol. Clin.* **2015**, *33*, 13–23. [CrossRef] [PubMed]
36. Amorati, R.; Zotova, J.; Baschieri, A.; Valgimigli, L. Antioxidant activity of magnolol and honokiol: Kinetic and mechanistic investigations of their reaction with peroxyl radicals. *J. Org. Chem.* **2015**, *80*, 10651–10659. [CrossRef] [PubMed]
37. Alonso, C.; Lucas, R.; Barba, C.; Marti, M.; Rubio, L.; Comelles, F.; Morales, J.C.; Coderch, L.; Parra, J.L. Skin delivery of antioxidant surfactants based on gallic acid and hydroxytyrosol. *J. Pharm. Pharmacol.* **2015**, *67*, 900–908. [CrossRef] [PubMed]
38. Takeuchi, H.; Gomi, T.; Shishido, M.; Watanabe, H.; Suenobu, N. Neutrophil elastase contributes to extracellular matrix damage induced by chronic low-dose UV irradiation in a hairless mouse photoaging model. *J. Dermatol. Sci.* **2010**, *60*, 151–158. [CrossRef] [PubMed]
39. Lombardi Borgia, S.; Schlupp, P.; Mehnert, W.; Schäfer-Korting, M. In vitro skin absorption and drug release—A comparison of six commercial prednicarbate preparations for topical use. *Eur. J. Pharm. Biopharm.* **2008**, *68*, 380–389. [CrossRef] [PubMed]
40. Al-Roujayee, A.S. Naringenin improves the healing process of thermally-induced skin damage in rats. *J. Intern. Med. Res.* **2017**, *45*, 570–582. [CrossRef] [PubMed]
41. Yao, K.; Chen, H.; Liu, K.; Langfald, A.; Yang, G.; Zhang, Y.; Yu, D.H.; Kim, M.O.; Lee, M.H.; Li, H.; et al. Kaempferol targets RSK2 and MSK1 to suppress UV radiation-induced skin cancer. *Cancer Prev. Res.* **2014**, *7*, 958–967. [CrossRef] [PubMed]

6

Influences of Orally Taken Carotenoid-Rich Curly Kale Extract on Collagen I/Elastin Index of the Skin

Martina C. Meinke [1,*,†], Ceylan K. Nowbary [1,†], Sabine Schanzer [1], Henning Vollert [2], Jürgen Lademann [1] and Maxim E. Darvin [1]

1 Charité-Universitätsmedizin Berlin, Corporate Member of Freie Universität Berlin, Humboldt-Universität zu Berlin, and Berlin Institute of Health, Center of Experimental and Applied Cutaneous Physiology (CCP), Department of Dermatology, Charité-Universitätsmedizin Berlin, 10117 Berlin, Germany; ceylan.nowbary@charite.de (C.K.N.); sabine.schanzer@charite.de (S.S.); juergen.lademann@charite.de (J.L.); maxim.darvin@charite.de (M.E.D.)

2 Bioactive Food GmbH, Am Ihlsee 36a, 23795 Bad Segeberg, Germany; henning_vollert@t-online.de

* Correspondence: martina.meinke@charite.de

† These authors contributed equally to this work.

Abstract: Two differently designed, spatially resolved reflectance spectroscopy-based scanners and two-photon tomography were used for noninvasive in vivo determination of cutaneous carotenoids, and collagen I/elastin aging index of dermis, respectively, in the skin of 29 healthy female volunteers between 40 and 56 years of age. The volunteers received a supplement in the form of a carotenoid-rich natural curly kale extract containing 1650 µg of carotenoids in total (three capsules of 550 µg), once a day. Measurements were taken before, after 5 months and after 10 months of daily supplementation. The results showed significantly increased values for the cutaneous carotenoids and the collagen I/elastin aging index of dermis 5 and 10 months after the beginning of the study. The obtained results show that a natural carotenoid-rich extract could prevent the aging-related collagen I degradation in the dermis and improve the extracellular matrix.

Keywords: skin aging; two photon tomography; reflectance spectroscopy; noninvasive methods; auto fluorescence; second harmonic generation; nutrition

---

1. Introduction

Nutrition rich in fruit and vegetables is beneficial to human health and wellbeing [1–4]. Secondary plant components, such as antioxidants [5], protect the cells and connective tissue against the development of oxidative stress, which is related to several pathological consequences, e.g., neurological [6], cardio-vascular [7], dermatological diseases [8] or aging [9]. Oxidative stress is induced by various factors, inter alia, solar radiation, smoking, alcohol consumption, lack of sleep, intensive physical activities and psychological stress [10–20], and therefore cannot be avoided in daily life. Oxidative stress is characterized by the generation of large amounts of reactive oxygen species (ROS), whose action is responsible for the development of premature skin aging and photo aging [7,21]. To counteract this effect, antioxidants should be available in sufficient concentration and composition to keep the balance and avoid tissue damage [22]. The majority of the essential antioxidants, including carotenoids, have to be consumed via dietary sources. The uptake and bioavailability of carotenoids can be measured in vivo by resonance Raman and reflectance spectroscopy [23,24]. Furthermore, it could be demonstrated that skin with a high amount of the carotenoid lycopene is less rough and therefore looks younger [21]. The physiologically relevant composition and concentration of antioxidants is important, as at very high concentrations, antioxidants might reverse their properties and become pro-oxidant [25,26]. This process is intricate and depends on many factors including oxygen tension and further antioxidants such as α-tocopherol in the tissue [27,28]. Taking this into account, a promising anti-aging strategy could be the physiologically relevant enhancement of carotenoids and other antioxidants in the tissue by nutrition and/or supplements [22].

The beneficial effects of such application on the skin status were studied based on skin parameters such as furrows and wrinkles, elasticity and skin hydration [29]. To understand such effects, more than roughness and wrinkle volume should be measured. The dermal proteins collagen I and elastin are related to the skin age and could serve as reliable parameters of the anti-aging effect of nutrition or a supplement [30,31]. Various studies have shown that the collagen I/elastin ratio, as well as the collagen I and elastin structures, change with age [32–35]. The elasticity of the skin increases with atrophy of the collagen I fiber bundles, the related flattening of the rete ridges, and the thickening of the dermal elastic fibers. Previously, biopsies had to be taken, but nowadays, noninvasive two-photon tomography is available to measure the collagen I by second harmonic generation (SHG) and the elastin by auto fluorescence (AF) signals in vivo in the dermis [36,37]. The SHG to AF aging index of dermis (SAAID) is a noninvasive objective parameter for determining the collagen I status in the dermis, which can be used for the description of the intrinsic and extrinsic aging on various skin areas in vivo [38,39], effect of skin protection [40], as well as efficacy of wound healing [41] and identification of disease affected skin [42,43]. The collagen I/elastin index can be quantified with the SAAID, which is defined according to [42]:

$$\text{SAAID} = (\text{SHG} - \text{AF})/(\text{SHG} + \text{AF}) \tag{1}$$

SAAID-scoring is a powerful method for analyzing the dermis dependent on AF and SHG signal intensities [43]. Other dermal collagens of types IV, VII and XVII are also known to reduce with age [44], but it is impossible to determine their concentrations in vivo in the skin. This can only be done by applying special algorithms [45].

The hypothesis is that systemically administered carotenoids will increase the collagen I synthesis or at least prevent its decrease, which usually occurs due to oxidative stress during our life, and results in skin aging. In the presented in vivo study, two different cutaneous carotenoid sensors, which were recently developed based on spatially resolved reflectance spectroscopy (SRRS), were applied to monitor the skin carotenoids noninvasively [46]. To increase the skin carotenoids, a vegetable curly kale extract rich in carotenoids, in comparison to a placebo, was systemically administered over a time period of 10 months. The curly kale extract was selected because previous studies had shown its positive effects on the skin in terms of bioavailability and radical scavenging activity [47,48]. The SAAID was measured as an objective skin aging parameter. The measurements were performed before, after 5, and after 10 months of intake of the carotenoid-rich curly kale supplement.

2. Material and Methods

2.1. Subjects

29 healthy female volunteers (10 smokers, 19 non-smokers) aged between 40 and 56 years (mean 49.2 years) of skin type II according to the Fitzpatrick classification [49] were enrolled in the study.

Exclusion criteria were subjects with skin diseases, admission to an institution due to an administrative or judicial order (according to § 29 MPG), known drug addiction or alcoholism, and expectant or lactating women. The investigations were carried out in accordance with the ethical guidelines of the Declaration of Helsinki and had been approved by the local Ethics Committee prior to starting the study (EA1/229/14). All volunteers gave their informed written consent.

2.2. Supplements

During the uptake study, the volunteers ingested three capsules of a curly kale extract, hereinafter called verum, once a day (provided by BioActive Food, Bad Segeberg, Germany). One capsule contained the following substances: 430 μg lutein, 70 μg beta-carotene, 30 μg lycopene, 20 μg zeaxanthin, i.e., 550 μg carotenoids, analyzed independently by Bioanalyt GmbH (Potsdam, Germany). As a control, a placebo capsule containing an olive oil without carotenoids was given. The content of the capsules was measured with resonance Raman spectroscopy and the placebo did not show any carotenoid values.

2.3. Study Protocol

The volunteers were randomly divided into placebo ($N = 15$) and verum groups ($N = 14$).

The measurements were performed on the palm, the inner forearm and the cheek. Carotenoids can be sensitively determined only at the palm as the stratum corneum is sufficiently thick there and the measurements are not influenced by blood and melanin. The SAAID was measured on the cheek and the inner forearm to have one sun exposed and one sun protected area.

2.4. Carotenoid Determination

For the investigations, two different sensors were applied. One optical sensor was based on multiple spatially resolved reflectance spectroscopy (MSRRS). This sensor is commercially available under the tradename biozoom (model Biozoom Portable, Kassel, Germany). It uses several differently positioned light sources and light detectors, exhibiting different distances between light source and detector and different angles for irradiation and detection, and has been described in detail elsewhere [23,46]. Briefly, the LED light sources cover a spectral range from approximately 350 nm to 1000 nm in wavelength in 16 steps, providing 118 light emitters. The sensor picks up the backscattered light at a total number of 152 light sensitive areas. This combination results in almost 18,000 raw data values, which are picked up several times during one measurement at a sensor surface area of 20 mm by 20 mm.

The second carotenoid sensor was a CaroLED sensor (Laser-und Medizin-Technologie Berlin, LMTB, Germany). The underlying measuring principle of CaroLED is based on SRRS, and was recently described by Meinke et al. [46]. Briefly, five light emitting diodes (LED) of different wavelengths in the visible and near infrared region illuminate the skin through a measurement window. While light propagates through the individual skin layers, and the spectral signature of carotenoids and of other skin constituents is obtained [50]. Four photodiodes, each of which is placed at a different lateral distance to the illumination site, measure the spectral signature at different depth sensitivities.

The measurements using both sensors were performed five times on the same palm area (thenar eminence) of the right hand for all subjects, and mean values were calculated for each subject and measurement method before the statistical analysis was applied. Because of the different initial values, the data were normalized to the initial values, dividing the values from visit after 5 and 10 months by the initial values.

Both sensors were calibrated before starting the study using resonance Raman spectroscopy on the palm of healthy volunteers in vivo using a resonant excitation at 488 nm [46].

2.5. Collagen I/Elastin Index SAAID

The collagen I and elastin structure of the skin can be characterized by the second harmonic generation (SHG) to autofluorescence (AF) aging index of dermis (SAAID). The SAAID can be determined in vivo using two-photon microscopy by calculation of the corresponding AF and SHG image intensities [51,52]. The SAAID is defined as described in Equation (1). In the dermis, the AF is mainly determined by the elastin concentration, while the SHG is determined by the collagen I concentration. In this nomenclature, the SAAID decreases with photo aging, approaching its minimal value-1 when the collagen is completely replaced by elastic fibers.

The investigations were carried out using a two-photon tomograph (JenLab GmbH, Jena, Germany) equipped with a femtosecond titanium sapphire laser (Mai Tai XF, Spectra-Physics, Santa Clara, CA, USA). The laser was operated at 760 nm and generated 100 fs pulses at a repetition rate of 80 MHz. For studying the structure of the dermis at different depths of the skin, sensitive photo multipliers were applied. The radiation collected from different depths was averaged over slices of 200×200 μm^2. The acquisition time was equal to 7 s for one slice, thus ensuring a satisfactory measurement stability and picture quality [41].

During the measurements, the laser focus was moved from the skin surface into deeper parts of the skin at 10 μm increments. The maximum measuring depth into the skin was 120 μm. For the whole depth, the SAAID was calculated and the profiles were normalized to the onset of the SHG signal. Four values after the SHG's onset were considered within the mean values to ensure data from the upper part of papillary dermis below the basal layer. The utilized two-photon tomograph has been described in detail elsewhere [40].

The measurements were performed in vivo at the lower inner arm and the cheek. For all subjects, the area at the forearm was selected at 30 cm from the middle finger tip. The cheek area was selected, as it had the best coupling possibility with the optical measuring head on the line between nose and ear.

2.6. Statistics

The data were statically analyzed using SPSS for Windows (IBM® SPSS® Statistics, version 19, Inc., Chicago, IL, USA). The data were analyzed to a normal distribution using explorative data analysis. An unpaired *t*-test was applied to determine differences in the mean values between the groups, and a paired *t*-test for changes within one group. For the correlation, the Pearson correlation coefficient was calculated. Values of $p \leq 0.05$ were considered to indicate a significant difference.

3. Results

Although 34 volunteers were enrolled, only 29 completed the study successfully. 5 dropouts occurred, 3 in the verum group and 2 in the placebo group. 2 volunteers quit the study due to problems with the stomach, and 3 did not come to the investigation after the 3rd visit and therefore were not replaced. All 29 volunteers underwent the carotenoid measurements and the two-photon tomography.

3.1. Carotenoids

The group-averaged cutaneous carotenoid concentrations measured using both carotenoid sensors are shown in Figure 1. The data are presented normalized to the initial value because the individual values show a high variation. The carotenoid values of the verum group measured with both devices increased significantly within the first 5 months, in which the volunteers ingested the carotenoid-rich extract, and decreased again over the next 5 months. But the values of the verum group after 10 months were still significantly higher than the initial value. The placebo values measured by CaroLED also increased and decreased, but the changes were not significant. The carotenoid concentration in the placebo group remained unchanged for the first 5 months and showed an insignificant decrease after 10 months of supplementation.

3.2. SAAID

The SAAID was measured at the inner forearm and at the cheek. The differences from the initial values are shown in Figure 2. After 5 months, all SAAID values had increased significantly ($p < 0.05$ for placebo and $p < 0.01$ for verum), but after 10 months, the increase had remained significant only for the verum group. The verum group consistently showed higher values than the placebo group, and the difference between the two groups was significant for the cheek after 10 months ($p < 0.05$).

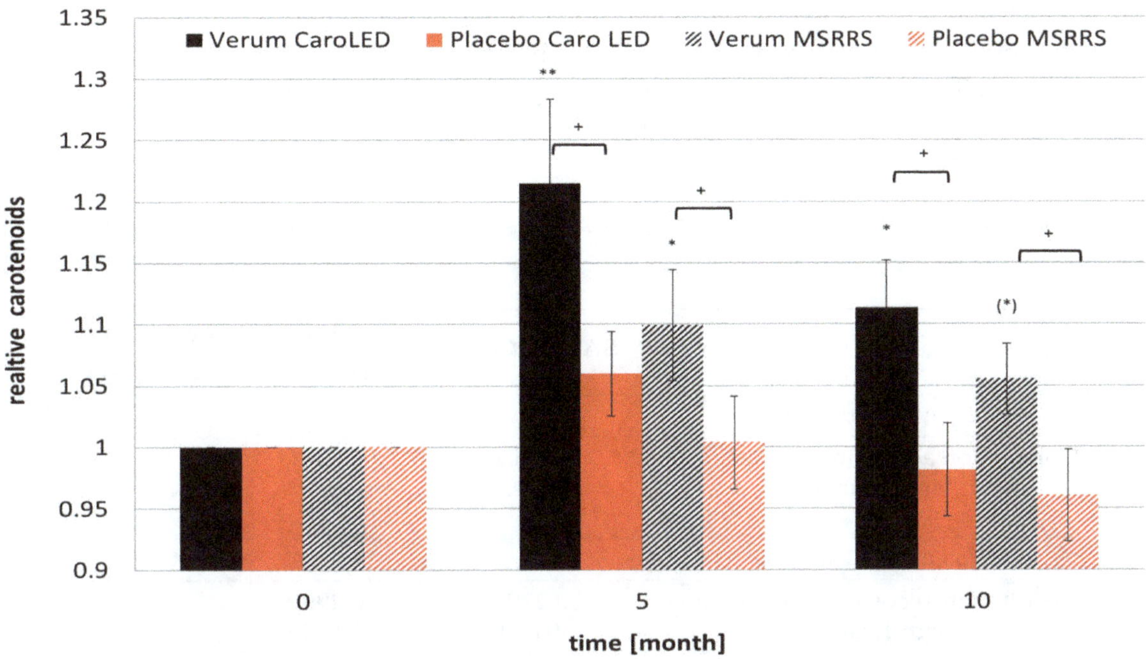

Figure 1. Carotenoid values relative to the initial values measured by two different carotenoid sensors obtained in the palm (mean ± SEM). + $p < 0.05$ between placebo and verum; (*) $p < 0.1$, * $p < 0.05$, ** $p < 0.01$ to initial value. $N = 15$ for placebo and $N = 14$ for verum.

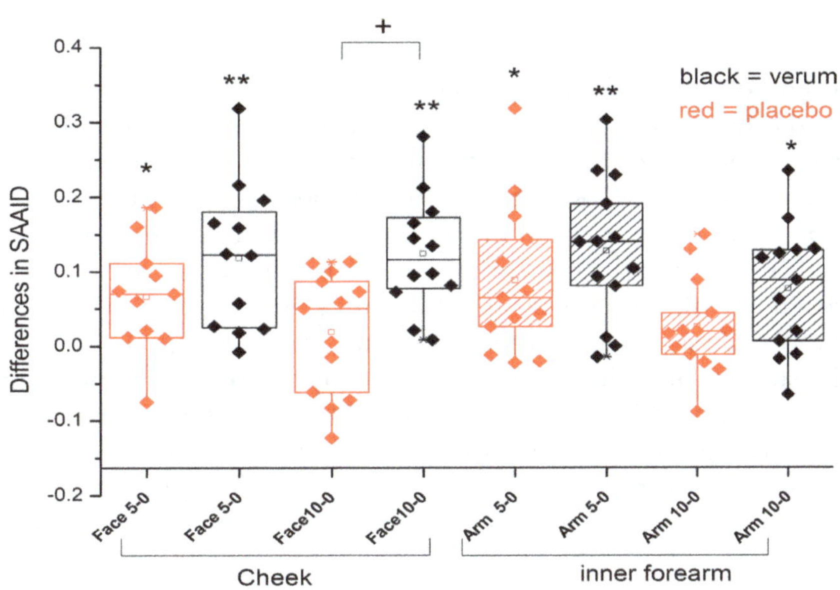

Figure 2. Box plot of the differences of SAAID to the initial values measured at the cheek and inner forearm. + $p < 0.05$ between placebo and verum; * $p < 0.05$, ** $p < 0.01$ to initial value. The box presents 50% of the data. The bottom and top of the box are always the first and third quartiles and the solid line box is always the second quartile, the median.

3.3. Correlations

If the hypothesis is correct that the SAAID increases during the intake of carotenoids, a correlation of these two values is possible. Therefore, the Pearson correlation coefficient of the SAAID values and the carotenoid values was calculated (Table 1) for all subjects from whom at least one SAAID value (cheek or arm) was obtained for all visits (max. $n_{subjects} = 27$, maximum measured values

$N = 81$). As a positive check, the correlation between the two carotenoid values was determined, as well. As expected, the two carotenoid values have a highly significant positive correlation. Furthermore, the two SAAID values show a moderately positive correlation, which is highly significant. The correlations between the carotenoid and the SAAID values are between slightly and moderately positive with an r of about 0.3, and are significant.

Table 1. Pearson correlation coefficient r with p-values and number of the SAAID and carotenoid values (N); * $p < 0.05$, ** $p < 0.01$.

	SAAID Cheek	SAAID Forearm	Carotenoids CaroLED
SAAID forearm			
Correlation according to Pearson	0.504 **	1	
Significance	<0.001		
N	76	77	
Carotenoids CaroLED			
Correlation according to Pearson	0.279 *	0.295 **	1
Significance	0.014	0.008	
N	77	80	81
Carotenoids MSRRS			
Correlation according to Pearson	0.328 **	0.225 *	0.853 **
Significance	0.004	0.023	<0.001
N	77	80	81

4. Discussion

Human nutrition is subject to seasonal variations, and the intake of secondary plant substances such as carotenoids and other antioxidants is related to it. From former investigations, it is known that the carotenoid status in humans is enhanced in the summer and autumn months due to the availability of regional fresh and ripe fruits and vegetables. This has been referred to as "seasonal increase" [53]. In the current study, the first measurements were performed in autumn and the second ones in the springtime. The last visit took place at the end of summer and mainly in autumn. This could explain the observed changes in the placebo group. Furthermore, infections, which occur very often in the wintertime, additionally decreased the carotenoid values in the skin [53].

As expected, the skin carotenoid values increased by 10 to 20% in the group that received the carotenoid-rich curly kale extract. This increase is below the data obtained in former studies because the dose of carotenoids in this long-term study was lower compared to former studies [47,48]. Nevertheless, the obtained enhancement was significantly higher than that of the placebo.

The investigations performed using two-photon tomography have shown that the SAAID also increased at the forearm and cheek in the placebo group. However, the enhancement of the SAAID of the verum group was always higher than the placebo. This indicates new collagen I production or a reduced thickening of the dermal elastic fibers. So far, it has not been observed in vivo that nutrition or supplementation results in such an effect. The more pronounced differences at the solar-exposed cheek compared to the protected inner forearm indicate not only a protection by the antioxidants and less degradation in the verum group, but also an improvement of the extracellular matrix compared to the first visit. Exposure to solar radiation induces free radicals, which interact with the extracellular matrix determinants once a critical threshold is reached [40]. This effect is called photo aging or premature skin aging [54–56]. The radical scavenging activity of the utilized curly kale extract has already been shown in a former in vivo study using electron paramagnetic resonance spectroscopy [48]. The verum group showed a higher radical scavenging activity in the skin and, as a result, an enhanced protection against VIS/NIR irradiation.

Interestingly, a correlation between the carotenoids and the SAAID values was obtained. These findings also suggest that the significant increase of SAAID values after 10 months could be due to the intake of the carotenoid-rich extract. The tendency towards correlation between SAAID and carotenoids has previously been reported [40], but such a supplementation-induced effect has not been observed so far.

The long-term study indicates that anti-aging effects are not easy to observe because many other factors could also influence the values. The measurements are only snapshots during this long-term investigation. Nevertheless, the SAAID could serve as a reliable parameter for the determination of the skin aging status, which is not so sensitive to short-term changes.

The above-mentioned skin parameters were measured noninvasively and in vivo, and do not interfere with each other.

5. Conclusions

In the performed placebo-controlled in vivo study, it was demonstrated with two different optical scanners that oral supplementation of the carotenoid-rich natural curly kale extract (1650 µg of total carotenoids) once a day had caused a statistically significant increase of carotenoids in the skin 5 and 10 months after the beginning of the study. In the cheek and forearm skin areas, the collagen I/elastin ratio (SAAID value) increased significantly in both the verum and placebo groups, although it was higher in the verum group. After 10 months of supplementation, the SAAID value in the verum group had remained significantly higher. Thus, the results show that a natural extract containing a mixture of carotenoids at physiological concentrations could prevent skin aging and improve the extracellular matrix. Therefore, a healthy lifestyle including a diet rich in carotenoids is the best prevention strategy against premature skin aging.

Acknowledgments: The study was supported by the German Federal Ministry of Education and Research (BMBF), funding code 13N12593.

Author Contributions: M.C.M. planned, analyzed and wrote the paper, C.K.N. performed the measurements and partly analyzed the data, S.S. partly performed the measurements, H.V. developed and provided the supplement. J.L. designed the study and M.D. analyzed the data und partly wrote the paper.

References

1. Fito, M.; Konstantinidou, V. Nutritional Genomics and the Mediterranean Diet's Effects on Human Cardiovascular Health. *Nutrients* **2016**, *8*. [CrossRef] [PubMed]
2. Li, S.; Zhu, Y.; Chavarro, J.E.; Bao, W.; Tobias, D.K.; Ley, S.H.; Forman, J.P.; Liu, A.; Mills, J.; Bowers, K.; et al. Healthful Dietary Patterns and the Risk of Hypertension Among Women With a History of Gestational Diabetes Mellitus: A Prospective Cohort Study. *Hypertension* **2016**. [CrossRef]
3. Sun, Y.; Li, Z.; Li, J.; Li, Z.; Han, J. A Healthy Dietary Pattern Reduces Lung Cancer Risk: A Systematic Review and Meta-Analysis. *Nutrients* **2016**, *8*. [CrossRef] [PubMed]
4. Dias, I.H.; Polidori, M.C.; Li, L.; Weber, D.; Stahl, W.; Nelles, G.; Grune, T.; Griffiths, H.R. Plasma levels of HDL and carotenoids are lower in dementia patients with vascular comorbidities. *J. Alzheimer's Dis.* **2014**, *40*, 399–408. [CrossRef]
5. Polidori, M.C.; De Spirt, S.; Stahl, W.; Pientka, L. Conflict of evidence: Carotenoids and other micronutrients in the prevention and treatment of cognitive impairment. *Biofactors* **2012**, *38*, 167–171. [CrossRef] [PubMed]
6. Xin, Y.J.; Yuan, B.; Yu, B.; Wang, Y.Q.; Wu, J.J.; Zhou, W.H.; Qiu, Z. Tet1-mediated DNA demethylation regulates neuronal cell death induced by oxidative stress. *Sci. Rep.* **2015**, *5*, 7645. [CrossRef] [PubMed]
7. Varga, Z.V.; Giricz, Z.; Liaudet, L.; Hasko, G.; Ferdinandy, P.; Pacher, P. Interplay of oxidative, nitrosative/nitrative stress, inflammation, cell death and autophagy in diabetic cardiomyopathy. *Biochim. Biophys. Acta* **2015**, *1852*, 232–242. [CrossRef] [PubMed]

8. Moretti, D.; Del Bello, B.; Allavena, G.; Corti, A.; Signorini, C.; Maellaro, E. Calpain-3 impairs cell proliferation and stimulates oxidative stress-mediated cell death in melanoma cells. *PLoS ONE* **2015**, *10*, e0117258. [CrossRef] [PubMed]
9. Kandola, K.; Bowman, A.; Birch-Machin, M.A. Oxidative stress—A key emerging impact factor in health, ageing, lifestyle and aesthetics. *Int. J. Cosmet. Sci.* **2015**, *37* (Suppl. S2), 1–8. [CrossRef] [PubMed]
10. Khoubnasabjafari, M.; Ansarin, K.; Jouyban, A. Reliability of malondialdehyde as a biomarker of oxidative stress in psychological disorders. *Bioimpacts* **2015**, *5*, 123–127. [CrossRef] [PubMed]
11. Mons, U.; Muscat, J.E.; Modesto, J.; Richie, J.P.J.; Brenner, H. Effect of smoking reduction and cessation on the plasma levels of the oxidative stress biomarker glutathione-Post-hoc analysis of data from a smoking cessation trial. *Free Radic. Biol. Med.* **2016**, *91*, 172–177. [CrossRef] [PubMed]
12. Varadinova, M.G.; Valcheva-Traykova, M.L.; Boyadjieva, N.I. Effect of Circadian Rhythm Disruption and Alcohol on the Oxidative Stress Level in Rat Brain. *Am. J. Ther.* **2015**, *23*, 6. [CrossRef] [PubMed]
13. Yoshida, A.; Shiotsu-Ogura, Y.; Wada-Takahashi, S.; Takahashi, S.S.; Toyama, T.; Yoshino, F. Blue light irradiation-induced oxidative stress in vivo via ROS generation in rat gingival tissue. *J. Photochem. Photobiol. B* **2015**, *151*, 48–53. [CrossRef] [PubMed]
14. Grether-Beck, S.; Marini, A.; Jaenicke, T.; Krutmann, J. French Maritime Pine Bark Extract (Pycnogenol(R)) Effects on Human Skin: Clinical and Molecular Evidence. *Skin Pharmacol. Physiol.* **2016**, *29*, 13–17. [CrossRef] [PubMed]
15. Schempp, C.M.; Ludtke, R.; Winghofer, B.; Simon, J.C. Effect of topical application of Hypericum perforatum extract (St. John's wort) on skin sensitivity to solar simulated radiation. *Photodermatol. Photoimmunol. Photomed.* **2000**, *16*, 125–128. [CrossRef] [PubMed]
16. Jung, S.; Darvin, M.E.; Chung, H.S.; Jung, B.; Lee, S.H.; Lenz, K.; Chung, W.S.; Yu, R.X.; Patzelt, A.; Lee, B.N.; et al. Antioxidants in Asian-Korean and caucasian skin: The influence of nutrition and stress. *Skin Pharmacol. Physiol.* **2014**, *27*, 293–302. [CrossRef] [PubMed]
17. Fluhr, J.W.; Caspers, P.; van der Pol, J.A.; Richter, H.; Sterry, W.; Lademann, J.; Darvin, M.E. Kinetics of carotenoid distribution in human skin in vivo after exogenous stress: Disinfectant and wIRA-induced carotenoid depletion recovers from outside to inside. *J. Biomed. Opt.* **2011**, *16*, 035002. [CrossRef] [PubMed]
18. Maeter, H.; Briese, V.; Gerber, B.; Darvin, M.E.; Lademann, J.; Olbertz, D.M. Case study: In vivo stress diagnostics by spectroscopic determination of the cutaneous carotenoid antioxidant concentration in midwives depending on shift work. *Laser Phys. Lett.* **2013**, *10*, 105701. [CrossRef]
19. Darvin, M.E.; Sterry, W.; Lademann, J.; Patzelt, A. Alcohol consumption decreases the protection efficiency of the antioxidant network and increases the risk of sunburn in human skin. *Skin Pharmacol. Physiol.* **2013**, *26*, 45–51. [CrossRef] [PubMed]
20. Vierck, H.B.; Darvin, M.E.; Lademann, J.; Reisshauer, A.; Baack, A.; Sterry, W.; Patzelt, A. The influence of endurance exercise on the antioxidative status of human skin. *Eur. J. Appl. Physiol.* **2012**, *112*, 3361–3367. [CrossRef] [PubMed]
21. Darvin, M.; Patzelt, A.; Gehse, S.; Schanzer, S.; Benderoth, C.; Sterry, W.; Lademann, J. Cutaneous concentration of lycopene correlates significantly with the roughness of the skin. *Eur. J. Pharm. Biopharm.* **2008**, *69*, 943–947. [CrossRef] [PubMed]
22. Darvin, M.; Zastrow, L.; Sterry, W.; Lademann, J. Effect of supplemented and topically applied antioxidant substances on human tissue. *Skin Pharmacol. Physiol.* **2006**, *19*, 238–247. [CrossRef] [PubMed]
23. Darvin, M.; Lademann, J.; Magnussen, B.; Köcher, W. Multiple Spatially Resolved Reflection Spectroscopy for non-invasive determination of carotenoids in human skin. *Laser Phys. Lett.* **2016**, *13*, 095601. [CrossRef]
24. Darvin, M.E.; Meinke, M.C.; Sterry, W.; Lademann, J. Optical methods for noninvasive determination of carotenoids in human and animal skin. *J. Biomed. Opt.* **2013**, *18*, 61230. [CrossRef] [PubMed]
25. Palozza, P.; Serini, S.; Di Nicuolo, F.; Piccioni, E.; Calviello, G. Prooxidant effects of beta-carotene in cultured cells. *Mol. Asp. Med.* **2003**, *24*, 353–362. [CrossRef]
26. Lambert, J.D.; Elias, R.J. The antioxidant and pro-oxidant activities of green tea polyphenols: A role in cancer prevention. *Arch. Biochem. Biophys.* **2010**, *501*, 65–72. [CrossRef] [PubMed]
27. Zhang, P.; Omaye, S.T. DNA strand breakage and oxygen tension: Effects of beta-carotene, alpha-tocopherol and ascorbic acid. *Food Chem. Toxicol.* **2001**, *39*, 239–246. [CrossRef]
28. Palozza, P.; Calviello, G.; Bartoli, G.M. Prooxidant activity of beta-carotene under 100% oxygen pressure in rat liver microsomes. *Free Radic. Biol. Med.* **1995**, *19*, 887–892. [CrossRef]

29. Heinrich, U.; Tronnier, H.; Stahl, W.; Bejot, M.; Maurette, J.M. Antioxidant supplements improve parameters related to skin structure in humans. *Skin Pharmacol. Physiol.* **2006**, *19*, 224–231. [CrossRef] [PubMed]
30. Gogly, B.; Godeau, G.; Gilbert, S.; Legrand, J.M.; Kut, C.; Pellat, B.; Goldberg, M. Morphometric analysis of collagen and elastic fibers in normal skin and gingiva in relation to age. *Clin. Oral Investig.* **1997**, *1*, 147–152. [PubMed]
31. Yasui, T.; Yonetsu, M.; Tanaka, R.; Tanaka, Y.; Fukushima, S.; Yamashita, T.; Ogura, Y.; Hirao, T.; Murota, H.; Araki, T. In vivo observation of age-related structural changes of dermal collagen in human facial skin using collagen-sensitive second harmonic generation microscope equipped with 1250-nm mode-locked Cr:Forsterite laser. *J. Biomed. Opt.* **2013**, *18*, 31108. [CrossRef] [PubMed]
32. Knott, A.; Reuschlein, K.; Lucius, R.; Stab, F.; Wenck, H.; Gallinat, S. Deregulation of versican and elastin binding protein in solar elastosis. *Biogerontology* **2009**, *10*, 181–190. [CrossRef] [PubMed]
33. Sanchez, W.Y.; Obispo, C.; Ryan, E.; Grice, J.E.; Roberts, M.S. Changes in the redox state and endogenous fluorescence of in vivo human skin due to intrinsic and photo-aging, measured by multiphoton tomography with fluorescence lifetime imaging. *J. Biomed. Opt.* **2013**, *18*, 061217. [CrossRef] [PubMed]
34. Koehler, M.J.; Preller, A.; Kindler, N.; Elsner, P.; Konig, K.; Buckle, R.; Kaatz, M. Intrinsic, solar and sunbed-induced skin aging measured in vivo by multiphoton laser tomography and biophysical methods. *Skin Res. Technol.* **2009**, *15*, 357–363. [CrossRef] [PubMed]
35. Karagas, M.R.; Zens, M.S.; Nelson, H.H.; Mabuchi, K.; Perry, A.E.; Stukel, T.A.; Mott, L.A.; Andrew, A.S.; Applebaum, K.M.; Linet, M. Measures of cumulative exposure from a standardized sun exposure history questionnaire: A comparison with histologic assessment of solar skin damage. *Am. J. Epidemiol.* **2007**, *165*, 719–726. [CrossRef] [PubMed]
36. Konig, K. Multiphoton microscopy in life sciences. *J. Microsc. (Oxf.)* **2000**, *200*, 83–104. [CrossRef]
37. Konig, K. Clinical multiphoton tomography. *J. Biophotonics* **2008**, *1*, 13–23. [CrossRef] [PubMed]
38. Sugata, K.; Osanai, O.; Sano, T.; Akiyama, M.; Fujimoto, N.; Tajima, S.; Takema, Y. Evaluation of unique elastic aggregates (elastic globes) in normal facial skin by multiphoton laser scanning tomography. *Eur. J. Dermatol.* **2015**, *25*, 138–144. [CrossRef] [PubMed]
39. Koehler, M.J.; Konig, K.; Elsner, P.; Buckle, R.; Kaatz, M. In vivo assessment of human skin aging by multiphoton laser scanning tomography. *Opt. Lett.* **2006**, *31*, 2879–2881. [CrossRef] [PubMed]
40. Darvin, M.E.; Richter, H.; Ahlberg, S.; Haag, S.F.; Meinke, M.C.; Le Quintrec, D.; Doucet, O.; Lademann, J. Influence of sun exposure on the cutaneous collagen/elastin fibers and carotenoids: Negative effects can be reduced by application of sunscreen. *J. Biophotonics* **2014**, *7*, 735–743. [CrossRef] [PubMed]
41. Springer, S.; Zieger, M.; Bottcher, A.; Lademann, J.; Kaatz, M. Examination of wound healing after curettage by multiphoton tomography of human skin in vivo. *Skin Res. Technol.* **2017**. [CrossRef] [PubMed]
42. Adur, J.; Carvalho, H.F.; Cesar, C.L.; Casco, V.H. Nonlinear optical microscopy signal processing strategies in cancer. *Cancer Inform.* **2014**, *13*, 67–76. [CrossRef] [PubMed]
43. Cicchi, R.; Kapsokalyvas, D.; De Giorgi, V.; Maio, V.; Van Wiechen, A.; Massi, D.; Lotti, T.; Pavone, F.S. Scoring of collagen organization in healthy and diseased human dermis by multiphoton microscopy. *J. Biophotonics* **2010**, *3*, 34–43. [CrossRef] [PubMed]
44. Langton, A.K.; Halai, P.; Griffiths, C.E.; Sherratt, M.J.; Watson, R.E. The impact of intrinsic ageing on the protein composition of the dermal-epidermal junction. *Mech. Ageing Dev.* **2016**, *156*, 14–16. [CrossRef] [PubMed]
45. Shirshin, E.A.; Gurfinkel, Y.I.; Priezzhev, A.V.; Fadeev, V.V.; Lademann, J.; Darvin, M.E. Two-photon autofluorescence lifetime imaging of human skin papillary dermis in vivo: Assessment of blood capillaries and structural proteins localization. *Sci. Rep. (UK)* **2017**, *7*, 1171. [CrossRef] [PubMed]
46. Meinke, M.C.; Lohan, S.B.; Kocher, W.; Magnussen, B.; Darvin, M.E.; Lademann, J. Multiple spatially resolved reflection spectroscopy to monitor cutaneous carotenoids during supplementation of fruit and vegetable extracts in vivo. *Skin Res. Technol.* **2017**. [CrossRef] [PubMed]
47. Meinke, M.C.; Darvin, M.E.; Vollert, H.; Lademann, J. Bioavailability of natural carotenoids in human skin compared to blood. *Eur. J. Pharm. Biopharm.* **2010**, *76*, 269–274. [CrossRef] [PubMed]
48. Meinke, M.C.; Friedrich, A.; Tscherch, K.; Haag, S.F.; Darvin, M.E.; Vollert, H.; Groth, N.; Lademann, J.; Rohn, S. Influence of dietary carotenoids on radical scavenging capacity of the skin and skin lipids. *Eur. J. Pharm. Biopharm.* **2013**, *84*, 365–373. [CrossRef] [PubMed]

49. Fitzpatrick, T.B. The validity and practicality of sun-reactive skin types I through VI. *Arch. Dermatol.* **1988**, *124*, 869–871. [CrossRef] [PubMed]
50. Andree, S.; Reble, C.; Helfmann, J. Spectral in vivo signature of carotenoids in visible light diffuse reflectance from skin in comparison to ex vivo absorption spectra. *Photonics Lasers Med.* **2013**, *2*, 3. [CrossRef]
51. Darvin, M.E.; Gersonde, I.; Meinke, M.; Sterry, W.; Lademann, J. Non-invasive in vivo determination of the carotenoids beta-carotene and lycopene concentrations in the human skin using the Raman spectroscopic method. *J. Phys. D Appl. Phys.* **2005**, *38*, 2696–2700. [CrossRef]
52. Lin, S.J.; Wu, R., Jr.; Tan, H.Y.; Lo, W.; Lin, W.C.; Young, T.H.; Hsu, C.J.; Chen, J.S.; Jee, S.H.; Dong, C.Y. Evaluating cutaneous photoaging by use of multiphoton fluorescence and second-harmonic generation microscopy. *Opt. Lett.* **2005**, *30*, 2275–2277. [CrossRef] [PubMed]
53. Darvin, M.E.; Patzelt, A.; Knorr, F.; Blume-Peytavi, U.; Sterry, W.; Lademann, J. One-year study on the variation of carotenoid antioxidant substances in living human skin: Influence of dietary supplementation and stress factors. *J. Biomed. Opt.* **2008**, *13*, 044028. [CrossRef] [PubMed]
54. Baillie, L.; Askew, D.; Douglas, N.; Soyer, H.P. Strategies for assessing the degree of photodamage to skin: A systematic review of the literature. *Br. J. Dermatol.* **2011**, *165*, 735–742. [CrossRef] [PubMed]
55. Proksch, E.; Schunck, M.; Zague, V.; Segger, D.; Degwert, J.; Oesser, S. Oral intake of specific bioactive collagen peptides reduces skin wrinkles and increases dermal matrix synthesis. *Skin Pharmacol. Physiol.* **2014**, *27*, 113–119. [CrossRef] [PubMed]
56. Manickavasagam, A.; Hirvonen, L.M.; Melita, L.N.; Chong, E.Z.; Cook, R.J.; Bozecc, L.; Festy, F. Multimodal optical characterisation of collagen photodegradation by femtosecond infrared laser ablation. *Analyst* **2014**, *139*, 6135–6143. [CrossRef] [PubMed]

7

Targeting NRF2 for Improved Skin Barrier Function and Photoprotection: Focus on the Achiote-Derived Apocarotenoid Bixin

Montserrat Rojo de la Vega, Andrea Krajisnik, Donna D. Zhang and Georg T. Wondrak *

Department of Pharmacology and Toxicology, College of Pharmacy & Arizona Cancer Center, University of Arizona, Tucson, AZ 85724, USA; emrvg@email.arizona.edu (M.R.d.l.V.); akrajisnik@email.arizona.edu (A.K.); dzhang@pharmacy.arizona.edu (D.D.Z.)

* Correspondence: wondrak@pharmacy.arizona.edu

Abstract: The transcription factor NRF2 (nuclear factor-E2-related factor 2) orchestrates major cellular defense mechanisms including phase-II detoxification, inflammatory signaling, DNA repair, and antioxidant response. Recent studies strongly suggest a protective role of NRF2-mediated gene expression in the suppression of cutaneous photodamage induced by solar UV (ultraviolet) radiation. The apocarotenoid bixin, a Food and Drug Administration (FDA)-approved natural food colorant (referred to as 'annatto') originates from the seeds of the achiote tree native to tropical America, consumed by humans since ancient times. Use of achiote preparations for skin protection against environmental insult and for enhanced wound healing has long been documented. We have recently reported that (i) bixin is a potent canonical activator of the NRF2-dependent cytoprotective response in human skin keratinocytes; that (ii) systemic administration of bixin activates NRF2 with protective effects against solar UV-induced skin damage; and that (iii) bixin-induced suppression of photodamage is observable in *Nrf2*$^{+/+}$ but not in *Nrf2*$^{-/-}$ SKH-1 mice confirming the NRF2-dependence of bixin-induced antioxidant and anti-inflammatory effects. In addition, bixin displays molecular activities as sacrificial antioxidant, excited state quencher, PPAR (peroxisome proliferator-activated receptor) α/γ agonist, and TLR (Toll-like receptor) 4/NFκB (nuclear factor kappa-light-chain-enhancer of activated B cells) antagonist, all of which might be relevant to the enhancement of skin barrier function and environmental stress protection. Potential skin photoprotection and photochemoprevention benefits provided by topical application or dietary consumption of this ethno-pharmacologically validated phytochemical originating from the Americas deserves further preclinical and clinical examination.

Keywords: skin photodamage; skin barrier function; solar ultraviolet (UV); NRF2; PPARα; bixin; achiote

---

1. Introduction: Solar Radiation, Photodamage, Photoaging, and Skin Photocarcinogenesis

Exposure to solar ultraviolet (UV) radiation is a causative factor in acute skin photodamage, chronic photoaging, and photocarcinogenesis [1–4]. More recently, a causative role of solar photons in the visible and infrared spectral range contributing to skin photodamage has been substantiated [5–8]. Moreover, cutaneous exposure to other environmental stressors including combustion pollutants, heavy metals, metalloids, and ozone has been shown to contribute to skin damage and carcinogenesis. Remarkably, nonmelanoma skin cancer (NMSC; also referred to as keratinocyte cancers (KC)) is the most common malignancy in the United States, and skin cancer incidence is increasing rapidly, presenting a public health burden of considerable magnitude [9]. Even though sunscreen-based photoprotection is an effective component of a sun-safe strategy to reduce cumulative lifetime exposure to UV light, much effort has been directed towards the development of more effective molecular strategies acting through mechanisms different from (or synergistic with) photon absorption [9–14].

2. NRF2: A Master Regulator of Skin Barrier Function, Cellular Defense Mechanisms against Environmental Stress, and Solar Radiation Response

The redox-sensitive transcription factor NRF2 (nuclear factor-E2-related factor 2) orchestrates major cellular defense mechanisms including phase-II detoxification, inflammatory signaling, DNA repair, and antioxidant response, and recent experimental evidence supports an important role of NRF2 in skin barrier function. NRF2 has therefore emerged as a promising molecular target for the pharmacological prevention of human pathologies resulting from exposure to environmental toxicants including solar UV-induced damage and carcinogenesis [15–18]. Moreover, the potential of NRF2 for modulation of skin chronological and photodamage-associated aging has attracted considerable attention [9,19,20].

3. NRF2: Molecular Biology and Pharmacological Modulation

NRF2 is ubiquitously expressed in all tissues, including the skin, but its protein levels and consequently its activity are tightly regulated (Figure 1). Under basal (homeostatic) conditions, NRF2 resides in the cytosol, where it binds to its negative regulator Kelch-ECH associated protein 1 (KEAP1), a substrate adaptor for a cullin 3-RING box protein 1 (CUL3-RBX1) E3 ubiquitin ligase complex [21]. Thus, NRF2 is ubiquitylated and degraded by the 26 S proteasome [22]. However, upon exposure to reactive oxygen species (ROS) or to electrophilic compounds, key sensor cysteine residues in KEAP1 (cysteine 151 in particular) are chemically modified, causing a conformational change in KEAP1 that prevents degradation of NRF2, which remains complexed to KEAP1 [23,24]. This allows newly synthesized NRF2 to accumulate and translocate to the nucleus, where it heterodimerizes with small MAF (musculoaponeurotic fibrosarcoma) proteins and binds to the antioxidant response elements (AREs) in the regulatory regions of its downstream genes [25]. This mode of canonical NRF2 regulation has been extensively studied in the context of skin protection and pathogenesis. In addition, other modes of NRF2 regulation, such as the p62-dependent non-canonical pathway that activates NRF2 in an autophagy-dependent manner [26,27] or the GSK3-βTrCP (glycogen synthase kinase 3/β-transducin repeat containing protein) degradation pathway [28,29], have been described. However, the involvement of these other modes of NRF2 regulation in skin barrier function and environmental stress protection remain to be determined.

Many natural chemopreventive compounds that have antioxidant properties exert their cytoprotective function through NRF2 activation. Classic examples of NRF2 inducers are sulforaphane (from cruciferous vegetables) [16], curcumin (from *Curcuma longa*) [30], cinnamaldehyde (from cinnamon) [31,32], and tanshinones (from *Salvia miltiorrhiza*) [33], among many others. These compounds are promiscuous electrophilic molecules that also react with cysteine 151 of KEAP1, induce NRF2, and confer protection against a number of chemical insults or radiation damage (including UV) observable in vitro and in vivo [34–36]. Recently, a synthetic triterpenoid NRF2 modulator and bardoxolone-derivative, RTA 408, has been tested for topical NRF2 activation in rat, murine, and human skin [37,38], but limited data on skin protection properties are available. Taken together, a significant opportunity for the development of cutaneous NRF2-dependent skin protection strategies using nutrient-derived molecular entities remains to be explored.

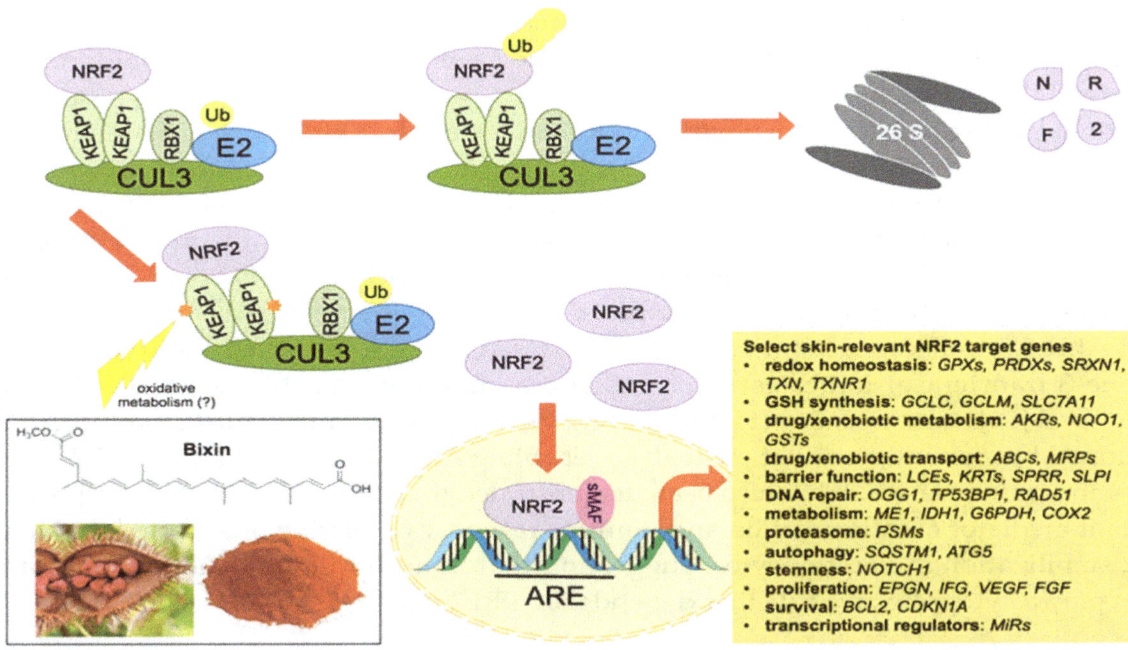

Figure 1. The nuclear factor-E2-related factor 2 (NRF2) pathway with a focus on skin barrier function and environmental stress protection. The transcription factor NRF2 binds to Kelch-ECH associated protein 1 (KEAP1), the substrate adaptor protein for the cullin 3-RING box protein 1 (CUL3-RBX1) E3 ubiquitin ligase complex. Under basal conditions, NRF2 is ubiquitylated and degraded by the 26S proteasome. Upon modification of reactive cysteines in KEAP1 by reactive oxygen species (ROS) and electrophiles (including bixin), NRF2 is no longer ubiquitylated. This allows for newly synthesized NRF2 to accumulate, translocate to the nucleus, and activate the transcription of antioxidant response element (ARE)-containing target genes by dimerizing with small MAF (sMAF) proteins. Select skin-relevant NRF2 target genes are displayed according to the cellular function they perform. *GPXs*, glutathione peroxidases; *PRDXs*, peroxiredoxins; *SRXN1*, sulfiredoxin 1; *TXN*, thioredoxin; *TXNR1*, thioredoxin reductase 1; *GCLC*, glutamate cysteine ligase, catalytic subunit; *GCLM*, glutamate cysteine ligase, modifier subunit; *SLC7A11*, glutamate/cystine antiporter (xCT); *AKRs*, aldoketoreductases; *NQO1*, NAD(P)H:quinone oxidoreductase 1; *GSTs*, glutathione S-transferases; *ABCs*, ATP-binding cassette family proteins; *MRPs*, multidrug resistance-associated proteins; *LCEs*, late cornified envelope family members; *KRTs*, keratins; *SPRR*, small proline rich proteins; *OGG1*, 8-oxo-guanine glycosylase; *TP53BP1*, p53 binding protein 1; *RAD51*, DNA repair protein RAD51 homolog 1; *ME1*, malic enzyme; *IDH1*, isocitrate dehydrogenase 1; *G6PDH*, glucose-6-phosphate dehydrogenase; *COX2*, cytochrome c oxidase subunit 2; *PSM*, proteasome subunit proteins; *SQSTM1*, sequestosome 1 (p62); *ATG5*, autophagy-related gene 5; *NOTCH1*, Notch homolog 1, translocation-associated; *EPGN*, epigen; *IGF*, insulin-like growth factor; *VEGF*, vascular endothelial growth factor; *FGF*, fibroblast growth factor; *BCL2*, B cell lymphoma 2; *CDKN1A*, cyclin dependent kinase inhibitor 1A (p21); *MiR*, microRNAs.

4. NRF2 Control of Skin Barrier Structure and Function

Recently, it has been shown that numerous genes encoding skin barrier structural and functional components are under NRF2 transcriptional control, including late cornified envelope 1 (LCE1) family members (*LCE1B*, *LCE1C*, *LCE1E*, *LCE1G*, *LCE1H*, *LCE1M*), keratins (*KRT6A*, *KRT16*, *KRT17*), small proline rich proteins (*SPRR2D*, *SPRR2H*), secretory leukocyte protease inhibitor (*SLPI*), and the EGF family member epigen (*EPGN*), some of which contain a validated ARE [39–43]. Moreover, a novel role of NRF2 in skin barrier and desmosome function has been attributed to transcriptional control of MiR-encoding genes (*MIR29AB1* and MIR29B2C) in keratinocytes, substantiating a novel NRF2-miR29-DSC2 (desmocollin-2) axis in control of desmosome function and cutaneous homeostasis [44]. In addition, much research has substantiated a role of NRF2 in epidermal redox control, stress response regulation, terminal differentiation, and barrier homeostasis, and a crucial role of NRF2 in the control of a cytoprotective glutathione gradient throughout the epidermis has been demonstrated [13,35,40,41,45].

Additional functional implications of NRF2 relevant to skin barrier maintenance, repair, and rejuvenation have recently emerged, including a role in metabolic control and mitochondrial homeostasis, proteasomal function and autophagy, and stem cell renewal and pluripotency [46–48].

Moreover, abundant functional crosstalk exists between NRF2 and other cutaneous stress response pathways including AhR (arylhydrocarbon receptor) and NFκB [49–51]. For example, the co-occurrence of ARE- and xenobiotic response element- (XRE-)sequences in the promoter region of several AhR-controlled genes (including NQO1 (NAD(P)H quinone oxidoreductase 1) and GST (glutathione-S-transferase) indicates mechanistic crosstalk between NRF2 and AhR at the gene expression level [52]. Likewise, direct AhR binding to XREs located in the NRF2 promoter region has been confirmed by immunoprecipitation analysis, enabling AhR agonists to induce NRF2 expression at the mRNA and protein levels. It has also been demonstrated that protease-activated receptor-2 (PAR-2), an important mediator of inflammation and immune responses by serine proteinases, activates NQO1 via NRF2 stabilization in keratinocytes, suggesting that in addition to induction of inflammation, PAR-2 can play a cytoprotective role that depends on NRF2 [53].

5. NRF2 in Skin Pathology

A substantial body of experimental evidence indicates that NRF2 dysregulation, either due to insufficient adaptive activation in response to environmental stressors or due to constitutive hyperactivation as a result of genetic alterations that may also involve KEAP1, has detrimental effects compromising skin barrier function and stress responses. Seminal research has documented that constitutive epidermal NRF2 overactivation through permanent genetic deletion of KEAP1-caused hyperkeratosis in murine skin [54]. It has also been demonstrated that forced constitutive NRF2 overactivation causes chloracne-like skin disease characterized by acanthosis, hyperkeratosis, and cyst formation in mice [43]. Likewise, oncogenic NRF2 mutations have been detected in squamous cell carcinomas of the esophagus and skin [55–57]. In contrast to compromised skin structure and function that may originate from both impaired NRF2 activation as well as forced hyperactivation, NRF2 activation in healthy skin is transient and subject to extensive feedback regulation and modulatory crosstalk. Pharmacological modulation of NRF2 in skin aiming at a therapeutic, preventive, or regenerative benefit must therefore be performed without causing prolonged hyperactivation of the pathway as has been discussed before [56,58].

Wound healing. Recent research indicates that a glutathione-NRF2-thioredoxin cross-talk enables keratinocyte survival and wound repair through modulation of inflammation, apoptosis, and oxidative stress [59]. Importantly, substantial research has identified an essential role of NRF2 in diabetic wound healing, amenable to therapeutic intervention using small molecule NRF2 activators such as sulforaphane and cinnamaldehyde [32,60].

Psoriasis. In psoriasis, NRF2 is an important driver of keratinocyte proliferation with up-regulation of Keratin 6, Keratin 16, and Keratin 17 [61]. However, NRF2-directed intervention in psoriasis is efficacious since the anti-psoriatic drug monomethylfumarate increases NRF2 levels and induces aquaporin-3 mRNA and protein expression, important for keratinocyte differentiation [62].

Allergic dermatitis. NRF2 activation has been identified as a key event triggered by common skin sensitizers known be cysteine-directed electrophiles [63–66]. However, pharmacological NRF2 activation using ginger-derived 6-shogaol has shown efficacy in allergic dermatitis-like skin lesions through anti-inflammatory redox modulation [67].

Atopic dermatitis. Redox dysregulation is an emerging causative factor contributing to compromised skin barrier function in atopic dermatitis, and pharmacological intervention targeting NRF2 has shown promise targeting atopic dermatitis-like skin lesions in 2,4-dinitrochlorobenzene (DNCB)-sensitized and challenged mice [68,69].

Melanocytic dysfunction. It is now understood that NRF2 also plays an essential role in the maintenance of melanocyte responses to environmental stressors. NRF2 has been implicated in cutaneous pigmentation disorders resulting from redox alterations relevant to vitiligo and stress-induced and chronological hair greying [70–73]. Interestingly, recent evidence suggests that NRF2 plays a role in facilitating glutathione-dependent chemoresistance of malignant melanoma cells [74].

Chronological aging and progeria. Increasing evidence indicates a role of NRF2 in the control of chronological cellular aging [75–77]. Recently, an unanticipated mechanistic role of NRF2 dysfunction as a key contributor to premature aging has been proposed in the genetic premature aging disorder Hutchinson-Gilford progeria syndrome (HGPS), attributed to increased chronic oxidative stress [78,79]. In HGPS, a de novo LMNA (lamin A/C) gene mutation encodes for progerin, a dysfunctional nuclear architectural protein variant of lamin A lacking 50 amino acids. Progerin formation is also observed during normal cellular aging, and chronic UVA exposure has been shown to induce progerin in cultured human dermal fibroblasts [80]. Recent experimental evidence suggests that progerin sequesters NRF2 and thereby causes its subnuclear mislocalization, resulting in impaired NRF2 transcriptional activity and consequently increased chronic oxidative stress. Importantly, reactivation of NRF2 activity in HGPS patient cells reverses progerin-associated nuclear aging defects, suggesting that progerin-dependent repression of NRF2-mediated antioxidant responses is a key factor underlying HGPS-type premature aging with potential relevance to chronological aging and UVA-induced photoaging.

NRF2 in skin photodamage. Recent studies strongly suggest a protective role of NRF2-mediated gene expression in the suppression of cutaneous photodamage induced by solar UV radiation (as evidenced by suppression of UV-induced apoptosis and inflammatory signaling), and NRF2 activation has been shown to protect cutaneous keratinocytes and fibroblasts against the cytotoxic effects of UVA and UVB [16,18,19,31,33,81–88]. Importantly, research performed in SKH-1 mice documents that genetic NRF2 activation protects mice against acute photodamage and photocarcinogenesis [36,89]. Therefore, pharmacological modulation of NRF2 has now attracted considerable attention as a novel approach to skin photoprotection, cancer photochemoprevention, and suppression of skin photoaging [13,33,34,86]. Indeed, protection of primary human keratinocytes from UVB-induced cell death by novel drug-like NRF2 activators has been reported, a photoprotective effect attributed in part to NRF2-dependent elevation of cellular glutathione levels [40,87,90].

Our own studies have demonstrated the photoprotective effects of pharmacological NRF2 activation in cultured human skin cells and reconstructed epidermal skin models [13,31,33]. Topical application of NRF2 inducers, e.g., the synthetic NRF2-activator TBE-31, has shown pronounced photoprotective and photochemopreventive activity in murine skin, and suppression of solar UV-induced human skin erythema was achieved by topical application of a standardized broccoli extract delivering the NRF2 inducer sulforaphane [36]. However, little research has explored the concept of cutaneous photoprotection and photochemoprevention achievable by systemic administration of NRF2 inducers [13,91].

6. Systemic Photoprotection by Dietary NRF2 Activators: Focus on the Apocarotenoid Bixin, an FDA-Approved Food Colorant and Spice Native to Tropical America

The dietary origin of numerous photochemopreventive factors suggests the possibility of achieving efficient skin delivery through oral systemic administration, an emerging concept referred to as 'nutritional' or 'systemic photoprotection' [9]. Indeed, clinical studies document feasibility of human skin photoprotection by dietary intake of lycopene from processed tomato and flavonoid-rich cocoa [10,92–94]. In an attempt to test for the first time the feasibility of NRF2-dependent systemic photoprotection by dietary constituents, we focused our photoprotection studies on the apocarotenoid bixin (Figures 1 and 2), an FDA-approved natural food colorant from the seeds of the achiote tree (*Bixa orellana*) native to tropical America [13,95,96]. A native spice derived from the Americas, annatto is an orange-red condiment and food coloring used to impart a yellow or orange color to signature foods of Latin America and the Caribbean.

Consumed by human populations in the Americas since ancient times, this apocarotenoid, derived from lycopene through oxidative cleavage, is now used worldwide as a spice, food colorant, and cosmetic and pharmaceutical ingredient (referred to as 'annatto'; E160b). Due to its unusual (linear/noncyclic) chemical structure, the apocarotenoid bixin displays characteristics different from all other carotenoids. Specifically, bixin is water soluble, does not display provitamin A activity, and is distinguished by an excellent safety record as well as established systemic bioavailability and pharmacokinetic profile upon oral administration as documented extensively in mice and humans [97–99]. Indeed, bixin is now one of the most consumed food colorants in the world distinguished by a long record of dietary and ethno-pharmacological use [95,96,100]. Chemical activities of bixin as sacrificial antioxidant, free radical scavenger, and efficient physical quencher of photoexcited states including singlet oxygen (surpassed only by lycopene) are documented [101]. Topical preparations of annatto extract have been in ethno-pharmacological use showing therapeutic efficacy for wound healing, mouth ulcers, and other pathologies associated with impaired epithelial barrier function [100,102]. It is also interesting that translational research documents the efficacy of bixin-loaded polycaprolactone nanofibers as an innovative delivery system accelerating wound healing and reducing scar tissue formation in diabetic mice [103]. Moreover, bixin-based systemic protection against environmental toxicants including methylmercury and carbon tetrachloride has been documented in vivo [104,105].

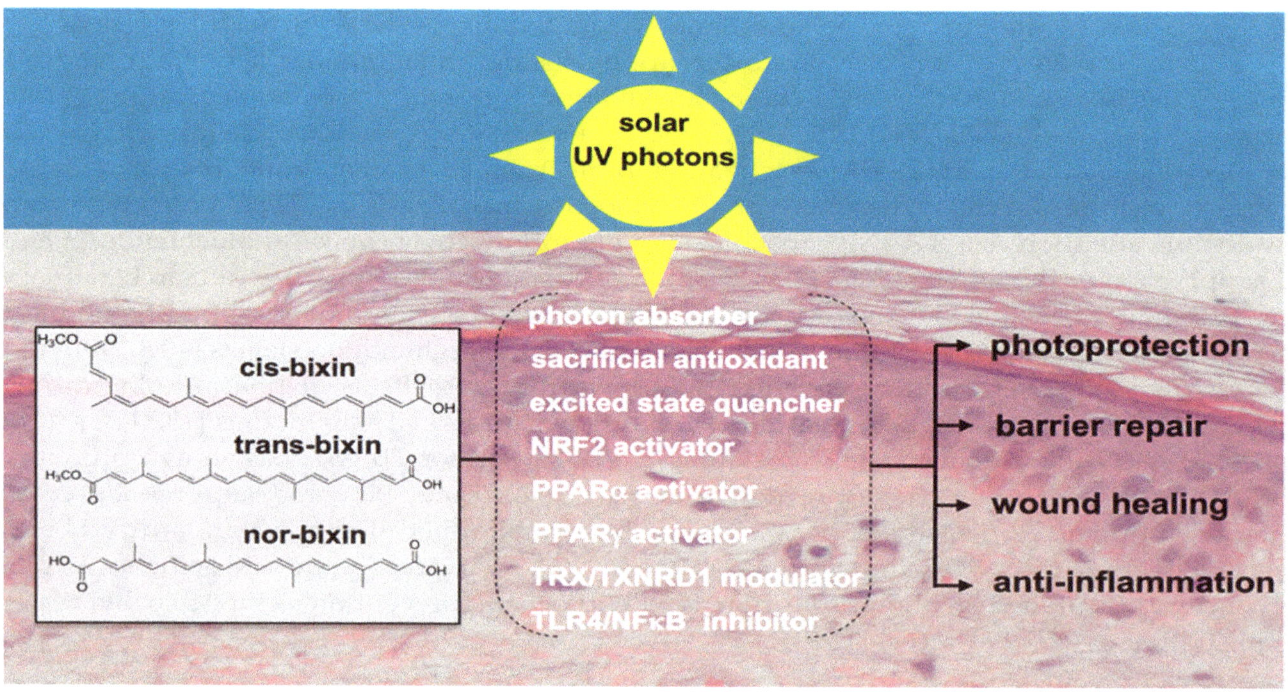

Figure 2. Bixin for improved skin barrier function and photoprotection. Based on pleiotropic activities including direct chemical and NRF2-dependent antioxidant modulation, cis-bixin and its physiologically relevant derivatives trans-bixin and nor-bixin enhance skin barrier structure and function with photoprotective and potentially photochemopreventive efficacy; thioredoxin (TRX), thioredoxin reductase 1 (TXNRD1).

In prior studies, bixin has demonstrated antigenotoxic and antioxidant cytoprotective activities, and systemic availability of oral bixin and its demethylated metabolite norbixin has been documented in rodent studies and healthy human subjects [97,98,106,107]. In long term murine feeding experiments, supplementation levels up to 5% (*w*/*w* food) were well tolerated. Importantly, acceptable daily intake (ADI) over a lifetime without an appreciable health risk (http://apps.who.int/food-additives-contaminants-jecfa-database/search.aspx) surpasses that of any other carotenoid approved as a food additive [ADI (bixin): 12 mg/kg body weight/day] [108].

7. Bixin for NRF2-Dependent Systemic Skin Photoprotection

Bixin was identified as the result of a screen for diet-derived small molecule NRF2 activators targeting oxidative stress and redox dysregulation in epithelial cells [13,109]. Using activity guided fractionation and bio-analytical tools for the quantitative detection of bixin and other small molecule constituents in annatto extracts, we were able to demonstrate that bixin is the active molecular entity in annatto total organic extracts responsible for NRF2 activation. Recently, we have reported for the first time that (i) bixin is a potent activator of the NRF2-dependent cytoprotective response in cultured human skin keratinocytes; (ii) systemic administration of bixin activates cutaneous NRF2 with potent protective effects against solar UV-induced skin damage in SKH-1 mice; and (iii) bixin-induced suppression of photodamage is observable in $Nrf2^{+/+}$ but not in $Nrf2^{-/-}$ SKH-1 mice confirming the NRF2-dependence of bixin-based antioxidant and anti-inflammatory cutaneous effects [13]. Based on its unique status as a FDA-approved food additive with an established safety profile and potent NRF2-inducing activity, we also have investigated and established efficacy of systemic NRF2 activation using intraperitoneal administration of bixin for lung protection against ventilation-induced oxidative stress [110]. Importantly, dietary carotenoids (including β-carotene, lycopene, lutein, 3,3′-dihydroxyisorenieratene, zeaxanthin, astaxanthin) and their biosynthetic precursor molecules (such as phytoene) have been under investigation for epithelial chemoprevention and cutaneous photoprotection before [10,92,111–113], and the systemic photoprotective activity of carotenoids, displayed only after dietary uptake and cutaneous accumulation, has largely been attributed to their activity as photon absorbers, sacrificial antioxidants, and excited state/singlet oxygen quenchers [101,113,114].

Interestingly, it has been shown that astaxanthin and its analogs (such as adonixanthin) activate NRF2, preventing light-induced ocular photoreceptor degeneration [115]. Moreover, fucoxanthin, another marine carotenoid from seaweed, has been shown to enhance the level of reduced glutathione via NRF2 in human keratinocytes [116]. Indeed, prior research has examined the specific mechanism of NRF2 activation by carotenoids, and oxidative metabolism leading to the generation of electrophilic unsaturated mono- and dialdehydes (such 10,10′-diapocarotene-10,10′-dial) has been identified as the mechanistic basis underlying upregulated antioxidant responses [117–119]. The specific structure-activity relationship of NRF2 upregulation by carotenoid-derived electrophilic metabolites has been explored before, and it is therefore likely that bixin-dependent NRF2 activation requires similar oxidative transformation to electrophilic intermediates, a subject of ongoing investigation. However, even though the concept of cutaneous photoprotection achieved by systemic administration of specific carotenoids and other phytochemicals has been explored in the past [10,92,111,112,120–122], prior to our own investigations, no research had investigated the NRF2-dependence of carotenoid-based systemic photoprotection [13]. However, the biological effects of prolonged cutaneous NRF2 activation as a consequence of oral/systemic delivery of a pharmacological molecular agent that may also affect NRF2 regulation in non-cutaneous tissue remain to be elucidated.

8. Other Molecular Targets of Bixin with Relevance to Skin Barrier Function and Protection

Beyond NRF2-directed activities, bixin has been demonstrated to cause specific modulation of the following molecular targets potentially relevant to skin barrier function and environmental stress responses (Figure 2).

8.1. PPARα and PPARγ

Interestingly, peroxisome proliferator-activated receptors (PPARs) have now been recognized as important determinants of keratinocyte responses to skin injury regulating skin homeostasis, epithelial repair, and morphogenesis [123,124]. Specifically, PPARα is a ligand-activated transcription factor that regulates the expression of genes involved in fatty acid oxidation.

Recently, it has been demonstrated that oral administration of bixin improves obesity-induced abnormalities of carbohydrate and lipid metabolism in mice, an affect attributed to PPARα activation confirmed by luciferase reporter assays [125]. Specifically, treatment with bixin- and norbixin-induced PPARα target gene expression upstream of fatty acid oxidation in PPARα-expressing HepG2 hepatocytes. Likewise, in obese KK-Ay mice, chronic nutritional supplementation using bixin suppressed the development of hyperlipidemia and hepatic lipid accumulation with improvement of hyperglycemia, hyperinsulinemia, and hypoadiponectinemia. This effect is consistent with upregulated mRNA expression levels of adiponectin (*ADIPOQ*), an adipocyte-derived adipokine with multiple beneficial effects such as anti-obesity and anti-insulin resistance roles as well as anti-apoptotic, anti-oxidative, and anti-inflammatory activities in skin [124]. Likewise, experimental evidence suggests that bixin also enhances adipocyte insulin sensitivity downstream of PPARγ activation [126]. It is therefore tempting to speculate that the documented beneficial effects of bixin on cutaneous barrier function and wound healing may be in part attributable to PPARα/γ-directed agonism operative in addition to NRF2 activation as discussed above. However, the effects of prolonged pharmacological PPARα- or γ-directed agonism on skin barrier function remain to be explored.

8.2. Thioredoxin/Thioredoxin Reductase

One of the key cellular antioxidant systems is regulated by the selenoproteins thioredoxin (TRX) and thioredoxin reductase (TXNRD1), which use NADPH as an electron donor to reduce oxidized substrates. TXNRD1 contains a very reactive selenocysteine in its active site that is prone to electrophilic or oxidative attack, making it another important sensor of the cellular redox state in addition to KEAP1 [127]. Thus, electrophilic compounds that typically activate NRF2 by KEAP1 cysteine modifications will also inhibit TXNRD1 [127]. The TRX/TXNRD1 system is essential for keratinocyte survival, UV protection, and wound healing [59]. Interestingly, one report indicates that at high (200 μM) concentrations bixin generates ROS, inhibiting both TRX and TXNRD1 with induction of cell death [128]. This could be due to an exacerbated redox imbalance caused by the inability of TRX/TXNRD1 to reduce their substrates, such as peroxiredoxins (PRX), as well as de-repression of proapoptotic proteins, such as apoptosis signaling kinase 1 (ASK1), apoptosis inducing factor (AIF), and caspase 3. Other important substrates of the TRX/TXNRD1 system are PTEN (phosphatase and tensin homolog), NF-κB, AP1 (activator protein 1), and p53 (tumor protein 53), with important implications for regulation of cell survival in response to TRX/TXNRD1 dysruption [129]. Interestingly, it has been proposed that the TRX/TXNRD1 system might reduce the oxidized cysteine residues in KEAP1 to restore its functionality [130]. Dual inactivation of these reactive proteins (KEAP1 and TRX/TXNRD1) could contribute to pronounced NRF2 activation achieved by bixin. However, since TRX and TXNRD1 are NRF2 target genes, reduced proteins might be restored by de novo synthesis and GSH synthesis.

8.3. TLR4/NFκB

It has been observed that nutrional bixin attenuates cardiac injury progression through inhibition of fibrosis, inflammation, and redox dysregulation, cytoprotective effects that were attributed to Toll-like receptor 4/nuclear factor kappa B (TLR4/NF-κB) antagonism in mice [131]. Likewise, bixin antagonized lipopolysaccharide (LPS)-induced pro-inflammatory cytokine over-expression in cultured cardiac muscle cells. Given the emerging importance of TLR4 signaling in skin inflammation and UV-induced photodamage, it is therefore tempting to speculate that nutritional bixin regimens may benefit human skin through TLR4 antagonism operative in addition to NRF2 activation [132,133].

9. Conclusions

The promising concept of achieving cutaneous solar protection through dietary intake of NRF2 activators remains largely unexplored, representing an innovative molecular strategy that deserves further exploration. Building on its excellent safety record as an FDA-approved natural food colorant and additive, its systemic availability upon oral administration in humans, and ability to activate NRF2 in skin, dietary consumption of bixin, an ethno-pharmacologically validated phytochemical originating from the Americas, warrants future preclinical and clinical evaluation for improved skin barrier function and photoprotection.

Acknowledgments: Funding through the following NIH grants contributed to this review: R03CA167580, R03CA212719, ES007091, ES006694.

References

1. Chen, H.; Weng, Q.Y.; Fisher, D.E. UV signaling pathways within the skin. *J. Investig. Dermatol.* **2014**, *134*, 2080–2085. [CrossRef] [PubMed]
2. Natarajan, V.T.; Ganju, P.; Ramkumar, A.; Grover, R.; Gokhale, R.S. Multifaceted pathways protect human skin from UV radiation. *Nat. Chem. Biol.* **2014**, *10*, 542–551. [CrossRef] [PubMed]
3. Brash, D.E. UV signature mutations. *Photochem. Photobiol.* **2015**, *91*, 15–26. [CrossRef] [PubMed]
4. Park, S.L.; Justiniano, R.; Williams, J.D.; Cabello, C.M.; Qiao, S.; Wondrak, G.T. The Tryptophan-Derived Endogenous Aryl Hydrocarbon Receptor Ligand 6-Formylindolo(3,2-b)Carbazole Is a Nanomolar UVA Photosensitizer in Epidermal Keratinocytes. *J. Investig. Dermatol.* **2015**, *135*, 1649–1658. [CrossRef] [PubMed]
5. Liebel, F.; Kaur, S.; Ruvolo, E.; Kollias, N.; Southall, M.D. Irradiation of skin with visible light induces reactive oxygen species and matrix-degrading enzymes. *J. Investig. Dermatol.* **2012**, *132*, 1901–1907. [CrossRef] [PubMed]
6. Nakashima, Y.; Ohta, S.; Wolf, A.M. Blue light-induced oxidative stress in live skin. *Free Radic. Biol. Med.* **2017**, *108*, 300–310. [CrossRef] [PubMed]
7. Schroeder, P.; Calles, C.; Benesova, T.; Macaluso, F.; Krutmann, J. Photoprotection beyond ultraviolet radiation—Effective sun protection has to include protection against infrared A radiation-induced skin damage. *Skin Pharmacol. Physiol.* **2010**, *23*, 15–17. [CrossRef] [PubMed]
8. Zastrow, L.; Groth, N.; Klein, F.; Kockott, D.; Lademann, J.; Renneberg, R.; Ferrero, L. The missing link—Light-induced (280–1600 nm) free radical formation in human skin. *Skin Pharmacol. Physiol.* **2009**, *22*, 31–44. [PubMed]
9. Wondrak, G.T. Sunscreen-Based Skin Protection Against Solar Insult: Molecular Mechanisms and Opportunities. In *Fundamentals of Cancer Prevention*; Alberts, D., Hess, L.M., Eds.; Springer: Berlin/Heidelberg, Garmany, 2014; pp. 301–320.
10. Gonzalez, S.; Astner, S.; An, W.; Goukassian, D.; Pathak, M.A. Dietary lutein/zeaxanthin decreases ultraviolet B-induced epidermal hyperproliferation and acute inflammation in hairless mice. *J. Investig. Dermatol.* **2003**, *121*, 399–405. [CrossRef] [PubMed]
11. Wondrak, G.T.; Jacobson, M.K.; Jacobson, E.L. Endogenous UVA-photosensitizers: Mediators of skin photodamage and novel targets for skin photoprotection. *Photochem. Photobiol. Sci.* **2006**, *5*, 215–237. [CrossRef] [PubMed]
12. Nichols, J.A.; Katiyar, S.K. Skin photoprotection by natural polyphenols: Anti-inflammatory, antioxidant and DNA repair mechanisms. *Arch. Dermatol. Res.* **2010**, *302*, 71–83. [CrossRef] [PubMed]
13. Tao, S.; Park, S.L.; de la Vega, M.R.; Zhang, D.D.; Wondrak, G.T. Systemic administration of the apocarotenoid bixin protects skin against solar UV-induced damage through activation of NRF2. *Free Radic. Biol. Med.* **2015**, *89*, 690–700. [CrossRef] [PubMed]

14. Diffey, B.L.; Norridge, Z. Reported sun exposure, attitudes to sun protection and perceptions of skin cancer risk: A survey of visitors to Cancer Research UK's SunSmart campaign website. *Br. J. Dermatol.* **2009**, *160*, 1292–1298. [CrossRef] [PubMed]
15. Suzuki, T.; Motohashi, H.; Yamamoto, M. Toward clinical application of the Keap1-Nrf2 pathway. *Trends Pharmacol. Sci.* **2013**, *34*, 340–346. [CrossRef] [PubMed]
16. Saw, C.L.; Huang, M.T.; Liu, Y.; Khor, T.O.; Conney, A.H.; Kong, A.N. Impact of Nrf2 on UVB-induced skin inflammation/photoprotection and photoprotective effect of sulforaphane. *Mol. Carcinog.* **2011**, *50*, 479–486. [CrossRef] [PubMed]
17. Ma, Q. Role of nrf2 in oxidative stress and toxicity. *Annu. Rev. Pharmacol. Toxicol.* **2013**, *53*, 401–426. [CrossRef] [PubMed]
18. Schafer, M.; Werner, S. Nrf2-A regulator of keratinocyte redox signaling. *Free Radic. Biol. Med.* **2015**, *88*, 243–252. [CrossRef] [PubMed]
19. Hirota, A.; Kawachi, Y.; Yamamoto, M.; Koga, T.; Hamada, K.; Otsuka, F. Acceleration of UVB-induced photoageing in nrf2 gene-deficient mice. *Exp. Dermatol.* **2011**, *20*, 664–668. [CrossRef] [PubMed]
20. Bosch, R.; Philips, N.; Suarez-Perez, J.A.; Juarranz, A.; Devmurari, A.; Chalensouk-Khaosaat, J.; Gonzalez, S. Mechanisms of Photoaging and Cutaneous Photocarcinogenesis, and Photoprotective Strategies with Phytochemicals. *Antioxidants* **2015**, *4*, 248–268. [CrossRef] [PubMed]
21. Kobayashi, A.; Kang, M.I.; Okawa, H.; Ohtsuji, M.; Zenke, Y.; Chiba, T.; Igarashi, K.; Yamamoto, M. Oxidative stress sensor Keap1 functions as an adaptor for Cul3-based E3 ligase to regulate proteasomal degradation of Nrf2. *Mol. Cell. Biol.* **2004**, *24*, 7130–7139. [CrossRef] [PubMed]
22. Zhang, D.D.; Lo, S.C.; Cross, J.V.; Templeton, D.J.; Hannink, M. Keap1 is a redox-regulated substrate adaptor protein for a Cul3-dependent ubiquitin ligase complex. *Mol. Cell. Biol.* **2004**, *24*, 10941–10953. [CrossRef] [PubMed]
23. Zhang, D.D.; Hannink, M. Distinct cysteine residues in Keap1 are required for Keap1-dependent ubiquitination of Nrf2 and for stabilization of Nrf2 by chemopreventive agents and oxidative stress. *Mol. Cell. Biol.* **2003**, *23*, 8137–8151. [CrossRef] [PubMed]
24. Baird, L.; Lleres, D.; Swift, S.; Dinkova-Kostova, A.T. Regulatory flexibility in the Nrf2-mediated stress response is conferred by conformational cycling of the Keap1-Nrf2 protein complex. *Proc. Natl. Acad. Sci. USA* **2013**, *110*, 15259–15264. [CrossRef] [PubMed]
25. Itoh, K.; Chiba, T.; Takahashi, S.; Ishii, T.; Igarashi, K.; Katoh, Y.; Oyake, T.; Hayashi, N.; Satoh, K.; Hatayama, I.; et al. An Nrf2/small Maf heterodimer mediates the induction of phase II detoxifying enzyme genes through antioxidant response elements. *Biochem. Biophys. Res. Commun.* **1997**, *236*, 313–322. [CrossRef] [PubMed]
26. Komatsu, M.; Kurokawa, H.; Waguri, S.; Taguchi, K.; Kobayashi, A.; Ichimura, Y.; Sou, Y.S.; Ueno, I.; Sakamoto, A.; Tong, K.I.; et al. The selective autophagy substrate p62 activates the stress responsive transcription factor Nrf2 through inactivation of Keap1. *Nat. Cell. Biol.* **2010**, *12*, 213–223. [CrossRef] [PubMed]
27. Lau, A.; Wang, X.J.; Zhao, F.; Villeneuve, N.F.; Wu, T.; Jiang, T.; Sun, Z.; White, E.; Zhang, D.D. A noncanonical mechanism of Nrf2 activation by autophagy deficiency: Direct interaction between Keap1 and p62. *Mol. Cell. Biol.* **2010**, *30*, 3275–3285. [CrossRef] [PubMed]
28. Salazar, M.; Rojo, A.I.; Velasco, D.; de Sagarra, R.M.; Cuadrado, A. Glycogen synthase kinase-3beta inhibits the xenobiotic and antioxidant cell response by direct phosphorylation and nuclear exclusion of the transcription factor Nrf2. *J. Biol. Chem.* **2006**, *281*, 14841–14851. [CrossRef] [PubMed]
29. Chowdhry, S.; Zhang, Y.; McMahon, M.; Sutherland, C.; Cuadrado, A.; Hayes, J.D. Nrf2 is controlled by two distinct beta-TrCP recognition motifs in its Neh6 domain, one of which can be modulated by GSK-3 activity. *Oncogene* **2013**, *32*, 3765–3781. [CrossRef] [PubMed]
30. Li, H.; Gao, A.; Jiang, N.; Liu, Q.; Liang, B.; Li, R.; Zhang, E.; Li, Z.; Zhu, H. Protective Effect of Curcumin Against Acute Ultraviolet B Irradiation-induced Photo-damage. *Photochem. Photobiol.* **2016**, *92*, 808–815. [CrossRef] [PubMed]
31. Wondrak, G.T.; Cabello, C.M.; Villeneuve, N.F.; Zhang, S.; Ley, S.; Li, Y.; Sun, Z.; Zhang, D.D. Cinnamoyl-based Nrf2-activators targeting human skin cell photo-oxidative stress. *Free Radic. Biol. Med.* **2008**, *45*, 385–395. [CrossRef] [PubMed]

32. Long, M.; Rojo de la Vega, M.; Wen, Q.; Bharara, M.; Jiang, T.; Zhang, R.; Zhou, S.; Wong, P.K.; Wondrak, G.T.; Zheng, H.; et al. An Essential Role of NRF2 in Diabetic Wound Healing. *Diabetes* **2016**, *65*, 780–793. [CrossRef] [PubMed]
33. Tao, S.; Justiniano, R.; Zhang, D.D.; Wondrak, G.T. The Nrf2-inducers tanshinone I and dihydrotanshinone protect human skin cells and reconstructed human skin against solar simulated UV. *Redox Biol.* **2013**, *1*, 532–541. [CrossRef] [PubMed]
34. Chun, K.S.; Kundu, J.; Kundu, J.K.; Surh, Y.J. Targeting Nrf2-Keap1 signaling for chemoprevention of skin carcinogenesis with bioactive phytochemicals. *Toxicol. Lett.* **2014**, *229*, 73–84. [CrossRef] [PubMed]
35. Mathew, S.T.; Bergstrom, P.; Hammarsten, O. Repeated Nrf2 stimulation using sulforaphane protects fibroblasts from ionizing radiation. *Toxicol. Appl. Pharmacol.* **2014**, *276*, 188–194. [CrossRef] [PubMed]
36. Knatko, E.V.; Ibbotson, S.H.; Zhang, Y.; Higgins, M.; Fahey, J.W.; Talalay, P.; Dawa, R.; Ferguson, J.; Huang, J.T.; Clarke, R.; et al. Nrf2 activation protects against solar-simulated ultraviolet radiation in mice and humans. *Cancer Prev. Res.* **2015**, *8*, 475–486. [CrossRef] [PubMed]
37. Reisman, S.A.; Goldsberry, A.R.; Lee, C.Y.; O'Grady, M.L.; Proksch, J.W.; Ward, K.W.; Meyer, C.J. Topical application of RTA 408 lotion activates Nrf2 in human skin and is well-tolerated by healthy human volunteers. *BMC Dermatol.* **2015**, *15*, 10. [CrossRef] [PubMed]
38. Nakagami, Y.; Masuda, K. A novel Nrf2 activator from microbial transformation inhibits radiation-induced dermatitis in mice. *J. Radiat. Res.* **2016**, *57*, 567–571. [CrossRef] [PubMed]
39. Ishitsuka, Y.; Huebner, A.J.; Rice, R.H.; Koch, P.J.; Speransky, V.V.; Steven, A.C.; Roop, D.R. Lce1 Family Members Are Nrf2-Target Genes that Are Induced to Compensate for the Loss of Loricrin. *J. Investig. Dermatol.* **2016**, *136*, 1656–1663. [CrossRef] [PubMed]
40. Schafer, M.; Farwanah, H.; Willrodt, A.H.; Huebner, A.J.; Sandhoff, K.; Roop, D.; Hohl, D.; Bloch, W.; Werner, S. Nrf2 links epidermal barrier function with antioxidant defense. *EMBO Mol. Med.* **2012**, *4*, 364–379. [CrossRef] [PubMed]
41. Kumar, V.; Bouameur, J.E.; Bar, J.; Rice, R.H.; Hornig-Do, H.T.; Roop, D.R.; Schwarz, N.; Brodesser, S.; Thiering, S.; Leube, R.E.; et al. A keratin scaffold regulates epidermal barrier formation, mitochondrial lipid composition, and activity. *J. Cell Biol.* **2015**, *211*, 1057–1075. [CrossRef] [PubMed]
42. Huebner, A.J.; Dai, D.; Morasso, M.; Schmidt, E.E.; Schafer, M.; Werner, S.; Roop, D.R. Amniotic fluid activates the nrf2/keap1 pathway to repair an epidermal barrier defect in utero. *Dev. Cell* **2012**, *23*, 1238–1246. [CrossRef] [PubMed]
43. Schafer, M.; Willrodt, A.H.; Kurinna, S.; Link, A.S.; Farwanah, H.; Geusau, A.; Gruber, F.; Sorg, O.; Huebner, A.J.; Roop, D.R.; et al. Activation of Nrf2 in keratinocytes causes chloracne (MADISH)-like skin disease in mice. *EMBO Mol. Med.* **2014**, *6*, 442–457. [CrossRef] [PubMed]
44. Kurinna, S.; Schafer, M.; Ostano, P.; Karouzakis, E.; Chiorino, G.; Bloch, W.; Bachmann, A.; Gay, S.; Garrod, D.; Lefort, K.; et al. A novel Nrf2-miR-29-desmocollin-2 axis regulates desmosome function in keratinocytes. *Nat. Commun.* **2014**, *5*, 5099. [CrossRef] [PubMed]
45. Piao, M.S.; Park, J.J.; Choi, J.Y.; Lee, D.H.; Yun, S.J.; Lee, J.B.; Lee, S.C. Nrf2-dependent and Nrf2-independent induction of phase 2 detoxifying and antioxidant enzymes during keratinocyte differentiation. *Arch. Dermatol. Res.* **2012**, *304*, 387–395. [CrossRef] [PubMed]
46. Jang, J.; Wang, Y.; Kim, H.S.; Lalli, M.A.; Kosik, K.S. Nrf2, a regulator of the proteasome, controls self-renewal and pluripotency in human embryonic stem cells. *Stem Cells* **2014**, *32*, 2616–2625. [CrossRef] [PubMed]
47. Holmstrom, K.M.; Kostov, R.V.; Dinkova-Kostova, A.T. The multifaceted role of Nrf2 in mitochondrial function. *Curr. Opin. Toxicol.* **2016**, *1*, 80–91. [CrossRef] [PubMed]
48. Hawkins, K.E.; Joy, S.; Delhove, J.M.; Kotiadis, V.N.; Fernandez, E.; Fitzpatrick, L.M.; Whiteford, J.R.; King, P.J.; Bolanos, J.P.; Duchen, M.R.; et al. NRF2 Orchestrates the Metabolic Shift during Induced Pluripotent Stem Cell Reprogramming. *Cell Rep.* **2016**, *14*, 1883–1891. [CrossRef] [PubMed]
49. Haarmann-Stemmann, T.; Abel, J.; Fritsche, E.; Krutmann, J. The AhR-Nrf2 pathway in keratinocytes: On the road to chemoprevention? *J. Investig. Dermatol.* **2012**, *132*, 7–9. [CrossRef] [PubMed]
50. Wakabayashi, N.; Slocum, S.L.; Skoko, J.J.; Shin, S.; Kensler, T.W. When NRF2 talks, who's listening? *Antioxid. Redox Signal.* **2010**, *13*, 1649–1663. [CrossRef] [PubMed]
51. Takei, K.; Hashimoto-Hachiya, A.; Takahara, M.; Tsuji, G.; Nakahara, T.; Furue, M. Cynaropicrin attenuates UVB-induced oxidative stress via the AhR-Nrf2-Nqo1 pathway. *Toxicol. Lett.* **2015**, *234*, 74–80. [CrossRef] [PubMed]

52. Miao, W.; Hu, L.; Scrivens, P.J.; Batist, G. Transcriptional regulation of NF-E2 p45-related factor (NRF2) expression by the aryl hydrocarbon receptor-xenobiotic response element signaling pathway: Direct cross-talk between phase I and II drug-metabolizing enzymes. *J. Biol. Chem.* **2005**, *280*, 20340–20348. [CrossRef] [PubMed]
53. Kim, J.Y.; Kim, D.Y.; Son, H.; Kim, Y.J.; Oh, S.H. Protease-activated receptor-2 activates NQO-1 via Nrf2 stabilization in keratinocytes. *J. Dermatol. Sci.* **2014**, *74*, 48–55. [CrossRef] [PubMed]
54. Wakabayashi, N.; Itoh, K.; Wakabayashi, J.; Motohashi, H.; Noda, S.; Takahashi, S.; Imakado, S.; Kotsuji, T.; Otsuka, F.; Roop, D.R.; et al. Keap1-null mutation leads to postnatal lethality due to constitutive Nrf2 activation. *Nat. Genet.* **2003**, *35*, 238–245. [CrossRef] [PubMed]
55. Kim, Y.R.; Oh, J.E.; Kim, M.S.; Kang, M.R.; Park, S.W.; Han, J.Y.; Eom, H.S.; Yoo, N.J.; Lee, S.H. Oncogenic NRF2 mutations in squamous cell carcinomas of oesophagus and skin. *J. Pathol.* **2010**, *220*, 446–451. [CrossRef] [PubMed]
56. Lau, A.; Villeneuve, N.F.; Sun, Z.; Wong, P.K.; Zhang, D.D. Dual roles of Nrf2 in cancer. *Pharmacol. Res.* **2008**, *58*, 262–270. [CrossRef] [PubMed]
57. Wang, X.J.; Sun, Z.; Villeneuve, N.F.; Zhang, S.; Zhao, F.; Li, Y.; Chen, W.; Yi, X.; Zheng, W.; Wondrak, G.T.; et al. Nrf2 enhances resistance of cancer cells to chemotherapeutic drugs, the dark side of Nrf2. *Carcinogenesis* **2008**, *29*, 1235–1243. [CrossRef] [PubMed]
58. Harder, B.; Jiang, T.; Wu, T.; Tao, S.; Rojo de la Vega, M.; Tian, W.; Chapman, E.; Zhang, D.D. Molecular mechanisms of Nrf2 regulation and how these influence chemical modulation for disease intervention. *Biochem. Soc. Trans.* **2015**, *43*, 680–686. [CrossRef] [PubMed]
59. Telorack, M.; Meyer, M.; Ingold, I.; Conrad, M.; Bloch, W.; Werner, S. A Glutathione-Nrf2-Thioredoxin Cross-Talk Ensures Keratinocyte Survival and Efficient Wound Repair. *PLoS Genet.* **2016**, *12*, e1005800. [CrossRef] [PubMed]
60. Zheng, H.; Whitman, S.A.; Wu, W.; Wondrak, G.T.; Wong, P.K.; Fang, D.; Zhang, D.D. Therapeutic potential of Nrf2 activators in streptozotocin-induced diabetic nephropathy. *Diabetes* **2011**, *60*, 3055–3066. [CrossRef] [PubMed]
61. Yang, L.; Fan, X.; Cui, T.; Dang, E.; Wang, G. Nrf2 Promotes Keratinocyte Proliferation in Psoriasis through Up-Regulation of Keratin 6, Keratin 16, and Keratin 17. *J. Investig. Dermatol.* **2017**, *137*, 2168–2176. [CrossRef] [PubMed]
62. Helwa, I.; Choudhary, V.; Chen, X.; Kaddour-Djebbar, I.; Bollag, W.B. Anti-Psoriatic Drug Monomethylfumarate Increases Nuclear Factor Erythroid 2-Related Factor 2 Levels and Induces Aquaporin-3 mRNA and Protein Expression. *J. Pharmacol. Exp. Ther.* **2017**, *362*, 243–253. [CrossRef] [PubMed]
63. Natsch, A. The Nrf2-Keap1-ARE toxicity pathway as a cellular sensor for skin sensitizers—Functional relevance and a hypothesis on innate reactions to skin sensitizers. *Toxicol. Sci.* **2010**, *113*, 284–292. [CrossRef] [PubMed]
64. Delaine, T.; Niklasson, I.B.; Emter, R.; Luthman, K.; Karlberg, A.T.; Natsch, A. Structure-activity relationship between the in vivo skin sensitizing potency of analogues of phenyl glycidyl ether and the induction of Nrf2-dependent luciferase activity in the KeratinoSens in vitro assay. *Chem. Res. Toxicol.* **2011**, *24*, 1312–1318. [CrossRef] [PubMed]
65. Natsch, A.; Emter, R. Nrf2 activation as a key event triggered by skin sensitisers: The development of the stable KeratinoSens reporter gene assay. *Altern. Lab. Anim.* **2016**, *44*, 443–451. [PubMed]
66. El Ali, Z.; Delomenie, C.; Botton, J.; Pallardy, M.; Kerdine-Romer, S. Dendritic cells' death induced by contact sensitizers is controlled by Nrf2 and depends on glutathione levels. *Toxicol. Appl. Pharmacol.* **2017**, *322*, 41–50. [CrossRef] [PubMed]
67. Park, G.; Oh, D.S.; Lee, M.G.; Lee, C.E.; Kim, Y.U. 6-Shogaol, an active compound of ginger, alleviates allergic dermatitis-like skin lesions via cytokine inhibition by activating the Nrf2 pathway. *Toxicol. Appl. Pharmacol.* **2016**, *310*, 51–59. [CrossRef] [PubMed]
68. Akram, M.; Shin, I.; Kim, K.A.; Noh, D.; Baek, S.H.; Chang, S.Y.; Kim, H.; Bae, O.N. A newly synthesized macakurzin C-derivative attenuates acute and chronic skin inflammation: The Nrf2/heme oxygenase signaling as a potential target. *Toxicol. Appl. Pharmacol.* **2016**, *307*, 62–71. [CrossRef] [PubMed]
69. Choi, J.H.; Jin, S.W.; Han, E.H.; Park, B.H.; Kim, H.G.; Khanal, T.; Hwang, Y.P.; Do, M.T.; Lee, H.S.; Chung, Y.C.; et al. Platycodon grandiflorum root-derived saponins attenuate atopic dermatitis-like skin

lesions via suppression of NF-kappaB and STAT1 and activation of Nrf2/ARE-mediated heme oxygenase-1. *Phytomedicine* **2014**, *21*, 1053–1061. [CrossRef] [PubMed]

70. Marrot, L.; Jones, C.; Perez, P.; Meunier, J.R. The significance of Nrf2 pathway in (photo)-oxidative stress response in melanocytes and keratinocytes of the human epidermis. *Pigment Cell Melanoma Res.* **2008**, *21*, 79–88. [CrossRef] [PubMed]
71. Denat, L.; Kadekaro, A.L.; Marrot, L.; Leachman, S.A.; Abdel-Malek, Z.A. Melanocytes as instigators and victims of oxidative stress. *J. Investig. Dermatol.* **2014**, *134*, 1512–1518. [CrossRef] [PubMed]
72. Jadkauskaite, L.; Coulombe, P.A.; Schafer, M.; Dinkova-Kostova, A.T.; Paus, R.; Haslam, I.S. Oxidative stress management in the hair follicle: Could targeting NRF2 counter age-related hair disorders and beyond? *Bioessays* **2017**, *39*. [CrossRef] [PubMed]
73. Jian, Z.; Li, K.; Song, P.; Zhu, G.; Zhu, L.; Cui, T.; Liu, B.; Tang, L.; Wang, X.; Wang, G.; Gao, T.; Li, C. Impaired activation of the Nrf2-ARE signaling pathway undermines H_2O_2-induced oxidative stress response: A possible mechanism for melanocyte degeneration in vitiligo. *J. Investig. Dermatol.* **2014**, *134*, 2221–2230. [CrossRef] [PubMed]
74. Rocha, C.R.; Kajitani, G.S.; Quinet, A.; Fortunato, R.S.; Menck, C.F. NRF2 and glutathione are key resistance mediators to temozolomide in glioma and melanoma cells. *Oncotarget* **2016**, *7*, 48081–48092. [CrossRef] [PubMed]
75. Kubo, E.; Chhunchha, B.; Singh, P.; Sasaki, H.; Singh, D.P. Sulforaphane reactivates cellular antioxidant defense by inducing Nrf2/ARE/Prdx6 activity during aging and oxidative stress. *Sci. Rep.* **2017**, *7*, 14130. [CrossRef] [PubMed]
76. Bruns, D.R.; Drake, J.C.; Biela, L.M.; Peelor, F.F., 3rd; Miller, B.F.; Hamilton, K.L. Nrf2 Signaling and the Slowed Aging Phenotype: Evidence from Long-Lived Models. *Oxid. Med. Cell. Longev.* **2015**, *2015*, 732596. [CrossRef] [PubMed]
77. Zhang, H.; Davies, K.J.A.; Forman, H.J. Oxidative stress response and Nrf2 signaling in aging. *Free Radic. Biol. Med.* **2015**, *88*, 314–336. [CrossRef] [PubMed]
78. Kubben, N.; Zhang, W.; Wang, L.; Voss, T.C.; Yang, J.; Qu, J.; Liu, G.H.; Misteli, T. Repression of the Antioxidant NRF2 Pathway in Premature Aging. *Cell* **2016**, *165*, 1361–1374. [CrossRef] [PubMed]
79. Gorbunova, V.; Rezazadeh, S.; Seluanov, A. Dangerous Entrapment for NRF2. *Cell* **2016**, *165*, 1312–1313. [CrossRef] [PubMed]
80. Takeuchi, H.; Runger, T.M. Longwave UV light induces the aging-associated progerin. *J. Investig. Dermatol.* **2013**, *133*, 1857–1862. [CrossRef] [PubMed]
81. Hirota, A.; Kawachi, Y.; Itoh, K.; Nakamura, Y.; Xu, X.; Banno, T.; Takahashi, T.; Yamamoto, M.; Otsuka, F. Ultraviolet A irradiation induces NF-E2-related factor 2 activation in dermal fibroblasts: Protective role in UVA-induced apoptosis. *J. Investig. Dermatol.* **2005**, *124*, 825–832. [CrossRef] [PubMed]
82. Dinkova-Kostova, A.T.; Jenkins, S.N.; Fahey, J.W.; Ye, L.; Wehage, S.L.; Liby, K.T.; Stephenson, K.K.; Wade, K.L.; Talalay, P. Protection against UV-light-induced skin carcinogenesis in SKH-1 high-risk mice by sulforaphane-containing broccoli sprout extracts. *Cancer Lett.* **2006**, *240*, 243–252. [CrossRef] [PubMed]
83. Benedict, A.L.; Knatko, E.V.; Dinkova-Kostova, A.T. The indirect antioxidant sulforaphane protects against thiopurine-mediated photooxidative stress. *Carcinogenesis* **2012**, *33*, 2457–2466. [CrossRef] [PubMed]
84. Gruber, F.; Mayer, H.; Lengauer, B.; Mlitz, V.; Sanders, J.M.; Kadl, A.; Bilban, M.; de Martin, R.; Wagner, O.; Kensler, T.W.; et al. NF-E2-related factor 2 regulates the stress response to UVA-1-oxidized phospholipids in skin cells. *FASEB J.* **2010**, *24*, 39–48. [CrossRef] [PubMed]
85. Tian, F.F.; Zhang, F.F.; Lai, X.D.; Wang, L.J.; Yang, L.; Wang, X.; Singh, G.; Zhong, J.L. Nrf2-mediated protection against UVA radiation in human skin keratinocytes. *Biosci. Trends* **2011**, *5*, 23–29. [CrossRef] [PubMed]
86. Kalra, S.; Knatko, E.V.; Zhang, Y.; Honda, T.; Yamamoto, M.; Dinkova-Kostova, A.T. Highly potent activation of Nrf2 by topical tricyclic bis(cyano enone): Implications for protection against UV radiation during thiopurine therapy. *Cancer Prev. Res.* **2012**, *5*, 973–981. [CrossRef] [PubMed]
87. Schafer, M.; Dutsch, S.; auf dem Keller, U.; Navid, F.; Schwarz, A.; Johnson, D.A.; Johnson, J.A.; Werner, S. Nrf2 establishes a glutathione-mediated gradient of UVB cytoprotection in the epidermis. *Genes Dev.* **2010**, *24*, 1045–1058. [CrossRef] [PubMed]

88. Rolfs, F.; Huber, M.; Kuehne, A.; Kramer, S.; Haertel, E.; Muzumdar, S.; Wagner, J.; Tanner, Y.; Bohm, F.; Smola, S.; et al. Nrf2 Activation Promotes Keratinocyte Survival during Early Skin Carcinogenesis via Metabolic Alterations. *Cancer Res.* **2015**, *75*, 4817–4829. [CrossRef] [PubMed]
89. Knatko, E.V.; Higgins, M.; Fahey, J.W.; Dinkova-Kostova, A.T. Loss of Nrf2 abrogates the protective effect of Keap1 downregulation in a preclinical model of cutaneous squamous cell carcinoma. *Sci. Rep.* **2016**, *6*, 25804. [CrossRef] [PubMed]
90. Lieder, F.; Reisen, F.; Geppert, T.; Sollberger, G.; Beer, H.D.; auf dem Keller, U.; Schafer, M.; Detmar, M.; Schneider, G.; Werner, S. Identification of UV-protective activators of nuclear factor erythroid-derived 2-related factor 2 (Nrf2) by combining a chemical library screen with computer-based virtual screening. *J. Biol. Chem.* **2012**, *287*, 33001–33013. [CrossRef] [PubMed]
91. Dinkova-Kostova, A.T.; Fahey, J.W.; Benedict, A.L.; Jenkins, S.N.; Ye, L.; Wehage, S.L.; Talalay, P. Dietary glucoraphanin-rich broccoli sprout extracts protect against UV radiation-induced skin carcinogenesis in SKH-1 hairless mice. *Photochem. Photobiol. Sci.* **2010**, *9*, 597–600. [CrossRef] [PubMed]
92. Sies, H.; Stahl, W. Nutritional Protection Against Skin Damage From Sunlight. *Annu. Rev. Nutr.* **2004**, *24*, 173–200. [CrossRef] [PubMed]
93. Heinrich, U.; Neukam, K.; Tronnier, H.; Sies, H.; Stahl, W. Long-term ingestion of high flavanol cocoa provides photoprotection against UV-induced erythema and improves skin condition in women. *J. Nutr.* **2006**, *136*, 1565–1569. [PubMed]
94. Stahl, W.; Heinrich, U.; Wiseman, S.; Eichler, O.; Sies, H.; Tronnier, H. Dietary tomato paste protects against ultraviolet light-induced erythema in humans. *J. Nutr.* **2001**, *131*, 1449–1451. [PubMed]
95. Ulbricht, C.; Windsor, R.C.; Brigham, A.; Bryan, J.K.; Conquer, J.; Costa, D.; Giese, N.; Guilford, J.; Higdon, E.R.; Holmes, K.; et al. An evidence-based systematic review of annatto (*Bixa orellana* L.) by the Natural Standard Research Collaboration. *J. Diet. Suppl.* **2012**, *9*, 57–77. [CrossRef] [PubMed]
96. Stohs, S.J. Safety and efficacy of Bixa orellana (achiote, annatto) leaf extracts. *Phytother. Res.* **2014**, *28*, 956–960. [CrossRef] [PubMed]
97. Levy, L.W.; Regalado, E.; Navarrete, S.; Watkins, R.H. Bixin and norbixin in human plasma: Determination and study of the absorption of a single dose of Annatto food color. *Analyst* **1997**, *122*, 977–980. [CrossRef] [PubMed]
98. Junior, A.C.; Asad, L.M.; Oliveira, E.B.; Kovary, K.; Asad, N.R.; Felzenszwalb, I. Antigenotoxic and antimutagenic potential of an annatto pigment (norbixin) against oxidative stress. *Genet. Mol. Res.* **2005**, *4*, 94–99. [PubMed]
99. World Health Organization. Evaluation of certain food additives and contaminants. *World Health Organ. Tech. Rep. Ser.* **2013**, *983*, 1–75.
100. Vilar Dde, A.; Vilar, M.S.; de Lima e Moura, T.F.; Raffin, F.N.; de Oliveira, M.R.; Franco, C.F.; de Athayde-Filho, P.F.; Diniz Mde, F.; Barbosa-Filho, J.M. Traditional uses, chemical constituents, and biological activities of *Bixa orellana* L.: A review. *Sci. World J.* **2014**, *2014*, 857292.
101. Di Mascio, P.; Kaiser, S.; Sies, H. Lycopene as the most efficient biological carotenoid singlet oxygen quencher. *Arch. Biochem. Biophys.* **1989**, *274*, 532–538. [CrossRef]
102. Piva, R.M.; Johann, A.C.; Costa, C.K.; Miguel, O.G.; Rosa, E.R.; de Azevedo-Alanis, L.R.; Trevilatto, P.C.; Ignacio, S.A.; Bettega, P.V.; Gregio, A.M. Bixin action in the healing process of rats mouth wounds. *Curr. Pharm. Biotechnol.* **2013**, *14*, 785–791. [CrossRef] [PubMed]
103. Pinzon-Garcia, A.D.; Cassini-Vieira, P.; Ribeiro, C.C.; de Matos Jensen, C.E.; Barcelos, L.S.; Cortes, M.E.; Sinisterra, R.D. Efficient cutaneous wound healing using bixin-loaded PCL nanofibers in diabetic mice. *J. Biomed. Mater. Res. B Appl. Biomater.* **2017**, *105*, 1938–1949. [CrossRef] [PubMed]
104. Barcelos, G.R.; Grotto, D.; Serpeloni, J.M.; Aissa, A.F.; Antunes, L.M.; Knasmuller, S.; Barbosa, F., Jr. Bixin and norbixin protect against DNA-damage and alterations of redox status induced by methylmercury exposure in vivo. *Environ. Mol. Mutagen.* **2012**, *53*, 535–541. [CrossRef] [PubMed]
105. Moreira, P.R.; Maioli, M.A.; Medeiros, H.C.; Guelfi, M.; Pereira, F.T.; Mingatto, F.E. Protective effect of bixin on carbon tetrachloride-induced hepatotoxicity in rats. *Biol. Res.* **2014**, *47*, 49. [CrossRef] [PubMed]
106. Somacal, S.; Figueiredo, C.G.; Quatrin, A.; Ruviaro, A.R.; Conte, L.; Augusti, P.R.; Roehrs, M.; Denardin, I.T.; Kasten, J.; da Veiga, M.L.; et al. The antiatherogenic effect of bixin in hypercholesterolemic rabbits is associated to the improvement of lipid profile and to its antioxidant and anti-inflammatory effects. *Mol. Cell. Biochem.* **2015**, *403*, 243–253. [CrossRef] [PubMed]

107. Roehrs, M.; Figueiredo, C.G.; Zanchi, M.M.; Bochi, G.V.; Moresco, R.N.; Quatrin, A.; Somacal, S.; Conte, L.; Emanuelli, T. Bixin and norbixin have opposite effects on glycemia, lipidemia, and oxidative stress in streptozotocin-induced diabetic rats. *Int. J. Endocrinol.* **2014**, *2014*, 839095. [CrossRef] [PubMed]
108. WHO (World Health Organization). Evaluation of Certain Food Additives and Contaminants. Thirty-fifth report of the Joint FAO/WHO Expert Committee on Food Additives. *Tech. Rep. Ser.* **1990**, *789*, 1–48.
109. Long, M.; Tao, S.; Rojo de la Vega, M.; Jiang, T.; Wen, Q.; Park, S.L.; Zhang, D.D.; Wondrak, G.T. Nrf2-dependent suppression of azoxymethane/dextran sulfate sodium-induced colon carcinogenesis by the cinnamon-derived dietary factor cinnamaldehyde. *Cancer Prev. Res.* **2015**, *8*, 444–454. [CrossRef] [PubMed]
110. Tao, S.; Rojo de la Vega, M.; Quijada, H.; Wondrak, G.T.; Wang, T.; Garcia, J.G.; Zhang, D.D. Bixin protects mice against ventilation-induced lung injury in an NRF2-dependent manner. *Sci. Rep.* **2016**, *6*, 18760. [CrossRef] [PubMed]
111. Astner, S.; Wu, A.; Chen, J.; Philips, N.; Rius-Diaz, F.; Parrado, C.; Mihm, M.C.; Goukassian, D.A.; Pathak, M.A.; Gonzalez, S. Dietary lutein/zeaxanthin partially reduces photoaging and photocarcinogenesis in chronically UVB-irradiated Skh-1 hairless mice. *Skin Pharmacol. Physiol.* **2007**, *20*, 283–291. [CrossRef] [PubMed]
112. Stahl, W.; Sies, H. beta-Carotene and other carotenoids in protection from sunlight. *Am. J. Clin. Nutr.* **2012**, *96*, 1179S–1184S. [CrossRef] [PubMed]
113. Fernandez-Garcia, E. Skin protection against UV light by dietary antioxidants. *Food Funct.* **2014**, *5*, 1994–2003. [CrossRef] [PubMed]
114. Di Mascio, P.; Devasagayam, T.P.; Kaiser, S.; Sies, H. Carotenoids, tocopherols and thiols as biological singlet molecular oxygen quenchers. *Biochem. Soc. Trans.* **1990**, *18*, 1054–1056. [CrossRef] [PubMed]
115. Inoue, Y.; Shimazawa, M.; Nagano, R.; Kuse, Y.; Takahashi, K.; Tsuruma, K.; Hayashi, M.; Ishibashi, T.; Maoka, T.; Hara, H. Astaxanthin analogs, adonixanthin and lycopene, activate Nrf2 to prevent light-induced photoreceptor degeneration. *J. Pharmacol. Sci.* **2017**, *134*, 147–157. [CrossRef] [PubMed]
116. Zheng, J.; Piao, M.J.; Kim, K.C.; Yao, C.W.; Cha, J.W.; Hyun, J.W. Fucoxanthin enhances the level of reduced glutathione via the Nrf2-mediated pathway in human keratinocytes. *Mar. Drugs* **2014**, *12*, 4214–4230. [CrossRef] [PubMed]
117. Ben-Dor, A.; Steiner, M.; Gheber, L.; Danilenko, M.; Dubi, N.; Linnewiel, K.; Zick, A.; Sharoni, Y.; Levy, J. Carotenoids activate the antioxidant response element transcription system. *Mol. Cancer Ther.* **2005**, *4*, 177–186. [PubMed]
118. Linnewiel, K.; Ernst, H.; Caris-Veyrat, C.; Ben-Dor, A.; Kampf, A.; Salman, H.; Danilenko, M.; Levy, J.; Sharoni, Y. Structure activity relationship of carotenoid derivatives in activation of the electrophile/antioxidant response element transcription system. *Free Radic. Biol. Med.* **2009**, *47*, 659–667. [CrossRef] [PubMed]
119. Linnewiel-Hermoni, K.; Khanin, M.; Danilenko, M.; Zango, G.; Amosi, Y.; Levy, J.; Sharoni, Y. The anti-cancer effects of carotenoids and other phytonutrients resides in their combined activity. *Arch. Biochem. Biophys.* **2015**, *572*, 28–35. [CrossRef] [PubMed]
120. Vayalil, P.K.; Mittal, A.; Hara, Y.; Elmets, C.A.; Katiyar, S.K. Green tea polyphenols prevent ultraviolet light-induced oxidative damage and matrix metalloproteinases expression in mouse skin. *J. Investig. Dermatol.* **2004**, *122*, 1480–1487. [CrossRef] [PubMed]
121. Gonzalez, S.; Gilaberte, Y.; Philips, N. Mechanistic insights in the use of a Polypodium leucotomos extract as an oral and topical photoprotective agent. *Photochem. Photobiol. Sci.* **2010**, *9*, 559–563. [CrossRef] [PubMed]
122. Chen, A.C.; Damian, D.L.; Halliday, G.M. Oral and systemic photoprotection. *Photodermatol. Photoimmunol. Photomed.* **2014**, *30*, 102–111. [CrossRef] [PubMed]
123. Icre, G.; Wahli, W.; Michalik, L. Functions of the peroxisome proliferator-activated receptor (PPAR) alpha and beta in skin homeostasis, epithelial repair, and morphogenesis. *J. Investig. Dermatol. Symp. Proc.* **2006**, *11*, 30–35. [CrossRef] [PubMed]
124. Kim, E.J.; Lee, D.H.; Kim, Y.K.; Eun, H.C.; Chung, J.H. Adiponectin Deficiency Contributes to Sensitivity in Human Skin. *J. Investig. Dermatol.* **2015**, *135*, 2331–2334. [CrossRef] [PubMed]
125. Goto, T.; Takahashi, N.; Kato, S.; Kim, Y.I.; Kusudo, T.; Taimatsu, A.; Egawa, K.; Kang, M.S.; Hiramatsu, T.; Sakamoto, T.; et al. Bixin activates PPARalpha and improves obesity-induced abnormalities of carbohydrate and lipid metabolism in mice. *J. Agric. Food Chem.* **2012**, *60*, 11952–11958. [CrossRef] [PubMed]

126. Takahashi, N.; Goto, T.; Taimatsu, A.; Egawa, K.; Katoh, S.; Kusudo, T.; Sakamoto, T.; Ohyane, C.; Lee, J.Y.; Kim, Y.I.; et al. Bixin regulates mRNA expression involved in adipogenesis and enhances insulin sensitivity in 3T3-L1 adipocytes through PPARgamma activation. *Biochem. Biophys. Res. Commun.* **2009**, *390*, 1372–1376. [CrossRef] [PubMed]
127. Cebula, M.; Schmidt, E.E.; Arner, E.S. TrxR1 as a potent regulator of the Nrf2-Keap1 response system. *Antioxid. Redox Signal.* **2015**, *23*, 823–853. [CrossRef] [PubMed]
128. Tibodeau, J.D.; Isham, C.R.; Bible, K.C. Annatto constituent cis-bixin has selective antimyeloma effects mediated by oxidative stress and associated with inhibition of thioredoxin and thioredoxin reductase. *Antioxid. Redox Signal.* **2010**, *13*, 987–997. [CrossRef] [PubMed]
129. Zhang, J.; Li, X.; Han, X.; Liu, R.; Fang, J. Targeting the Thioredoxin System for Cancer Therapy. *Trends Pharmacol. Sci.* **2017**, *38*, 794–808. [CrossRef] [PubMed]
130. Dinkova-Kostova, A.T.; Kostov, R.V.; Canning, P. Keap1, the cysteine-based mammalian intracellular sensor for electrophiles and oxidants. *Arch. Biochem. Biophys.* **2017**, *617*, 84–93. [CrossRef] [PubMed]
131. Xu, Z.; Kong, X.Q. Bixin ameliorates high fat diet-induced cardiac injury in mice through inflammation and oxidative stress suppression. *Biomed. Pharmacother.* **2017**, *89*, 991–1004. [CrossRef] [PubMed]
132. Dickinson, S.E.; Wondrak, G.T. TLR4-directed Molecular Strategies Targeting Skin Photodamage and Carcinogenesis. *Curr. Med. Chem.* **2017**. [CrossRef] [PubMed]
133. Janda, J.; Burkett, N.B.; Blohm-Mangone, K.; Huang, V.; Curiel-Lewandrowski, C.; Alberts, D.S.; Petricoin, E.F., 3rd; Calvert, V.S.; Einspahr, J.; Dong, Z.; et al. Resatorvid-based Pharmacological Antagonism of Cutaneous TLR4 Blocks UV-induced NF-kappaB and AP-1 Signaling in Keratinocytes and Mouse Skin. *Photochem. Photobiol.* **2016**, *92*, 816–825. [CrossRef] [PubMed]

8

Dietary Management of Skin Health: The Role of Genistein

Natasha Irrera [1,†], Gabriele Pizzino [1,†], Rosario D'Anna [2], Mario Vaccaro [1], Vincenzo Arcoraci [1], Francesco Squadrito [1,*], Domenica Altavilla [3] and Alessandra Bitto [1]

1 Department of Clinical and Experimental Medicine, University of Messina, Messina 98125, Italy; nirrera@unime.it (N.I.); cgpizzino@unime.it (G.P.); vaccaro@unime.it (M.V.); varcoraci@unime.it (V.A.); abitto@unime.it (A.B.)
2 Department of Human Pathology, University of Messina, Messina 98125, Italy; rdanna@unime.it
3 Department of Biomedical Sciences, Dentistry and Morphological and Functional Images, University of Messina, Messina 98125, Italy; daltavilla@unime.it
* Correspondence: fsquadrito@unime.it
† N.I. and G.P. equally contributed to this paper.

Abstract: In women, aging and declining estrogen levels are associated with several cutaneous changes, many of which can be reversed or improved by estrogen supplementation. Two estrogen receptors—α and β—have been cloned and found in various tissue types. Epidermal thinning, declining dermal collagen content, diminished skin moisture, decreased laxity, and impaired wound healing have been reported in postmenopausal women. Experimental and clinical studies in postmenopausal conditions indicate that estrogen deprivation is associated with dryness, atrophy, fine wrinkling, and poor wound healing. The isoflavone genistein binds to estrogen receptor β and has been reported to improve skin changes. This review article will focus on the effects of genistein on skin health.

Keywords: genistein; skin; estrogen receptor beta

1. Introduction

Aging is associated with a reduction in skin thickness and in the number of epithelial cells, with a concurrent decrease in stromal collagen [1]. The skin ageing process may intensify after menopause, and estrogen deficiency seems to have a direct effect on the epidermis. It seems that estrogen stimulation could encourage the proliferation of keratinocytes, leading to thickening of the epidermis, preventing its atrophy [2]. In the dermis, blood vessels would be stimulated again, and fibroblast production would also be stepped up, thus preserving the components that they secrete (e.g., collagen, elastic fibres, and glycosaminoglycans) [2,3]. Estrogen exerts its actions through two different receptors (estrogen receptors, ERs), also found in the skin. Both ERs are distinct proteins encoded by separate genes on different chromosomes. ERβ is located on human chromosome 14, whereas ERα is found on chromosome 6. Ligand binding activates the receptors that act as transcription factors by binding conserved estrogen response elements in the regulatory regions of target genes. Interestingly, many genes that are induced by estrogens lack estrogen response elements, including epidermal growth factor, epidermal growth factor receptor, and the cell cycle-associated cyclin D1. These genes belong to the group of secondary estrogen responsive genes, and estrogen affects their transcription/expression through activation of cytoplasmic signaling pathways such as Src/Shc/ERK. These secondary messengers are known to be activated by many transmembrane tyrosine kinase growth factor receptors, suggesting that estrogen effect may sometimes augment growth factor receptor activation [4]. In some cells, ERβ counteracts ERα, in some cases acting as an ERα heterodimer to inhibit the transactivating function of ERα, and in other cases acting as a homodimer to regulate specific genes, many of which are anti-proliferative [5]. The binding of estrogens to the ERs triggers specific responses in terms of proliferation activation and apoptosis arrest; nonetheless, some estrogen actions require the intervention of other hormones, such as progesterone and androgens. The variation in the distribution of receptors within the skin suggests that each has a different, cell-specific role. ERβ is the predominant estrogen receptor in adult human skin; it is strongly expressed in the stratum basale and stratum spinosum of the epidermis [6,7]. The same receptor is also found activated in fibroblasts from female skin, suggesting a strong involvement of ERβ in maintaining skin homeostasis [7]. Furthermore, estrogens prolong the anagen phase of scalp hair growth by increasing cell proliferation rates and postponing their transition to the telogen phase. ERα expression is limited to the dermal papilla cells of the hair follicle, whereas ERβ is found in the outer root sheath cells, epithelial matrix cells, dermal papilla cells, and the cells of the specialized bulge region of the outer root sheath [8]. It has been collectively demonstrated that ERα expression is quite low in the epidermis, while ERβ is abundantly represented.

Considering the presence and distribution of estrogen receptors within the skin and its annexes, it is not difficult to understand that hormone replacement therapy (HRT) can improve the menopause-related alterations. However, given the serious side effects of HRT (e.g., an increased risk of blood clots and certain types of cancer), a number of alternatives have been explored during the last decades, and the most intriguing seems to be the use of phytoestrogens. Isoflavones and lignans are the two main groups of phytoestrogens; their activity is generally weaker than endogenous estrogens, and they are not stored within the tissues [9]. Many phytoestrogens possess both agonist and antagonist estrogen properties, and their estrogenic activity is demonstrated through interaction with both ERα and ERβ [10]. Genistein (5,7,4′-trihydroxyisoflavone) is an isoflavone abundantly found in soy and other legumes, and acts as a selective estrogen receptor modulator (SERM), mainly binding to ERβ [11]. Genistein has a ~30-fold higher affinity for ERβ than ERα; when genistein is bound to ERβ, helix 12 does not adopt an agonist conformation, but instead has a position more similar to that seen with an antagonist. This result is unexpected because the molecular shape and volume of genistein and estradiol are very similar, and because genistein is a partial (60–70% of E2) agonist of ERβ. The conformation of helix 12 in the ERβ-genistein structure may account for the different effects exerted by genistein compared to estradiol.

Besides the specific estrogen receptor-related effects, genistein also acts as an antioxidant and as a specific inhibitor of tyrosine kinases, affecting many signaling pathways [12]. Genistein—as with all the other isoflavones—exists in two different forms: the glycosylated (genistin) and the aglycone (genistein). The aglycone genistein is absorbed from the intestine and conjugated with glucuronic acid during transport across the intestinal epithelial cells. After transport to the liver, the glucuronide may be excreted in the bile, whereafter it could re-enter the small intestine, allowing genistein to be deconjugated, absorbed, and metabolized for the second time [13]. In vivo bioavailability of genistein and its glycoside genistin indicates that genistein is readily bioavailable, while the glycoside derivative is poorly absorbed in the small intestine due to the higher molecular weight and hydrophilicity [14]. For this reason, the most studied form of genistein is the aglycone, which so far has been used in preclinical and clinical studies. Genistein supplementation in postmenopausal women is quite popular; in fact, several nutraceutical preparations have been launched in the market with very different amounts of genistein alone or combined with other isoflavones. However, the beneficial effects of genistein on menopausal features can be achieved at very specific dosage (54 mg/day), and only few preparations fulfill this requirement. In this review article are summarized the main effects of genistein on skin health from preclinical and clinical observations. This is a narrative review focusing on studies performed using genistein in vitro or in vivo to demonstrate an effect on skin. As search terms on Pubmed, we used "genistein and skin", "genistein and fibroblast", "genistein and wound healing", and we selected all those articles with available full text. As a further criterion, articles using mixes of isoflavones without clear indications of genistein's dose were not included.

2. In Vitro Evidence

2.1. Genistein Effects on Fibroblasts

Wound healing and scar formation are dynamic biological processes involving numerous cell–cell and cell–matrix interactions in a complex milieu of both local and systemic influences. In abnormal hyper-proliferating fibroblasts from hypertrophic scars, an important role is played by altered growth factors expression, dysfunctional receptors, and tyrosine kinase signaling dysregulation [15]. Fibroblasts obtained from hypertrophic burn scars were cultured with genistein at different concentrations (25, 50, 100 μmol/L) to inhibit their growth and proliferation through the blockade of the RAS (Rat sarcoma), Raf, ERK, and p38 proteins [16]. Genistein inhibited cell proliferation and activity by affecting nuclear translocation of phosphorylated ERK molecules; ERK mainly regulates cell proliferation, growth, and differentiation, while p38 is mainly related to stress and inflammatory reactions. These pathways are interconnected, and genistein may exert its suppressing effects on cells' proliferation by interfering with them [16].

Abnormal scarring can also result in keloid formation, characterized by an imbalanced extracellular matrix (ECM) synthesis and degradation, a CTGF (connective tissue growth factor)-dependent fibroblast proliferation, and resistance to apoptosis. Normal human dermal fibroblasts (NHDF, Adult) and keloid fibroblasts (KEL FIB) were tested with different concentrations of genistein; the keloid fibroblast culture revealed an increase of CTGF mRNA and an increase of CTGF protein expression compared to normal fibroblast, confirming the contribution of CTGF in keloid fibroblast pathology [17]. Genistein decreased mRNA and protein expression of CTGF in keloid fibroblast in a concentration-dependent manner. Moreover, genistein decreases TGFβ1, β2, and β3 gene expression in keloid fibroblast, but its potential application as an antifibrotic factor in keloids treatment requires further research. Genistein did not induce p53 and p21 expression, and therefore it seems that it does not induce apoptosis in monoculture of keloids fibroblast. However, it revealed a cytoprotective effect, stimulating BCL-2 gene expression [17]. In another study, normal human epidermal keratinocytes (NHEK), NHDF, and KEL FIB were tested to investigate genistein as a potential regulator of C-JUN, C-FOS, and FOS-B of AP-1 subunits expression. C-JUN and C-FOS expression was lower in keloid fibroblast compared to normal fibroblasts cultured in control conditions. The study demonstrated that genistein modulated C-JUN expression in dermal keratinocytes and fibroblasts in a dose-dependent manner. The expression of C-JUN was significantly higher in keratinocytes treated with genistein compared to control cells [18]. These data further corroborate the potential efficacy of genistein for treating keloid scars.

Collagen synthesis by fibroblast is also crucial for maintaining skin homeostasis and healing of wounds. Genistein effects on collagen biosynthesis and the signaling pathways involved in its regulation were investigated in human dermal fibroblasts [19] under the oxidative stress conditions evoked by *t*-BHP (*t*-butylhydroperoxide). Genistein exerts biphasic effects on collagen biosynthesis; at 1 μM, it counteracted collagen biosynthesis inhibition evoked by *t*-BHP in fibroblasts. At 10 μM, it exerted a significantly diminished protective effect on collagen biosynthesis, whereas at 100 μM, it potentiated the inhibitory action of *t*-BHP. The study suggested that at nutritionally attainable concentrations (1 μM), genistein protects human dermal fibroblasts from oxidative stress-induced collagen biosynthesis inhibition. The mechanism of the protective effect of genistein on collagen biosynthesis in *t*-BHP-treated fibroblasts may be due to the prevention of disturbances in the IGF-I receptor-mediated, ERK1/ERK2-associated signaling pathway evoked by the oxidant [19].

2.2. Genistein Affects Glycosaminoglycan Synthesis

Aside from the tyrosine kinase inhibitory effect of genistein, another modulating activity was identified on glycosaminoglycan (GAG) synthesis by blocking the tyrosine kinase activity of the epidermal growth factor receptor [20] in fibroblasts from patients with mucolipidosis II (a mucopolysaccharidosis caused by deficiencies in enzymes involved in degradation of GAG). In this experimental condition, genistein—despite causing a significant reduction in GAG synthesis rate—ensures the maintenance of sufficient amounts of GAG, which is necessary for the proper functioning of cells and tissues [21]. In another mucopolysaccharidosis, the Sanfilippo disease, genistein was tested and compared to other flavonoids to reduce GAG synthesis and accumulation in fibroblasts obtained by affected subjects [22]. An inhibition of GAG synthesis was found in the presence of all tested compounds, though the most pronounced impairment of production of GAGs was observed in the presence of kaempferol, daidzein, and genistein; thus, the authors concluded by suggesting that these flavonoids alone or in combination might be a safe treatment option for mucopolysaccharidosis [22].

2.3. Genistein Effects on ultraviolet (UV)-Protection

Genistein was also tested for protection against UV-light exposure and prevented the UV radiation-dependent expression of cyclooxygenase-2 (COX-2) in HaCaT cells cultures suppressing both the basal and stimulated expression of cyclooxygenase-2, which suggests that it exerts anti-inflammatory activity [23]. In UVB-irradiated BJ-5ta cells are human skin fibroblast cells immortalized with hTERT, and besides reducing COX-2 expression, genistein also induced Gadd45 gene expression, thereby activating the DNA repair system [24]. The protective effect of genistein against senescence-like characteristics was also tested on human dermal fibroblasts (HDFs) following repeated subcytotoxic exposures to UVB to cause senescence. Genistein reversed the senescence process in HDFs, acting as an antioxidant through the down-regulation of p66Shc protein that involves forkhead protein suppression [25]. These data further suggest that genistein could be a good candidate ingredient for protective agents against UV-induced photodamage.

The effects reported by these in vitro studies have been summarized in Table 1.

Table 1. Genistein effects on in vitro experimental models.

In Vitro Experimental Models	Genistein Effects
Fibroblasts from hypertrophic burn scars, normal human dermal fibroblasts (NHDF) keloid fibroblasts (KEL FIB), normal human epidermal keratinocytes (NHEK), NHDF stimulated with *t*-BHP (*t*-butylhydroperoxide) [16–19]	↓ RAS, RAF, ERK, p38 ↓ CTGF, TGFβ1, β2 and β3 ↑ BCL-2 ↑ C-JUN
Fibroblasts from patients with mucolipidosis II and Sanfilippo disease [21,22]	↓ GAG
HaCaT, BJ-5ta, and human dermal fibroblasts exposed to UV radiation [23–25]	↓ COX-2 ↑ Gadd45 gene expression ↓ p66Shc protein

↑ and ↓ respectively indicate an increase or a reduction of the expression of the molecules. RAS, Rat Sarcoma; RAF, Rapidly Accelerated Fibrosarcoma; ERK, Extracellular signal-regulated Kinase; CTGF, Connective Tissue Growth Factor; TGFβ, Transforming Growth Factor beta, BCL-2, B cell leukemia 2.

3. In Vivo Studies

3.1. Genistein Effect on Photodamage

Most of the in vivo studies carried out in rodents evaluated the effect of genistein alone or combined with other flavonoids in reducing the damages associated with UV-light exposure. In a long-term (8 weeks) dietary supplementation study with isoflavone-rich fermented soybean (0.2083 μg genistein/mg of soybean), hairless albino mice exposed to UVB demonstrated a markedly reduced skin inflammation [26]. Topically applied genistein was shown to reduce the incidence and multiplicity of skin tumors in the dimethylbenz(a)anthracene initiated and 12-*O*-tetradecanoyl phorbol-13-acetate promoted mouse models [27,28]. In the UVB light-induced complete carcinogenesis model, topical pretreatment of mice with 10 μmol genistein significantly reduced the formation of H_2O_2 and 8-hydroxy-2-deoxyguanosine [27,28]. Because these are the precursors for free radicals, their attenuation is a significant step for chemoprevention.

The possible anti-nitrosative effect of genistein (10 mg/kg or 15 mg/kg, i.p.) in the prevention of skin injury and in the modulation of cell proliferation were tested in Hairless HRS/J mice following

24 h of UVB irradiation [29]. The most effective dose (10 mg/kg) demonstrated a reduction in lipid peroxides and nitrotyrosine, accompanied by upregulation of both PCNA and Ki67, which indicated that prevention of nitrosative skin injury promoted cell proliferation and DNA repair [29]. In another study, genistein potently inhibited the UVB-induced skin carcinogenesis and photodamage in hairless mice. The possible mechanisms of the anticarcinogenic action hypothesized by the authors include scavenging of reactive oxygen species, blocking of oxidative and photodynamic damage to DNA, inhibition of tyrosine protein kinase, downregulation of EGF-receptor phosphorylation and MAPK activation, and suppression of oncoprotein expression [30].

3.2. Genistein Effect on Wound Healing

In wound healing models, genistein was tested in excisional and incisional wound models. ICR mice receiving a genistein-enriched diet (0.025% and 0.1% genistein) for 2 weeks before wounding demonstrated a faster wound repair, likely stimulated by a modulated production of reactive oxygen species (ROS), which in turn downregulated the activity of NF- κB and TNF-α within the first 72 h following wounding. In ovariectomized 10-week-old C57/Bl6 mice, full thickness skin incisional wounds were systemically treated with 17-estradiol (0.05 mg, 21-day, slow-release 17-estradiol pellet, subcutaneously implanted) or genistein (50 mg/kg/day). Genistein substantially accelerated wound repair, associated with a dampened inflammatory response. Unexpectedly, co-treatment with the ER antagonist ICI had little impact on the anti-inflammatory and healing promoting effects of genistein [31,32]. Thus, the authors speculated that genistein's actions are only partially mediated via classical estrogen receptor-dependent signaling pathways.

In ovariectomized rats chronically (6 months) treated with genistein (1 and 10 mg/kg/day, subcutaneously), full thickness incisional wounds were made and analyzed after 7 and 14 days [33]. Genistein was able to counteract the delayed wound healing, improving extracellular matrix remodeling and turn-over in OVX rats. Moreover, genistein (1 mg/kg) was more effective than estradiol or raloxifene on all skin parameters tested at days 7 and 14 after wounding [33]. The same authors also evaluated skin aging in 9-month-old OVX rats chronically treated with genistein, raloxifene, and estradiol [34]. OVX rats showed a decrease in TGF-b1, VEGF, MMP-2, MMP-9, tissue inhibitor of metalloproteinase (TIMP)-1 and TIMP-2 compared with sham OVX rats. All the treatments significantly restored this depressed molecular profile, but genistein (1 mg/kg) also significantly increased collagen thickness and skin breaking strength [34].

Collectively (Table 2), these data suggest that dosages as low as 1 mg/kg could be beneficial for treating skin disorders during estrogen deprivation, while higher dosages (up to 50 mg/kg) are needed where a normal estrogenic milieu is present.

Table 2. Genistein effects on in vivo experimental models.

In Vivo Model	Dose	Outcomes	Genistein Effects
UVB-irradiation and carcinogenesis models [26,27,29]	Dietary supplementation 0.2083 µg/mg of fermented soy beans 1, 5, 10, 20 µmol genistein topically applied Intraperitoneal injections 10–15 mg/kg	Anti-inflammatory effect in hairless mice with photodamage Reduction of skin tumorigenesis in mice Anti-nitrosative effect in hairless mice	↓ skin inflammation ↓ H_2O_2 ↓ 8-hydroxy-2-deoxyguanosine ↓ lipid peroxides ↓ nitrotyrosine ↓ tyrosine protein kinase ↓ EGF-receptor phosphorylation ↓ MAPK activation ↓ oncoprotein expression ↑ PCNA ↑ Ki67
Wound healing models [31–34]	Dietary supplementation 0.25–1 g/kg Subcutaneous injections 50 mg/kg Subcutaneous injections 1–10 mg/kg Subcutaneous injections 1–10 mg/kg	Improving wound healing in intact mice Wound healing in OVX mice Wound healing in OVX rats Skin aging in OVX rats	↑ wound repair ↓ ROS ↓ NF-κB ↓ TNF-α ↑ TGF-β1 ↑ VEGF ↑ MMP-2 and MMP-9 ↑ TIMP-1 and TIMP-2 ↑ collagen thickness ↑ skin breaking strength

4. Human Studies

In addition to all of the aforementioned preclinical evidence, it was also reported that the use of soy isoflavones may induce proliferation of the epidermis and increase dermal collagen [35].

In a double-blind placebo-controlled trial, 26 women in their late 30s and early 40s were randomly assigned to receive either an oral intake of 40 mg soy isoflavone aglycones per day or placebo for 12 weeks. It was observed that the isoflavones improved fine wrinkles and malar skin elasticity at the end of the study period [36]. Based on this observation, a randomized, double-blind, estrogen-controlled trial evaluated in 36 postmenopausal women the effect of a topical gel applied on the face, containing either isoflavone (4% genistein) or estrogen for 24 weeks [37]. Facial skin biopsies were taken from the preauricular area before and after the 24-week gel treatment; the cutaneous effects of isoflavone gel at six months were limited to an increase in dermal thickness and in the number of blood vessels, but the increments were smaller than those in the estradiol group. Furthermore, no change in hormonal vaginal cytology at 3 and 6 months was observed in comparison to baseline, suggesting the absence of a significant systemic effect [37]. Genistein was also tested in UVB-induced erythema (sunburn) in the dorsal skin of six men with skin type II to skin type IV. Genistein 5 $\mu mol/cm^2$ was topically applied 60 min before and 5 min after UVB irradiation. The skin was photographed and quantitated for erythema, and genistein effectively blocked UVB-induced skin burns, suggesting its use as UV-protective agent [30].

Genistein was also used in an open-label study, where a group of 19 children with different subtypes of mucopolysaccharidosis type III, Sanfilippo syndrome, and different degrees of disability received genistein supplementation (5 mg/kg/day) for 1 year [38]. Treatment with genistein produced improvement in skin texture and hair morphology, reduced CoQ10, but did not modify GAG urinary excretion or the severity of the underlying disease. The treatment was generally well-tolerated and no secondary effects were observed. This study is of great importance because it demonstrates that genistein can also be safely administered to young subjects [38].

5. The Problem of Delivery

Topical delivery should help overcome the discrepancies associated with the relative bioavailability of genistein after oral administration, which has been observed in certain studies [39,40], but not in others [41]. However, genistein use in creams and topical applications may be affected by a low permeability rate, as reported by some authors [42]. To overcome this problem, drug delivery systems based on lipid nanoparticles have been employed. The most widely studied lipid nanoparticles are solid lipid nanoparticles (SLN) and nanostructured lipid carriers (NLC). Both have a solid lipid matrix, but NLC are prepared with a mixture of solid lipid and oil, which can increase drug loading and stability [43]. An experimental study compared SLN and NLC nanoparticles combined with genistein for controlled release in skin, and increased penetration in deeper skin layers. The genistein–NLC formulation was the most effective in favoring the penetration in to the deeper skin layers, suggesting that NLC could be a promising nanocarrier for the topical delivery of genistein [44].

Another well-studied approach exploited the use of polymeric gels—in particular, polyethylene glycol 400 (PEG 400). The formulation was tested for skin permeation from a saturated solution of dry soy extract [45]. Genistein flux increased significantly when pure genistein was used as a suspension in PEG 400, and resulted in significant skin retention. To further investigate the transdermal delivery of genistein, studies were conducted using pH 6 and pH 10.8 buffers and soybean oil as vehicles [46]. Of these, the calibrated deposition of genistein into nude mice and pig skin for a saturated solution in pH 6 buffer was higher than the other vehicles. Pretreatment of skin for 2 h with either oleic acid or α-terpineol as penetration enhancers did not increase the permeation of genistein at pH 6. It was reported that topical delivery was promising for genistein use against photoaging and photodamage, providing a possible application of these gels as skin protection agents for UV-induced damage and chemoprevention of melanoma [47].

Another approach exploited to improve isoflavone delivery into the skin was tried with microemulsions. The effects accumulation as well as the solubility of genistein were tested on pig skin using a water/oil-type microemulsion, and a significant protection against UV-induced oxidative damage was observed [48]. Genistein inhibited lipid peroxidation in guinea pig dorsal skin, as well as UV-B-induced erythema formation.

6. Conclusions

During menopause, as estrogen levels decrease, testosterone stimulates sebaceous glands to secrete thicker sebum, giving the appearance of oily skin; in addition, some women may develop facial hair, particularly in the chin area. As estrogen levels drop during menopause, fat deposits tend to redistribute over the abdomen and/or on the thighs and buttocks. The result is a loss of supportive fat below the skin of the face, neck, hands, and arms; this allows sagging wrinkles to appear, and the skin over these areas is less easily compressed as it loses its mobility. The lowered estrogen levels also result in less production and repair of collagen and elastin in the dermis (particularly if the skin is exposed to UV rays), resulting in elastosis. Estrogens also temper melanin production; their lack can result in brown "age spots" appearing on the face, hands, neck, arms, and chest of many women. All these changes lead to a faster aging of skin. Estrogen replacement prevents and ameliorates these features, but too many side effects have been related to their use. Over the past decades, genistein has been used as an alternative treatment for menopausal symptoms [49–53], and in light of the effects reported on skin aging (Figure 1), it could be considered as an effective alternative treatment for menopause. In conclusion, genistein might be a new potential therapy for the management of skin disorders as well as age- and menopause-related skin changes commonly observed in postmenopausal women. Considering the bioavailability following oral assumption and the permeability after topical application, it seems that oral administration of at least 50 mg/day of pure genistein without other isoflavones could be the best dosing strategy to obtain clinical efficacy.

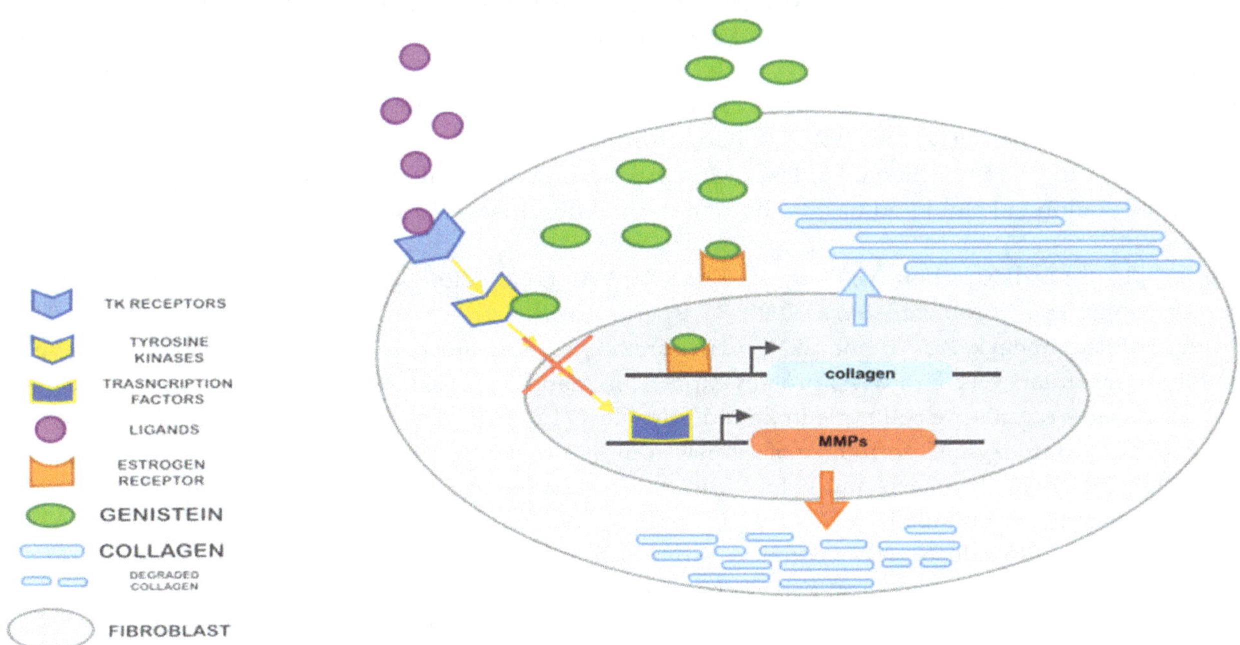

Figure 1. Mechanism of action of genistein in fibroblasts.

Acknowledgments: No specific funds have been received for experiments or covering the costs to publish in open access.

References

1. Hall, G.; Phillips, T.J. Estrogen and skin: The effects of estrogen, menopause, and hormone replacement therapy on the skin. *J. Am. Acad. Dermatol.* **2005**, *53*, 555–568. [CrossRef]
2. Verdier-Sevrain, S.; Bontè, F.; Gilchrest, B. Biology of estrogens in skin: Implications for skin aging. *Exp. Dermatol.* **2006**, *15*, 83–94. [CrossRef]
3. Wolff, E.F.; Narayan, D.; Taylor, H.S. Long-term effects of hormone therapy on skin rigidity and wrinkles. *Fertil. Steril.* **2005**, *84*, 285–288. [CrossRef]
4. Albertazzi, P.; Purdie, D.W. The life and times of the estrogen receptors: An interim report. *Climacteric* **2001**, *4*, 194–202. [CrossRef]
5. Younes, M.; Honma, N. Estrogen receptor β. *Arch. Pathol. Lab. Med.* **2011**, *135*, 63–66.
6. Thornton, M.J.; Taylor, A.H.; Mulligan, K.; Al-Azzawi, F.; Lyon, C.C.; O'Driscoll, J.B.; Messenger, A.G. Estrogen receptor beta (ERβ) is the predominant estrogen receptor in human scalp. *Exp. Dermatol.* **2003**, *12*, 181–190. [CrossRef]
7. Thornton, M.J.; Taylor, A.H.; Mulligan, K.; Al-Azzawi, F.; Lyon, C.C.; O'Driscoll, J.B.; Messenger, A.G. The distribution of estrogen receptor beta (ERβ) is distinct to that of ER alpha and the androgen receptor in human skin and the pilosebaceous unit. *J. Investig. Dermatol. Symp. Proc.* **2003**, *8*, 100–103. [CrossRef]
8. Thornton, M.J. The biological actions of estrogens on skin. *Exp. Dermatol.* **2002**, *11*, 487–502. [CrossRef]
9. Fitzpatrick, L.A. Selective estrogen receptor modulators and phytoestrogens: New therapies for the postmenopausal women. *Mayo Clin. Proc.* **1999**, *74*, 601–607. [CrossRef]
10. Beck, V.; Unterrieder, E.; Krenn, L.; Kubelka, W.; Jungbauer, A. Comparison of hormonal activity (estrogen, androgen and progestin) of standardized plant extracts for large scale use in hormone replacement therapy. *J. Steroid Biochem. Mol. Biol.* **2003**, *84*, 259–268. [CrossRef]
11. Kuiper, G.G.; Lemmen, J.G.; Carlsson, B.; Corton, J.C.; Safe, S.H.; van der Saag, P.T.; van der Burg, B.; Gustafsson, J.A. Interaction of estrogenic chemicals and phytoestrogens with estrogen receptor beta. *Endocrinology* **1998**, *139*, 4252–4263. [CrossRef]
12. Akiyama, T.; Ishida, J.; Nakagawa, S.; Ogawara, H.; Watanabe, S.; Itoh, N.; Shibuya, M.; Fukami, Y. Genistein, a specific inhibitor of tyrosine-specific protein kinases. *J. Biol. Chem.* **1987**, *262*, 5592–5595.
13. Steensma, A.; Faassen-Peters, M.A.; Noteborn, H.P.; Rietjens, I.M. Bioavailability of genistein and its glycoside genistin as measured in the portal vein of freely moving unanesthetized rats. *J. Agric. Food Chem.* **2006**, *54*, 8006–8012. [CrossRef]
14. Cederroth, C.R.; Zimmermann, C.; Nef, S. Soy, phytoestrogens and their impact on reproductive health. *Mol. Cell. Endocrinol.* **2012**, *355*, 192–200. [CrossRef]
15. Chin, G.S.; Liu, W.; Steinbrech, D.; Hsu, M.; Levinson, H.; Longaker, M.T. Cellular signaling by tyrosine phosphorylation in keloid and normal human dermal fibroblasts. *Plast. Reconstr. Surg.* **2000**, *106*, 1532–1540. [CrossRef]
16. Cao, C.; Li, S.; Dai, X.; Chen, Y.; Feng, Z.; Zhao, Y.; Wu, J. Genistein inhibits proliferation and functions of hypertrophic scar fibroblasts. *Burns* **2009**, *35*, 89–97. [CrossRef]
17. Jurzak, M.; Adamczyk, K.; Antończak, P.; Garncarczyk, A.; Kuśmierz, D.; Latocha, M. Evaluation of genistein ability to modulate CTGF mRNA/protein expression, genes expression of TGFβ isoforms and expression of selected genes regulating cell cycle in keloid fibroblasts in vitro. *Acta Pol. Pharm.* **2014**, *71*, 972–986.
18. Jurzak, M.; Adamczyk, K. Influence of genistein on c-Jun, c-Fos and Fos-B of AP-1 subunits expression in skin keratinocytes, fibroblasts and keloid fibroblasts cultured in vitro. *Acta Pol. Pharm.* **2013**, *70*, 205–213.
19. Sienkiewicz, P.; Surazyński, A.; Pałka, J.; Miltyk, W. Nutritional concentration of genistein protects human dermal fibroblasts from oxidative stress-induced collagen biosynthesis inhibition through IGF-I receptor-mediated signaling. *Acta Pol. Pharm.* **2008**, *65*, 203–211.
20. Piotrowska, E.; Jakóbkiewicz-Banecka, J.; Barańska, S.; Tylki-Szymańska, A.; Czartoryska, B.; Wegrzyn, A.; Wegrzyn, G. Genistein-mediated inhibition of glycosaminoglycan synthesis as a basis for gene expression-targeted isoflavone therapy for mucopolysaccharidoses. *Eur. J. Hum. Genet.* **2006**, *14*, 846–852. [CrossRef]
21. Otomo, T.; Hossain, M.A.; Ozono, K.; Sakai, N. Genistein reduces heparan sulfate accumulation in human mucolipidosis II skin fibroblasts. *Mol. Genet. Metab.* **2012**, *105*, 266–269. [CrossRef]

22. Kloska, A.; Jakóbkiewicz-Banecka, J.; Narajczyk, M.; Banecka-Majkutewicz, Z.; Węgrzyn, G. Effects of flavonoids on glycosaminoglycan synthesis: Implications for substrate reduction therapy in Sanfilippo disease and other mucopolysaccharidoses. *Metab. Brain Dis.* **2011**, *26*, 1–8. [CrossRef]
23. Isoherranen, K.; Punnonen, K.; Jansen, C.; Uotila, P. Ultraviolet irradiation induces cyclooxygenase-2 expression in keratinocytes. *Br. J. Dermatol.* **1999**, *140*, 1017–1022. [CrossRef]
24. Iovine, B.; Iannella, M.L.; Gasparri, F.; Monfrecola, G.; Bevilacqua, M.A. Synergic Effect of Genistein and Daidzein on UVB-Induced DNA Damage: An Effective Photoprotective Combination. *J. Biomed. Biotechnol.* **2011**, *2011*, 692846:1–692846:8. [CrossRef]
25. Wang, Y.N.; Wu, W.; Chen, H.C.; Fang, H. Genistein protects against UVB-induced senescence-like characteristics in human dermal fibroblast by p66Shc down-regulation. *J. Dermatol. Sci.* **2010**, *58*, 19–27. [CrossRef]
26. Lee, T.H.; Do, M.H.; Oh, Y.L.; Cho, D.W.; Kim, S.H.; Kim, S.Y. Dietary fermented soybean suppresses UVB-induced skin inflammation in hairless mice via regulation of the MAPK signaling pathway. *J. Agric. Food Chem.* **2014**, *62*, 8962–8972. [CrossRef]
27. Wei, H.; Bowen, R.; Zhang, X.; Lebwohl, M. Isoflavone genistein inhibits the initiation and promotion of two-stage skin carcinogenesis in mice. *Carcinogenesis* **1998**, *19*, 1509–1514. [CrossRef]
28. Khan, N.; Afaq, F.; Mukhtar, H. Cancer chemoprevention through dietary antioxidants: Progress and promise. *Antioxid. Redox Signal.* **2008**, *10*, 475–510. [CrossRef]
29. Terra, V.A.; Souza-Neto, F.P.; Frade, M.A.; Ramalho, L.N.; Andrade, T.A.; Pasta, A.A.; Conchon, A.C.; Guedes, F.A.; Luiz, R.C.; Cecchini, R.; et al. Genistein prevents ultraviolet B radiation-induced nitrosative skin injury and promotes cell proliferation. *J. Photochem. Photobiol. B* **2015**, *144*, 20–27. [CrossRef]
30. Wei, H.; Saladi, R.; Lu, Y.; Wang, Y.; Palep, S.R.; Moore, J.; Phelps, R.; Shyong, E.; Lebwohl, M.G. Isoflavone genistein: Photoprotection and clinical implications in dermatology. *J. Nutr.* **2003**, *133* (Suppl. 1), 3811S–3819S.
31. Park, E.; Lee, S.M.; Jung, I.K.; Lim, Y.; Kim, J.H. Effects of genistein on early-stage cutaneous wound healing. *Biochem. Biophys. Res. Commun.* **2011**, *410*, 514–519. [CrossRef]
32. Emmerson, E.; Campbell, L.; Ashcroft, G.S.; Hardman, M.J. The phytoestrogen genistein promotes wound healing by multiple independent mechanisms. *Mol. Cell. Endocrinol.* **2010**, *321*, 184–193. [CrossRef]
33. Marini, H.; Polito, F.; Altavilla, D.; Irrera, N.; Minutoli, L.; Calò, M.; Adamo, E.B.; Vaccaro, M.; Squadrito, F.; Bitto, A. Genistein aglycone improves skin repair in an incisional model of wound healing: A comparison with raloxifene and oestradiol in ovariectomized rats. *Br. J. Pharmacol.* **2010**, *160*, 1185–1194. [CrossRef]
34. Polito, F.; Marini, H.; Bitto, A.; Irrera, N.; Vaccaro, M.; Adamo, E.B.; Micali, A.; Squadrito, F.; Minutoli, L.; Altavilla, D. Genistein aglycone, a soy-derived isoflavone, improves skin changes induced by ovariectomy in rats. *Br. J. Pharmacol.* **2012**, *165*, 994–1005. [CrossRef]
35. Kessel, B. Alternatives to estrogen for menopausal women. *Soc. Exp. Biol. Med.* **1998**, *217*, 38–44. [CrossRef]
36. Izumi, T.; Saito, M.; Obata, A.; Arii, M.; Yamaguchi, H.; Matsuyama, A. Oral intake of soy isoflavone aglycone improves the aged skin of adult women. *J. Nutr. Sci. Vitaminol. (Tokyo)* **2007**, *53*, 57–62. [CrossRef]
37. Moraes, A.B.; Haidar, M.A.; Soares Júnior, J.M.; Simões, M.J.; Baracat, E.C.; Patriarca, M.T. The effects of topical isoflavones on postmenopausal skin: Double-blind and randomized clinical trial of efficacy. *Eur. J. Obstet. Gynecol. Reprod. Biol.* **2009**, *146*, 188–192. [CrossRef]
38. Delgadillo, V.; O'Callaghan Mdel, M.; Artuch, R.; Montero, R.; Pineda, M. Genistein supplementation in patients affected by Sanfilippo disease. *J. Inherit. Metab. Dis.* **2011**, *34*, 1039–1044. [CrossRef]
39. Setchell, K.D.; Brown, N.M.; Desai, P.; Zimmer-Nechemias, L.; Wolfe, B.E.; Brashear, W.T.; Kirschner, A.S.; Cassidy, A.; Heubi, J.E. Bioavailability of pure isoflavones in healthy humans and analysis of commercial soy isoflavone supplements. *J. Nutr.* **2001**, *131*, 1362S–1375S.
40. Setchell, K.D.; Brown, N.M.; Desai, P.B.; Zimmer-Nechimias, L.; Wolfe, B.; Jakate, A.S.; Creutzinger, V.; Heubi, J.E. Bioavailability, disposition, and dose-response effects of soy isoflavones when consumed by healthy women at physiologically typical dietary intakes. *J. Nutr.* **2003**, *133*, 1027–1035.
41. Zubik, L.; Meydani, M. Bioavailability of soybean isoflavones from aglycone and glucoside forms in American women. *Am. J. Clin. Nutr.* **2003**, *77*, 1459–1465.
42. Georgetti, S.R.; Casagrande, R.; Verri, W.A., Jr.; Lopez, R.F.; Fonseca, M.J. Evaluation of in vivo efficacy of topical formulations containing soybean extract. *Int. J. Pharm.* **2008**, *352*, 189–196. [CrossRef]

43. Müller, R.H.; Petersen, R.D.; Hommoss, A.; Pardeike, J. Nanostructured lipid carriers (NLC) in cosmetic dermal products. *Adv. Drug Deliv. Rev.* **2007**, *59*, 522–530. [CrossRef]
44. Andrade, L.M.; de Fátima Reis, C.; Maione-Silva, L.; Anjos, J.L.; Alonso, A.; Serpa, R.C.; Marreto, R.N.; Lima, E.M.; Taveira, S.F. Impact of lipid dynamic behavior on physical stability, in vitro release and skin permeation of genistein-loaded lipid nanoparticles. *Eur. J. Pharm. Biopharm.* **2014**, *88*, 40–47. [CrossRef]
45. Minghetti, P.; Cilurzo, F.; Casiraghi, A.; Montanari, L. Evaluation of ex vivo human skin permeation of genistein and daidzein. *Drug Deliv.* **2006**, *13*, 411–415. [CrossRef]
46. Huang, Z.R.; Hung, C.F.; Lin, Y.K.; Fang, J.Y. In vitro and in vivo evaluation of topical delivery and potential dermal use of soy isoflavones genistein and daidzein. *Int. J. Pharm.* **2008**, *364*, 36–44. [CrossRef]
47. Chadha, G.; Sathigari, S.; Parsons, D.L.; Jayachandra Babu, R. In vitro percutaneous absorption of genistein from topical gels through human skin. *Drug Dev. Ind. Pharm.* **2011**, *37*, 498–505. [CrossRef]
48. Kitagawa, S.; Inoue, K.; Teraoka, R.; Morita, S.Y. Enhanced skin delivery of genistein and other two isoflavones by microemulsion and prevention against UV irradiation-induced erythema formation. *Chem. Pharm. Bull. (Tokyo)* **2010**, *58*, 398–401. [CrossRef]
49. Arcoraci, V.; Atteritano, M.; Squadrito, F.; D'Anna, R.; Marini, H.; Santoro, D.; Minutoli, L.; Messina, S.; Altavilla, D.; Bitto, A. Antiosteoporotic Activity of Genistein Aglycone in Postmenopausal Women: Evidence from a Post-Hoc Analysis of a Multicenter Randomized Controlled Trial. *Nutrients* **2017**, *9*, 179. [CrossRef]
50. Bitto, A.; Polito, F.; Squadrito, F.; Marini, H.; D'Anna, R.; Irrera, N.; Minutoli, L.; Granese, R.; Altavilla, D. Genistein aglycone: A dual mode of action anti-osteoporotic soy isoflavone rebalancing bone turnover towards bone formation. *Curr. Med. Chem.* **2010**, *17*, 3007–3018. [CrossRef]
51. Marini, H.; Bitto, A.; Altavilla, D.; Burnett, B.P.; Polito, F.; Di Stefano, V.; Minutoli, L.; Atteritano, M.; Levy, R.M.; D'Anna, R.; et al. Breast safety and efficacy of genistein aglycone for postmenopausal bone loss: A follow-up study. *J. Clin. Endocrinol. Metab.* **2008**, *93*, 4787–4796. [CrossRef] [PubMed]
52. Marini, H.; Minutoli, L.; Polito, F.; Bitto, A.; Altavilla, D.; Atteritano, M.; Gaudio, A.; Mazzaferro, S.; Frisina, A.; Frisina, N.; et al. Effects of the phytoestrogen genistein on bone metabolism in osteopenic postmenopausal women: A randomized trial. *Ann. Intern. Med.* **2007**, *146*, 839–847. [CrossRef] [PubMed]
53. D'Anna, R.; Cannata, M.L.; Marini, H.; Atteritano, M.; Cancellieri, F.; Corrado, F.; Triolo, O.; Rizzo, P.; Russo, S.; Gaudio, A.; et al. Effects of the phytoestrogen genistein on hot flushes, endometrium, and vaginal epithelium in postmenopausal women: A 2-year randomized, double-blind, placebo-controlled study. *Menopause* **2009**, *16*, 301–306. [CrossRef] [PubMed]

9

Claimed Effects, Outcome Variables and Methods of Measurement for Health Claims Proposed Under European Community Regulation 1924/2006 in the Framework of Maintenance of Skin Function

Daniela Martini [1,†], Donato Angelino [1,†], Chiara Cortelazzi [2], Ivana Zavaroni [3,4], Giorgio Bedogni [5], Marilena Musci [6], Carlo Pruneti [7], Giovanni Passeri [8], Marco Ventura [9], Daniela Galli [10], Prisco Mirandola [10], Marco Vitale [10], Alessandra Dei Cas [3,4], Riccardo C. Bonadonna [3,4], Sergio Di Nuzzo [2], Maria Beatrice De Felici [2] and Daniele Del Rio [1,*]

1 The Laboratory of Phytochemicals in Physiology, Department of Food and Drug, University of Parma, 43125 Parma, Italy; daniela.martini@unipr.it (D.M.); donato.angelino@unipr.it (D.A.)
2 Department of Medicine and Surgery, Section of Dermatology, University of Parma, 43125 Parma, Italy; chiara.cortelazzi@gmail.com (C.C.); sergio.dinuzzo@unipr.it (S.D.N.); bea.defelici@gmail.com (M.B.D.F.)
3 Department of Medicine and Surgery, Division of Endocrinology, University of Parma, 43125 Parma, Italy; ivana.zavaroni@unipr.it (I.Z.); alessandra.deicas@unipr.it (A.D.C.); riccardo.bonadonna@unipr.it (R.C.B.)
4 The Azienda Ospedaliera Universitaria of Parma, Division of Endocrinology, 43125 Parma, Italy
5 Clinical Epidemiology Unit, Liver Research Center, Basovizza, 34149 Trieste, Italy; giorgiobedogni@gmail.com
6 Department of Food and Drug, University of Parma, 43125 Parma, Italy; marilena.musci@unipr.it
7 Department of Medicine and Surgery, Clinical Psychology Unit, University of Parma, 43125 Parma, Italy; carlo.pruneti@unipr.it
8 Department of Medicine and Surgery, University of Parma, Building Clinica Medica Generale, 43125 Parma, Italy; giovanni.passeri@unipr.it
9 Laboratory of Probiogenomics, Department of Chemistry, Life Sciences and Environmental Sustainability, University of Parma, 43125 Parma, Italy; marco.ventura@unipr.it
10 Department of Medicine and Surgery, Sport and Exercise Medicine Centre (SEM), University of Parma, 43125 Parma, Italy; daniela.galli@unipr.it (D.G.); prisco.mirandola@unipr.it (P.M.); marco.vitale@unipr.it (M.V.)
* Correspondence: daniele.delrio@unipr.it
† Authors equally contributed to the study.

Abstract: Evidence suggests a protective role for several nutrients and foods in the maintenance of skin function. Nevertheless, all the requests for authorization to use health claims under Article 13(5) in the framework of maintenance of skin function presented to the European Food Safety Authority (EFSA) have received a negative opinion. Reasons for such failures are mainly due to an insufficient substantiation of the claimed effects, including the choice of inappropriate outcome variables (OVs) and methods of measurement (MMs). The present paper reports the results of an investigation aimed at collecting, collating and critically analyzing the information with relation to claimed effects (CEs), OVs and MMs related to skin health compliance with Regulation 1924/2006. CEs, OVs and MMs were collected from both the EFSA Guidance document and from the authorization requests of health claims under Article 13(5). The critical analysis of OVs and MMs was based on a literature review, and was aimed at defining their appropriateness (alone or in combination with others) in the context of a specific CE. The results highlight the importance of an adequate choice of OVs and MMs for an effective substantiation of the claims.

Keywords: health claim; outcome variable; method of measurement; skin health

1. Introduction

Skin represents the most external layer of the organism, and forms an effective barrier between the body and the environment [1]. Skin functions are extremely important and fall in several different categories: resistance to chemical and physical insults, defense from parasites and general poisons, regulation of body water, body temperature, oxygen absorption, and excretion of potentially toxic compounds (i.e., urea) [2,3]. All these functions are possible because of the particular structure of the skin, which consists of at least three main layers: (i) The epidermis, the most external layer, in direct contact with the environment, is formed by a *stratum germinativum* that constantly produces melanin and renews keratinocytes, and a *stratum corneum* consisting of dead cells, where keratin is stored, and which protects the layers underneath; (ii) The dermis, formed by epithelial tissue containing hair follicles, lymph and blood vessels; (iii) The subcutis, where blood vessels, nerves, glands and muscle fibers reside [1]. The cells in the structure are strictly connected by junctions (tight, gap, desmosomes, etc.), which allow the crosslinking of layers, thereby creating a strict and resistant mesh with selective permeability to nutrients and other compounds.

A wide range of diseases, including psoriasis, dermatitis, burns, ulcers, autoimmune disorders and cancer, can originate from alterations of the skin barrier induced by physical or chemical insults, by microorganisms, and by inflammatory processes that activate the immune system [4].

It has been estimated that at least 20% of the world population is affected by some sort of skin disorder requiring medical attention, i.e., viral or bacterial eczema, acne and infections [5]. Hay et al. highlighted that skin disorders are the fourth leading cause of non-fatal burden diseases in terms of years lost in disability [6], and statistics evidenced an 8.5% increase of death from skin disorders, and a 58.4% increase from malignant skin melanoma during the period 1990–2010 [7].

Lifestyle has been recognized as a relevant factor influencing the onset and the development of skin disorders. A major focus has been given to the relationship of body weight and lipid-related skin disease development. Randomized clinical trials (RCTs) have shown that physical activity and diet are strictly related to a decrease of psoriasis severity [8], as well as an improvement in the "dermatology life quality index" [9]. Dietary patterns, i.e., low glycemic load diets, enhanced the reduction of follicular sebum overflow and skin surface triglycerides, and increased the ratio of saturated/monounsaturated fatty acids [10]. However, as authors have concluded that it was not possible to attribute these effects to diet composition or weight loss, the role of the diet on sebum composition needs to be further investigated.

Some investigations have focused on the role of individual components of food, such as bioactive compounds, in skin health RCTs that have considered a lycopene-enriched tomato paste [11], a high flavanol-3-ols drink [12], or a green tea polyphenol beverage [13], showing significant reductions of erythema formation in healthy volunteers. Nevertheless, evidence of a direct effect of both single components and the whole diet in affecting skin-related outcomes is still extremely weak.

The current scientific evidence has convinced stakeholders to submit requests for authorization of health claims to the European Food Safety Authority (EFSA). Some health claims pertinent to Article 13(1) of the Regulation 1924/2006 have been approved (ec.europa.eu/nuhclaims/), whereas all the requests related to Article 13(5) regarding skin function have received a negative opinion. The main reasons for the negative opinions concern the insufficient characterization of the food item and its constituents, the choice of an inappropriate (e.g., vague) claimed effect and/or target population, and most of all the inadequate substantiation of the claim through well-designed and well-performed RCTs [14,15]. Many parameters may affect the quality of an RCT, such as the use of a placebo-controlled approach, the calculation of the sample size, the statistical analysis, and the choice of outcome variables (OVs) and/or their methods of measurements (MMs). For these reasons, the present work aims to collect, collate and critically analyze the information in relation to claimed effects (CEs), OVs and MMs, in the context of maintenance of normal skin function.

2. Search Strategy

This manuscript refers to the critical analysis of OVs and MMs collected from the EFSA Guidance on the scientific requirements for health claims related to bone, joints, skin, and oral health (EFSA 2011), from the requests for authorization of health claims under Articles 13(5) and 14 of Regulation 1924/2006 related to skin health (ec.europa.eu/nuhclaims/), and from comments received during public consultations. Adopting the decision tree described in Martini et al. (2016) [14], 3 claimed effects with 21 OVs were evaluated under Article 13(5). No disease risk reduction claims and no health claims referring to children's development had been proposed under the Article 14. For each OV, a database of references was created on PubMed based on the keywords defined by each OV, allowing a specific critical analysis of the OVs and the MMs (Table 1). The literature databases were reviewed and used for the critical evaluation of each OV and MM. The critical evaluation of OVs and MMs was performed taking into account their relevance in the framework of randomized controlled trials. For MMs, the two main parameters that were considered were (i) being a gold standard method; and (ii) the field acceptance. Moreover, we considered the following parameters in agreement with Fitzpatrick et al. [16].

- Appropriateness
- Reliability
- Validity
- Responsiveness
- Precision
- Interpretability
- Acceptability
- Feasibility

Each OV and related MM was ranked in one of the following categories: (i) appropriate alone; (ii) appropriate only in combination with other OVs or MMs; (iii) not appropriate per se; (iv) not appropriate in relation to the specific claimed effect proposed by the applicant(s); (v) not appropriate alone, but useful as supportive evidence for the scientific substantiation of the claimed effect. The index at the beginning of this paper lists the OVs and the respective MMs from the most to the least appropriate, if a ranking was applicable. The flow chart of the project is shown in Figure 1.

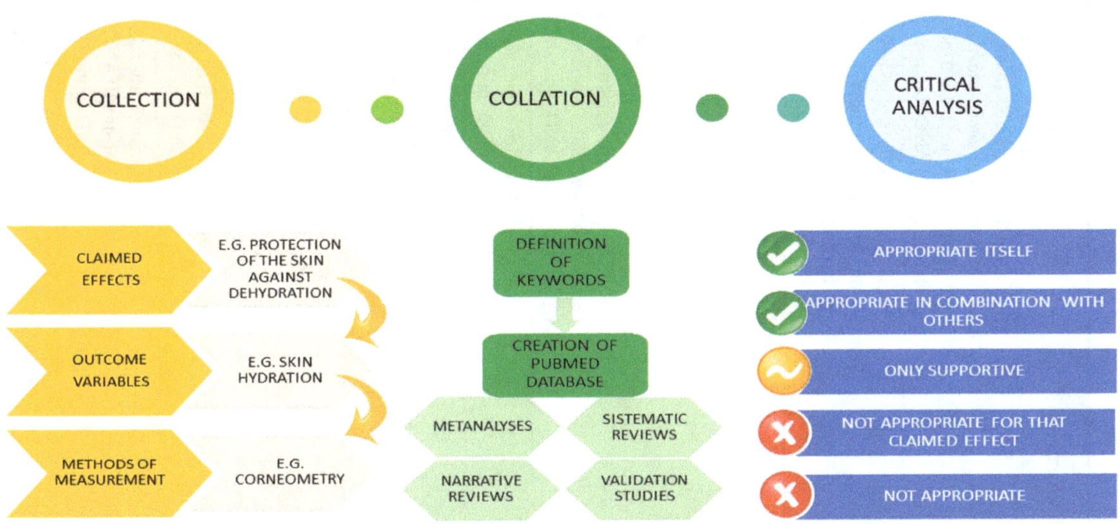

Figure 1. Collection, collation and critical evaluation of information in relation to claimed effects, outcome variables and methods of measurement in the framework of maintenance of skin function: flow chart of the project.

Table 1. Strategies used for retrieving the literature pertinent with outcome variables and methods of measurement related to maintenance of skin function.

DB Number	Syntax	Total Articles	Narrative Reviews	Systematic Reviews/Metanalyses	Validation Studies	Outcome Variables
1	"water loss, insensible" (mesh) OR "transepidermal water loss" (title/abstract) OR "twl" (title/abstract) OR "tewl" (title/abstract)) AND "english" (language) AND "humans" (mesh)"	2007	149	10	19	TEWL Water-holding capacity
2	"skin" (mesh) AND ("water" (mesh) OR "dehydration" (mesh) OR "dryness" (title/abstract) OR "hydration" (title/abstract)) AND "english" (language) AND "humans" (mesh)	1821	146	5	22	Skin hydration Skin dryness
3	"skin" (mesh) AND "elasticity" (mesh) AND "english" (language) AND "humans" (mesh)	585	35	3	18	Skin elasticity
4	("corneocyte" (title/abstract) AND "adhesion" (title/abstract)) AND "english" (language) AND "humans" (mesh)	14	2	0	0	Corneocyte adhesion
5	("Ceramide" (title/abstract) OR "*Stratum corneum*" (title/abstract)) AND "english" (language) AND "humans" (mesh)	260	31	0	2	Ceramide concentration of the *SC*
6	("pruritus" (mesh) OR "itch" (title/abstract)) AND "english" (language) AND "humans" (mesh)	8746	1186	131	32	Pruritus
7	"skin" (mesh) AND ("smooth*" (title/abstract) OR "rough*" (title/abstract)) AND "english" (language) AND "humans" (mesh)	1144	77	4	0	Skin smoothness and roughness
8	"skin aging" (mesh) OR ("skin" (mesh) AND "wrinkles" (title/abstract)) AND "english" (language) AND "humans" (mesh)	5185	1277	83	40	Skin wrinkles
9	"skin" (mesh) AND ("scal*" (title/abstract) OR "desquamate*" (title/abstract) OR "flak*" (title/abstract) OR "peel*" (title/abstract)) AND "english" (language) AND "humans" (mesh)	93	13	1	0	Skin scaling
10	"skin" (mesh) AND ("tight*" (title/abstract) OR "soft*" (title/abstract)) AND "english" (language) AND "humans" (mesh)	1620	203	16	7	Skin tightness and softness
11	("erythema" (mesh) OR ("skin" (mesh) AND "redness" (title/abstract) OR "reddening" (title/abstract))) AND "english" (language) AND "humans" (mesh)	15,702	1479	93	29	Skin reddening and erythema formation

Table 1. *Cont.*

DB Number	Syntax	Total Articles	Narrative Reviews	Systematic Reviews/Metanalyses	Validation Studies	Outcome Variables
12	"capillaries" (mesh) AND "english" (language) AND "humans" (mesh)	11,390	1110	26	40	Capillary blood flow
13	"skin" (mesh) AND ("oxidative stress"(mesh) OR "oxidative damage" (title/abstract)) AND "english" (language) AND "humans" (mesh)	818	126	4	1	Oxidative damage to DNA Oxidative damage to lipids Oxidative damage to proteins
14	"skin" (mesh) AND "dna damage" (mesh) AND "english" (language) AND "humans" (mesh)	739	123	3	1	DNA damage after UV exposure
15	"langerhans cells" (mesh) AND "english" (language) AND "humans" (mesh)	3338	500	3	2	Depletion of Langherans cells after UV light exposure
16	"erythema" (mesh) OR ("skin" (mesh) AND "redness" (title/abstract) OR "reddening" (title/abstract)) AND "english" (language) AND "humans" (mesh)	15,702	1479	93	29	UV-induced erythema and erythema grade
17	"hypersensitivity, delayed" (mesh) AND "english" (language) AND "humans" (mesh)	15,141	2001	73	17	DTH immune response to recall antigens in the skin

Legend: DB: Database; DTH: delayed type hypersensitivity; SC: *stratum corneum;* TEWL: Transepidermal water loss; UV: ultraviolet.

3. Critical Evaluation for Function Claims 13(5)

3.1. Protection of the Skin Against Dehydration

Skin is the largest organ of our body, and represents a physical barrier capable of holding water, as well as limiting the penetration of chemical substances, microorganisms and radiation from the environment. The ability of the skin to prevent the loss of body fluids is mainly attributed to the role of the *stratum corneum* (SC), an outer layer of the epidermis, formed by several deposits of dead keratinocytes, which acts as a physical barrier, limiting the loss of water and avoiding skin dehydration [1,17]. In particular, the presence of keratine and ceramides allows the formation of a compact layer that prevents the entrance of external particles and at the same time retains the body fluids under the epidermal layer [17].

Nevertheless, the use of aggressive products, such as detergents and surfactants, or exposure to environmental agents (e.g., sun, wind, cold) may compromise the structure and the function of SC, leading to a visible onset of the appearance of dehydration, e.g., dry and rough skin, desquamation. For these reasons, a compromised skin barrier may enhance the penetration of a wide range of substances/pathogens leading to pathological processes. Consequently, the maintenance of its permeability is essential and highly beneficial.

3.1.1. Transepidermal Water Loss

Transepidermal water loss (TEWL) has been recognized for over half a century as an in vivo parameter for assessing the skin barrier function. TEWL can be defined as the outward permeation of condensed water across the SC via diffusion, excluding other forms of water loss, such as perspiration [17]. It is expressed as grams of water per unit area of skin per unit of time ($g/m^2/h$).

To evaluate the appropriateness of TEWL as an OV for the protection of skin against dehydration, database 1 was generated (see Table 1).

TEWL is one of the most important parameters for evaluating the permeability function of the skin. A low TEWL is generally a characteristic feature of an intact skin function and a high hydration of the SC. Conversely, an elevated TEWL value is typically correlated with low hydration of the SC, and with an impaired epidermal barrier. This can be associated to several skin diseases, such as atopic dermatitis, or to contact with aggressive substances, such as solvents and detergents [18].

Based on these considerations, TEWL is an appropriate outcome measure to use for the substantiation of health claims in the context of protection of the skin against dehydration.

Tewameter®

Being the flux of condensed water diffusing through the skin, there are no direct methods for measuring TEWL. Nevertheless, there are two different indirect methods of measurement: open-chamber and closed-chamber methods [19]. Open chambers are open to the surrounding atmosphere. The closed-chamber method is a more recent methodology/procedure, developed to avoid the effect of external air convection and turbulence but, compared to the open chambers, have the disadvantage of requiring a purge after each measurement because of the accumulation of humidity and water vapor.

TEWL assessment can be performed using different instruments and, among them, the Tewameter® (Courage-Khazaka Electronic, Cologne, Germany), an open-chamber instrument, is one of the most widely accepted and employed methods for the measurement of TEWL. Therefore, most of the scientific literature on TEWL refers to this apparatus.

Open-chamber methods are preferable for the evaluation of skin barrier function, but must occur in a room with standardized conditions (i.e., with standardized temperature and relative humidity) [19].

In these open-chamber methods, TEWL is calculated by measuring the water vapor pressure (VP) gradient immediately above the surface of the skin, calculated as the difference in VP between two distinct points aligned perpendicularly to the skin surface.

The measuring principle of the instrument is that the vapor pressure gradient above the skin surface is proportional to the difference between the vapor pressures measured at two different heights located perpendicularly above the skin surface. With this aim, a probe, consisting of an open cylinder, is placed on the skin. The probe indirectly measures the density gradient of the water evaporation from the skin by two pairs of sensors inside the hollow cylinder. A microprocessor analyzes the values, and expresses the evaporation rate in $g/h/m^2$.

TEWL is one of the most measured parameters used in cosmetology to assess the efficacy of moisturizing cosmetics. It can be evaluated in combination with the use of irritants like sodium lauryl sulphate, sodium hydroxide or dimethylsulfoxide, to identify irritant reactions.

It is also worth noting that several and various conditions can influence the value of TEWL, such as ambient temperature, relative humidity, topical products, skin damage or diseases, probe position, sweating, smoking, age, sex, and skin sites [17,18]. Nevertheless, many of these factors can be controlled or minimized by using a well-developed study design. The Tewameter® allows an accurate and quick measurement of the TEWL. Limitations of the Tewameter® include the slight overestimation of the resulting values in comparison to other methods [17], and the variations of results among different instruments of the same type. Despite these limitations, the Tewameter® is one of the most used instruments in RCT.

In conclusion, the Tewameter® is an appropriate method to use for the measurement of TEWL.

3.1.2. Skin Hydration

Skin hydration is defined as the water content of the epidermis and the dermis. An adequate skin hydration is considered a very important factor in skin health. The epithelium remains flexible when it contains 10–20% water, and several substances may contribute to maintaining a balance in the skin homeostasis, such as natural moisturizing factor and some intercellular lipids of the SC [20,21]. All these factors synergize to preserve the adequate skin hydration and the barrier function of the epidermis as well as to prevent TEWL.

Superficial lipids create a filter for interaction with the external environment, and have been found to serve as water modulators in the SC.

The correct amount of water in the SC plays an important role on softness, smoothness and elasticity of the skin and allows maintenance of the typical barrier function of the skin, thus avoiding penetration of substances and microbes. Conversely, dry skin is generally linked to a reduced water content of the SC, and is associated with a rough surface, modifications of the lipid content or profile and of the permeability of the skin [21].

To evaluate the appropriateness of skin hydration as an OV for the protection of skin against dehydration, database 2 was generated (see Table 1).

An appropriate amount of water in the skin is important for the maintenance of its normal structure and properties, including adequate hydration and elasticity of the skin [22]. Moreover, skin hydration has been used extensively as an index of skin barrier function. An altered skin barrier function may modify the permeability function of the skin and facilitate the loss of body fluids and the penetration of chemicals and allergens.

Several diseases are associated to an impaired epidermal barrier, including atopic dermatitis, psoriasis, eczema, ichthyosis, and sensitive skin/rosacea [21]. Skin hydration can also decrease after the contact with aggressive cosmetics or professional substances leading to desiccation of SC with alteration of the normal epidermal barrier.

In conclusion, skin hydration is an appropriate outcome variable to use for the substantiation of health claims in the context of protection of the skin against dehydration. However, the simultaneous measure of TEWL is preferable, and provides a more complete and accurate measure of the hydration state of the skin.

Corneometry

Parameters related to skin hydration may be measured by considering the electrical properties that are dependent on the water content of the SC. Many commercially available instruments, based on principles of measuring skin capacitance, conductance, or impedance, have been widely used for this purpose [18,23].

Corneometry is one of the most commonly used techniques for measuring skin hydration, as well as water-holding capacity, as a surrogate measure of skin hydration.

The Corneometer® (Courage-Khazaka Electronic, Cologne, Germany) measures skin hydration by determining the skin capacitance with the use of probes [23]. The measurement is based on the difference between the dielectric constant of water and other substances by measuring the capacitance of a dielectric medium. The Corneometer® measures the change in the dielectric constant due to skin surface hydration by modulating the capacitance of a precision capacitor. The depth of measurement is quite low, as it reaches the first 10–20 μm of the SC.

One of the techniques that can be used is the water sorption-desorption test, which consists of the hydration of the skin with water followed by the observation of the subsequent dehydration activity by means of serial recording with electrical instruments.

The instrument delivers values expressed in arbitrary units (AU) varying from 0 to 120, where a higher value indicates a more hydrated skin with values >40 indicating adequate skin hydration [24].

Similar to other electrical measurements, corneometry has become very popular because of the relative low cost and ease of use; in fact, corneometry measurements are very rapid, and the modern probes enable temperature stability. In addition, the technique minimizes the subjectivity typical of visual scoring methods, and therefore allows greater accuracy and reproducibility [25,26].

Moreover, although several experimental and instrumentation-related factors also influence measurements (e.g., skin temperature, sweating, ambient temperature and humidity), many of these factors can be controlled or minimized by using a well-developed study design and specific standardized-condition rooms.

In conclusion, corneometry is an appropriate non-invasive method that can be used for the measurement of skin hydration and water-holding capacity, especially if in association with other skin parameter measurements, e.g., TEWL. In fact, as these are all indirect parameters, their association can lead to more meaningful results.

3.1.3. Skin Dryness

Skin dryness is a common condition in which skin loses its homeostasis, and there is an impaired epidermal barrier. Many causes can contribute to this condition, such as exposure to aggressive solvents, frequent hand washing, specific occupational activities, or skin diseases (allergic or atopic dermatitis). Aging and hormonal changes can determine skin dryness, too.

Skin dryness is often called "xerosis", a term used in dermatology to indicate any condition of abnormal dry skin [27].

Pruritus is the most important symptom of skin dryness.

To evaluate the appropriateness of evaluation of skin dryness by an expert evaluator as an OV for the protection of skin against dehydration, database 2 was generated (see Table 1).

Daily insults from the environment can lower the water content of the *stratum corneum*, which impairs the enzymatic function required for normal desquamation, leading to a dry and flaky skin. Therefore, skin dryness can be considered to be an indirect measure of skin hydration.

However, dry skin is associated with major signs such as scaling, roughness, cracks and redness, and thus the evaluation of skin dryness cannot disregard the evaluation of these signs to obtain the overall dry skin score (ODS), a scoring scale combining all these major and minor signs of dry skin [28].

In conclusion, the skin dryness score is an appropriate outcome measure to be used for the substantiation of health claims in the context of protection of the skin against dehydration.

However, the combination with additional outcome measures such as TEWL is essential to obtain a more reliable and objective result.

Evaluation of Skin Dryness by an Expert Evaluator

The evaluation of skin dryness can be self-assessed by the subject or performed by an expert evaluator. In the first case, the evaluation can be influenced by subjective feelings, such as itching, while the evaluation by experts is based on objective criteria.

Usually, as recommended in the guidance published by The European Group on Efficacy Measurement of Cosmetics and other Topical Products, the expert evaluator can use a scoring scale combining all the effects of dry skin and judging it from 0 (absent) to 4 (advanced roughness, redness and cracks) [28]. If necessary, a specified symptom sum score can be used, using an evaluation of the main signs of xerosis (scaling, roughness, redness and cracks) in selected anatomical regions. Finally, an evaluation of the whole skin, as well as specifically at different sites (e.g., head/neck, upper and lower extremities, trunk), can be performed.

Moreover, dryness is a condition often associated with several dermatological diseases, in particular atopic dermatitis (also known as atopic eczema). Different scores have been developed to evaluate and classify disease grade: Eczema Area and Severity Index, Scoring Atopic Dermatitis, Objective Component of Score, Investigator Global Assessment, Atopic Dermatitis Severity Index and Body Surface Area [29]. Simultaneous use of two or more scores is a reliable assessment of disease severity.

The evaluation of dry skin by an expert evaluator is preferable compared to self-evaluation, because it is not influenced by subjective feelings such as itching and thus is more reproducible. Nevertheless, most of these scores consider patient's symptoms (as pruritus) and the effect of the disease on quality of life.

In conclusion, the evaluation of dry skin by an expert evaluator is an appropriate method to use for the measurement of skin dryness.

3.1.4. Skin Elasticity

Skin elasticity represents the ability of the skin to resume its original shape once it is stretched [30]. This property is determined by elastic and collagen fibers, arranged as a mesh in the dermis, which are responsible for the elastic and mechanical properties of the skin, respectively. Specifically, collagen fibers determine the mechanical stability of the tissue and its resistance to deformation; meanwhile, elastic fibers restore deformed collagen bundles to a more relaxed state. As with all organs, skin health is affected by aging, but in two ways: chrono-aging (the physiological aging of the skin genetically determined) and photo-aging (due to ultraviolet (UV) exposure). These processes are also influenced by many other factors (e.g., smoke, alcohol, pollution), which lead to degradation of collagen and elastin with a more stiffness of the skin [31]. The resulting loss of elasticity, with consequent reduction in moisture and formation of wrinkles, typically occurs in sun-exposed areas, such as facial skin.

To evaluate the appropriateness of skin elasticity as an OV for the protection of skin against dehydration, database 3 was generated (see Table 1).

The measurement of the viscoelastic properties of the skin can be an indicator for the biological age of the skin. Being an elastic material, skin is subject to the mechanical laws defining its properties, which are modified by some factors. One of the most important is the process of skin aging (i.e., intrinsic and extrinsic). In fact, tensile functions of the skin and subcutaneous tissues contribute to the appearance of the aged and photo-damaged skin, and to the effects of various other pathophysiological processes [32]. Moreover, the depth of skin wrinkles can appear deeper in less moisturized skin.

Therefore, skin elasticity is not an appropriate outcome variable to be used alone for the substantiation of health claims in the context of protection of the skin against dehydration. However, it can be used in combination with more significant skin measures, such as TEWL, in order to provide significant and descriptive information about the hydration of the skin.

Cutometer®

To date, several methods based on different principles have been proposed for evaluating skin elasticity.

Among these, the Cutometer® (Courage-Khazaka Electronic, Cologne, Germany) is probably the most commonly used instrument, and is considered the tool against which innovative or pilot instruments are to be compared. It is a handle device able to measure the viscoelastic properties of human skin using the suction/elongation method [33]. In detail, it can determine the elasticity of the upper skin layer using negative pressure, which is created in the device, and which mechanically deforms the skin. Skin is drawn into the aperture of the probe, and is released after a defined time. The depth of penetration of the skin inside the probe is determined using a non-contact optical measuring system.

The elasticity, i.e., the skin's ability to return to its original position when deformed, is displayed as a strain-time curve that can be analyzed by software. The many parameters that can be measured include the ability to return to the original state, the overall elasticity, and the net elasticity of the skin [34]. In addition, F- and Q-parameters can be measured, giving additional indications on skin age and elasticity [35].

These parameters have been widely used in studies both on normal skin (including cosmetological applications) and in skin disease (e.g., psoriasis and scleroderma), reflecting both the state of the skin and the change in the skin structure.

Because of significant regional variations in the viscoelastic properties of the skin, skin elasticity should be measured in the same area within a RCT [36].

In conclusion, the Cutometer is an appropriate method for the measurement of skin elasticity.

3.1.5. Corneocyte Adhesion

The major purpose of epidermal differentiation is generating the *stratum corneum* (the superficial skin layer), whose primary function is to protect the internal organs from desiccation and from external injuries.

Moreover, *stratum corneum* functions as a protective barrier against the outside, because of its well-organized structure. The structural integrity of the *stratum corneum* is guaranteed by corneocytes—dead differentiated keratinocytes, in which the cytoplasm is constituted by specialized proteins (keratins, filaggrin)—while the interstices between the corneocytes are enriched by lipids [37].

Stratum corneum lipids are nearly devoid of phospholipids, and are selectively enriched in sphingolipids (ceramides), free sterols and not-esterified fatty acids, with lesser quantities of nonpolar lipids and cholesterol sulphate. Ceramides are hydrophobic, and are ideal for preventing excess water loss. Corneocyte adhesion is possible because they are bridged together through particularly modified desmosomes, named corneodesmosomes, which ensure the stability and integrity of the *stratum corneum*. As corneocytes migrate towards the upper layer of the *stratum corneum*, corneodesmosomes weaken their adhesive function, allowing cells to be disrupted, and promoting the physiological desquamation process for the renewal of the *stratum corneum* layer. Accelerated corneodesmosome degradation leads to an enhanced desquamation process, leaving the outer layer exposed to the environment, xerosis, desquamation, and possible penetration by microbes or allergens [38]. Abnormality of the normal corneodesmosome structure is also related to common skin disease (e.g., psoriasis, atopic dermatitis, lichen planus).

To evaluate the appropriateness of corneocyte adhesion as an OV for the protection of skin against dehydration, database 4 was generated (see Table 1).

Ultraviolet, the outermost epidermal layer, plays a critical role in the physical protection of the body. To maintain a constant SC thickness, as observed in normal epidermis, the continuous generation of corneocytes is balanced by cell shedding at the external surface in the tightly regulated process of desquamation. Cohesion of the SC is largely dependent on modified desmosomes or corneodesmosomes. Corneodesmosome degradation is of major importance in the desquamation process [39]. Several skin conditions are related to an altered skin scaling. In xerosis and various hyperkeratotic states, including psoriasis, accumulation of scales is observed, and the number of corneodesmosomes persisting over the corneocyte surface in the upper SC is greatly increased [40]. Moreover, some of the disorders of cornification, such as congenital ichthyosiform erythroderma, shows other alterations of the epidermal features, such as increased TEWL. Perturbed barrier function, abnormal desquamation, and hyperproliferation appear to be intimately linked.

In conclusion, corneocyte adhesion is not appropriate to be used alone for the substantiation of health claims in the context of protection of the skin against dehydration. Nevertheless, it can be used as supportive evidence when combined with other appropriate outcome measures (e.g., TEWL).

Squamometry

The assessment of scaling and dryness is difficult to standardize. Nowadays, several methods based on different principles have been proposed for the evaluation of skin scaling. The most common technique is based on the sampling of the superficial scaling portion of the *stratum corneum* using various kinds of adhesive tapes (for example D-Squame®, CuDerm, Dallas, TX, USA) [41]. The quantification of scales or squames is made by using low-power imaging techniques [42], which allow the calculation of the squame size, number, optical density, and heterogeneity in relation to different aspects of the desquamation process. Image analysis can be performed using appropriate video-cameras such as the Visioscan® (Courage-Khazaka Electronic, Cologne, Germany), an ultraviolet A (UVA)-light video camera with high resolution. The images show the skin structure and the level of dryness, but it can also be used on spots of hair and scalp. The camera can be connected to the computer, and several skin surface parameters can be determined, including desquamation, sebum production, scaliness, smoothness and roughness [43]. The technique is repeatable and reproducible.

In conclusion, squamometry is an appropriate method to use for the evaluation of corneocyte adhesion.

3.1.6. Ceramide Concentration of the *Stratum Corneum*

In the *stratum corneum,* the matrix between corneocytes is composed of lipids arranged in numerous lamellar sheets, creating an impermeable barrier against external pathogens, and preventing water loss. More than 50% of the lipids of the intercellular space is represented by ceramides, which chemically belong to the sphingolipid class, as they are produced following the hydrolysis of sphingomyelin. Ceramides allow the formation of a barrier against cell permeability, and play a role in signal transduction, cell regulation, cell differentiation and immune response [44]. In human cells and tissues, there are commonly three ceramide classes, and human *stratum corneum* is known to contain even more complex ceramides. At least nine classes of ceramides have been classified on the basis of the characteristic fatty acid chain: non-hydroxy, α-hydroxy, ester-linked ω-hydroxy fatty acids, etc. [45] A lower level of ceramides, due to fatty acid hydrolysis, has been related to a loss in permeability of the skin surface, enhancing the skin inflammation by external agents. In fact, the loss of ceramides allows the pauperization of the intercellular lipid content, triggering water loss, as well as inflammation due to parasites and the grime accumulation between corneocytes. Although the causes of the decreased concentration of the ceramides in the *stratum corneum* due to skin lesions have been established, there is still a debate on the causes of the loss in non-lesioned skin, such as dermatitis, psoriasis or xerosis. However, it is widely recognized that skin disorders involving diminished barrier function show also a decrease in total ceramide content with some differences in the ceramide pattern.

To evaluate the appropriateness of ceramide concentration of the SC as an OV for the protection of skin against dehydration, database 4 was generated (see Table 1).

SC lipids are selectively enriched in sphingolipids (ceramides), free sterols, and free fatty acids, with lower quantities of non-polar lipids and cholesterol sulphate. Ceramide critical components of the barrier are hydrophobic, and are ideal for preventing excessive water loss. For this reason, SC water retention is improved by the addition of ceramides to damaged skin and a loss of these lipids causes profound barrier damage with a TEWL increase [44]. However, damage is also due to other mechanisms, such as a simultaneous, passive loss of extracellular calcium and potassium ions, and other lipids, including cholesterol and fatty acids, are also implicated.

In conclusion, ceramide concentration of the SC cannot be used alone as an outcome variable for the substantiation of health claims in the context of protection of the skin against dehydration. However, it can be used as supporting evidence when appropriate outcome measures (e.g., TEWL) are also considered. In fact, all of these values are indirect values, so it is better to combine different measurements for a more reliable and sensitive result.

HPLC (High Performance Liquid Chromatography)

The most common method for detection and quantification of the different classes of ceramides is based on liquid chromatography techniques [46].

Biological samples that can be used for the analyses include epidermis collected by tape-stripping method, as well as blood or tissue samples (e.g., liver or adipose). Ceramides are chemically derivatized with benzoyl chloride or anhydride, depending on the fatty acid chain bound to sphingosine [47]. This step leads to the production of the *N*-acyl derivatives, which strongly absorb in the range 230–280 nm, depending on the ceramide type. Then, direct-phase HPLC is performed by using silica gels resins, while the mobile phase for the elution is based on organic solvents, such as hexane, pentane or ethyl acetate. The method is simple, sensitive and accurate. However, due to the instability of the derivatization product, samples should not be stored for prolonged periods, and analysis must be performed just after derivatization. Another limit of the HPLC method is that ceramide classes targeted for quantification are restricted to only few types.

In conclusion, HPLC is an appropriate method to be used for the measurement of the ceramide concentration of the *stratum corneum*.

3.1.7. Pruritus

Pruritus, or itching, can be defined as an unpleasant sensation of the skin causing the desire to scratch the affected area. The mechanisms of pruritus have not yet been totally understood. It may be both localized and generalized and can occur as an acute or chronic condition. Itching can be the result of a dermatological disease (such as atopic dermatitis, eczema or urticaria), but can also be the result of several systemic diseases (e.g., thyroid or liver dysfunctions, important hormonal changes, hematological diseases, and nerve or psychiatric disorders) [48]. Nevertheless, itching can also be quite a common sign of simple skin conditions, such as dehydrated skin, and it can be exacerbated by cold and dry weather or increase with age. Moreover, if severe, itching can affect the quality of life of individuals and it has also important psychological implications [49,50]. Evaluating pruritus is very difficult due to the absolute subjectivity of the symptoms.

To evaluate the appropriateness of pruritus as an OV for the protection of skin against dehydration, database 6 was generated (see Table 1).

Pruritus is the most common symptom in dermatology. As mentioned above, pruritus can be related to several pathological conditions, but it can also indicate a lack of the normal skin integrity and correct hydration. For this reason, it is a frequent symptom in aged people [50]. Due to the large amount of pruritus-associated conditions, to the difficulties in identifying symptoms and the psychological components, and to the difficult quantification for its subjectivity, pruritus cannot be used alone as an outcome variable for the substantiation of health claims in the context of protection of the skin against dehydration. However, it can be used as supporting evidence when appropriate outcome measures (e.g., TEWL) are also considered.

Questionnaires

Itching is a subjective condition difficult to quantify. Moreover, its multifactorial etiology is difficult to characterize.

Several scales and scores have been proposed, both monodimensional and multidimensional. The former, including the visual analogue scale, numerical rating scale, and verbal rating scale, report information about intensity of itching in a specific moment. Conversely, multidimensional scales can provide different information including affected areas, progression of itch throughout the day and its evolution during the time, disability induced by the pruritus, improvement during treatment. This is why multidimensional scales can also be used as an instrument for evaluating treatment.

One of the most used methods are the visual analog scales (VAS), both vertical and horizontal [51]. Different authors have proposed different categorizations of VAS, such as: 0 = no pruritus, >0–<4 points = mild pruritus, ≥4–<7 points = moderate pruritus, 7–8.9 points = severe pruritus, and ≥9 points = very severe pruritus. The VAS is a valuable, easy and rapid method for estimating pruritus, and has shown good reproducibility and reliability [52]. In addition, VAS results have proven to be reproducible even in different populations and ethnic groups. However, similar to other monodimensional methodologies, VAS has some drawbacks. For example, it only measures intensity, without considering the impact on quality of life, or other parameters such as duration and distribution of itching. For this reason, a 5-D itch scale has been developed as a multidimensional questionnaire [53,54]. The five dimensions are degree, duration, direction, disability and distribution, with a scale specifically designed to facilitate the use of pruritus as an outcome variable in RCTs and clinical trials.

In conclusion, questionnaires are an appropriate method to be used for the measurement of pruritus. The use of VAS is appropriate, although the use of multidimensional methods is preferable, allowing a thorough comprehension of the pruritus condition.

3.1.8. Water-Holding Capacity

The water in the skin is present as both free and bound (to macromolecules) water.

The ability of the skin to hold water is primarily related to the SC, which acts as a barrier to water loss. Although the SC is a thin biological membrane, it is an essential part of the body, allowing it to survive even in a dry atmosphere by protecting our body from desiccation. The barrier function and the water-holding capacity of the SC depend on the presence of well-differentiated corneocytes with cornified envelope-associated proteins. These proteins bind the ceramide containing intercellular lipids and large amounts of moisturizing factors mainly consisting of water-soluble amino acids produced by enzymatic degradation of filaggrin [55].

Lipids and keratins play a key role in the formation of the permeability barrier, and are responsible for the water-holding capacity, which can be defined as the ability of the SC to retain water.

Because the SC is the interface between the fully hydrated viable epidermis and the dry atmosphere, there is a gradient of water in this thin biological membrane [56]. However, when the uppermost portion of the SC loses water, even normal individuals develop dry skin. This condition leads to a fine cracking in the SC, which deteriorates its barrier function focally, allowing permeation of external substances as well as TEWL.

To evaluate the appropriateness of water-holding capacity as an OV for the protection of skin against dehydration, database 6 was generated (see Table 1).

Skin hydration can depend on the water-holding capacities of the SC, but it is not a unique parameter for correctly assessing skin hydration. That is why the combination with other variables is important for a more accurate assessment of skin conditions and of potential alterations and changes. In conclusion, the water-holding capacity is not appropriate to be used alone for the substantiation of health claims in the context of protection of the skin against dehydration. However, it can be used as supporting evidence when other appropriate outcome measures (e.g., TEWL) are considered.

Corneometry

See "Corneometry" in Section 3.1.2.

3.1.9. Skin Smoothness and Roughness

Due to the three-dimensional organization of cutis and subcutaneous tissue, skin surface is not perfectly smooth and is characterized by folds, furrows, orifices, and crests. In particular, some morphological characteristics of the epidermis (thickness of the cornified layer) and dermis (collagen content) can determine skin surface. However, pathological issues such as dermatitis, eczema, and other conditions, such as chronic light exposure, pollution and aggressive substances, may change the balance between skin smoothness and roughness, and may enhance the hardening process of the skin, leading to the coarsening of the skin surface structure with an increase of the wrinkle number and depth and, in general, of the roughness.

Skin smoothness and roughness, together with skin scaling and wrinkles, are considered to be the qualitative and quantitative parameters of skin physiological conditions, and represent the four clinical parameters that, if considered together, allow the Surface Evaluation of the Living Skin (SELS) [57].

To evaluate the appropriateness of skin smoothness and roughness as an OV for the protection of skin against dehydration, database 7 was generated (see Table 1).

With aging, skin texture undergoes several changes. Epidermal thickness decreases with a flattening of dermal-epidermal junction, while wrinkles increase due to loss of collagen content. This process is typical of aging, and it is more evident in photo-exposed areas. As the skin ages, changes in the texture and roughness or smoothness of the skin become apparent [58]. This is the result of loss of barrier integrity, which leads to increased water loss, but it is also due to changes in the collagen-supporting matrices showing visibly on the skin surface [59]. In fact, skin aging is a multifactorial process involving different mechanisms with a modification of different skin parameters, such as an increase in epidermal water loss.

In conclusion, skin smoothness and roughness are not appropriate to be used alone for the substantiation of health claims in the context of protection of the skin against dehydration. However, they can be used as supporting evidence when other appropriate outcome measures are considered (e.g., TEWL). In addition, the simultaneous evaluation of all 4 parameters, allowing the SELS (e.g., skin wrinkles and scaling), is preferable, in order to have a more reliable value.

UV Camera

Skin topography can be directly evaluated by using appropriate video-cameras. Among these, Visioscan®—a UVA-light video camera with high resolution—has been widely and successfully used as an alternative to the conventional color video cameras.

Visioscan® consists of a black and white video sensor chip, an objective and an UVA-light, and is equipped with two special halogenide lights that illuminate the skin.

Visioscan® can be used to measure the SELS, which has been proposed as a qualitative and quantitative measure of the skin surface. SELS includes evaluation of skin smoothness and roughness, skin scaling and wrinkles [57]. Other parameters can be analyzed with Visioscan®, such as skin desquamation and scalp and sebum production. With this method, skin can be optically monitored using an image-digitalization process. The grey level distribution is analyzed, making it possible to calculate the four SELS parameters, both quantitatively and qualitatively. This is useful to describe the skin surface as an index [60].

Visioscan® is small, easy-to-handle, and economical, and makes it possible to have multi-frame pictures of the skin and to store these images for subsequent evaluation; it is therefore useful in elaborating different parameters throughout the time.

In conclusion, UV cameras such as Visioscan® are an appropriate method for measuring skin smoothness and roughness, wrinkles and scaling. However, it is worth noting that none of these outcome measures is appropriate to be used alone for the substantiation of health claims in the context of maintenance of skin function.

3.1.10. Skin Wrinkles

Skin surface is not flat, but is characterized by several grooves, classified according to their depth. For this reason, the skin surface exhibits a network called microrelief or texture. This microrelief is very important for the mechanical properties of the skin, as it forms a complex system of small lines intersecting each other. On fingers and toes, these lines assume a characteristic disposition, and determine the fingerprint. As a result of age and UV exposure, skin microrelief changes, and some lines become more marked—being defined as wrinkles [58]. An example of wrinkles are so called "crow's-feet", which are localized on the forehead or around the eye circles, and may vary in amplitude and marking severity.

Age, diseases (including psoriasis or atopic dermatitis) and the loss of hydration of the skin may alter the physiological desquamation of the skin, giving some roughness to the touch.

As already mentioned, skin wrinkles, together with skin scaling, roughness and smoothness, are considered to be qualitative and quantitative parameters of skin physiological conditions, and represent the four clinical parameters that, if considered together, allow the SELS [57].

To evaluate the appropriateness of skin wrinkles as an OV for the protection of skin against dehydration, database 8 was generated (see Table 1).

Wrinkle formation is a genetically-determined process (a process called "chrono-aging" or intrinsic aging). Several environmental factors contribute to wrinkle formation and/or worsening, such as smoking, UV-exposure, age, pollution ("photo-aging" or extrinsic aging) [58]. These mechanisms lead to a loss of elasticity that contributes to the worsening of wrinkles through decreased skin hydration.

Even if skin wrinkles are a reliable parameter of skin structure, they are an indirect parameter of skin hydration [61]. For this reason, skin wrinkles are not appropriate to be used alone for the substantiation of health claims in the context of protection of the skin against dehydration. However, they can be used as supportive evidence when appropriate outcome measures are also considered (e.g., TEWL).

In addition, the simultaneous evaluation of all 4 parameters that allow the SELS (e.g., skin smoothness, roughness and scaling) is preferable, in order to obtain more accurate results.

UV Camera

See "UV Camera" In Section 3.1.9.

3.1.11. Skin Scaling

Skin scaling, also known as skin peeling or desquamation, is the loss of the outer layer of the epidermis (*stratum corneum*) in large flakes. This layer consists of 18–20 layers of flattened dead keratinocytes with no nuclei and cell organelles, which have a defensive role against pathogens and environmental insults [62]. Skin scaling is a physiological process occurring when keratinocytes shed in an inappreciable way because of the new ones located in the underneath layer. In contrast, it is considered pathological when induced by disease or pathological causes, such as atopic dermatitis, contact dermatitis/eczema, or extreme cases of severe drug reactions, which can lead to a real exfoliation with loss of several layers of epidermis [63]. In these cases, keratinocytes scale down, leaving the outer layer of the skin unprotected. For these reasons, the pathological peeling of the epidermis may be accompanied by itch, dryness or irritating phenomena, which enhance the loss of the keratinocytes.

As already mentioned, skin scaling, together with skin wrinkles, roughness, and smoothness are considered to be qualitative and quantitative parameters of the skin physiological conditions, and represent the four clinical parameters that, if considered together, allow the SELS [57].

To evaluate the appropriateness of skin scaling as an OV for the protection of skin against dehydration, database 9 was generated (see Table 1).

Skin scaling is a sign frequently observed on the skin surface. It usually suggests an alteration in skin homeostasis and an alteration of the *stratum corneum*. During their transit through the epidermal layers toward the skin surface, keratinocytes follow a well predetermined differentiation program in order to originate the *stratum corneum*. Several conditions can lead to skin scaling. As cited above, some dermatological diseases are characterized by scaling. However, scaling can be also determined by a transient state of skin dehydration or other particular conditions. For example, being elderly is accompanied by an epidermal barrier impaired with TEWL increase, xerosis and skin scaling [64].

In conclusion, skin scaling is not appropriate to be used alone for the substantiation of health claims in the context of protection of the skin against dehydration. However, it can be used as supporting evidence when appropriate outcome measures are also considered (e.g., TEWL).

In addition, the simultaneous evaluation of all 4 parameters allowing the SELS (e.g., skin smoothness, roughness and wrinkles) is preferable.

UV Camera

See "UV Camera" in Section 3.1.9.

3.1.12. Skin Tightness and Softness

Tightness and softness are skin conditions mainly dependent on skin compactness and elasticity, which may be influenced by several factors: diet; exposure to chemicals such as soaps or detergents; and atmospheric conditions, i.e., sun or wind. Pathological conditions, such as scleroderma, or diseases of collagen and subcutaneous tissue can modify skin tightness and softness [65].

To evaluate the appropriateness of skin tightness and softness as an OV for the protection of skin against dehydration, database 10 was generated (see Table 1).

Skin tightness and softness are features more typical of the deep tissue of the cutis (connective tissue) than the epidermis. They are determined by changes of deep components of the dermis, in particular, collagen and elastic fibers. Intrinsic and extrinsic aging leads to a degradation of collagen and elastic fibers with a consequent intensification of skin wrinkles, dryness and scaling.

However, skin texture can also be modified by pathological conditions of the connective tissue, which is characterized by changes in composition and/or tridimensional organization of collagen. In particular, systemic sclerosis (also known as scleroderma) or morphea (a localized form of sclerosis) are the result of an excessive activation of the repair process known as fibrosis leading to a severe skin tightening [66]. On the other hand, an increased softness is the main feature of elastic fiber disease, such as cutis laxa, in which the skin becomes inelastic and hangs loosely in folds. Patients develop a prematurely aged appearance. Nevertheless, a loss of skin elasticity is often associated with changes in other skin features, such as a decreased water content of the skin.

In conclusion, skin tightness and softness are not appropriate to be used alone for the substantiation of health claims in the context of protection of the skin against dehydration. However, they can be used as supporting evidence when appropriate outcome measures are also considered (e.g., TEWL).

Self-Assessment

Skin tightness or softness is evaluated by using the Modified Rodnan Score [67]. This score consists of an evaluation of skin thickness rated by clinical palpation using a 0–3 scale (0 = normal skin; 1 = mild thickness; 2 = moderate thickness; 3 = severe thickness with inability to pinch the skin into a fold) for each of the 17 surface anatomic areas of the body: face, anterior chest, abdomen, (right and left separately) fingers, forearms, upper arms, tights, lower legs, dorsum of hands and feet. These individual values are added, and the sum is defined as the total skin score, ranging from 0 to 51.

Modified Rodnan score is frequently utilized to evaluate the systemic sclerosis (or scleroderma), characterized by a progressive increase in skin tightness [68], and to monitor the efficacy of treatments. Skin thickness is used as a surrogate measure of disease activity, severity and mortality in patients with diffuse cutaneous systemic sclerosis, and higher skin thickness progression rates are predictive of internal organ involvement and mortality. This score can be used by physicians, but can also be self-assessed by the subjects, due to the high level of correlation between subject self-assessment and physician-assessment. In conclusion, the self-assessment with Modified Rodnan Score is an appropriate method to be used for the measurement of the skin tightness and softness.

3.1.13. Skin Reddening and Erythema Formation

Erythema is a skin condition characterized by redness and is typically caused by vasodilation of superficial capillaries in the dermis [69]. It is a major feature of inflammatory skin reactions elicited by irritants or allergens. Erythema is often associated with an impaired barrier function, such as in the case of "sensitive skin" and rosacea, atopic dermatitis, psoriasis, allergic reactions, autoimmune disease [70]. Erythema is one of the most frequent signs of a pathological skin, with or without an impaired epidermal barrier function.

To evaluate the appropriateness of skin reddening and erythema formation as an OV for the protection of skin against dehydration, database 11 was generated (see Table 1).

If severe, reddening and erythema may lead to the loss of the barrier function of the skin. Moreover, an impaired epidermal barrier (as measured by an increase in TEWL) can be associated with clinical symptoms like redness and erythema.

Nevertheless, erythema is not directly and unequivocally related to an impaired structure or hydration or permeability function of the skin.

Therefore, skin reddening and erythema formation are not appropriate to be used for the substantiation of health claims in the context of protection of the skin against dehydration.

3.1.14. Capillary Blood Flow

The total blood flow within the systemic circulation is about 5 L/min. Most of the cardiac output is received by the gastrointestinal system and the skeletal muscle, while only ~5% goes to the skin. Cutaneous microcirculation is organized into two horizontal plexuses: one more superficial, situated in the upper dermis (1 ± 1.5 mm below the skin surface) and one deeper, at the dermal-subcutaneous junction [71]. Several factors can induce an alteration of cutaneous microcirculation with a vasodilation such as drugs or chemicals, UV, cutaneous inflammatory disease (e.g., psoriasis, eczema, allergic reactions, rosacea), and vascular disorders (i.e., Raynaud's phenomenon or peripheral circulating disorders) [72]. A preserved microcirculation is essential for the proper delivery of oxygen and nutritive substances to the biological tissue as well as for the removal of toxins.

To evaluate the appropriateness of capillary blood flow as an OV for the protection of skin against dehydration, database 12 was generated (see Table 1).

A normal blood flow allows an appropriate delivery of nutrients and a simultaneous removal of products of metabolism. This is why an inappropriate removal of these waste products, which may occur in cases of reduced blood flow, could have negative effects on both the body and the skin.

Therefore, the measurement of blood flow might provide useful information on skin health. For instance, blood flow in the capillaries can be directly associated with wrinkle formation by a reduction of the flow and of the delivery of nutritional compounds to the cells [73].

However, there is no strong scientific evidence suggesting that a reduced capillary blood flow is unequivocally related to an impaired structure/hydration or elasticity of the skin. There are several other mechanisms that contribute to unhealthy skin. Erythema and altered blood flow are also not always associated with either an impaired of barrier or with a decrease in hydration.

In conclusion, capillary blood flow is not an appropriate outcome variable to be used for the substantiation of health claims in the context of protection of the skin against dehydration.

3.2. Protection of the Skin against Oxidative (Including UV-Induced) Damage

In physiological conditions, the skin cellular redox processes constantly produce free radicals, such as reactive oxygen species (ROS) and reactive nitrogen species (RNS), which are finely counteracted by endogenous and exogenous systems. When these antioxidant defenses are inadequate to fully inactivate the ROS (because of excessive production of ROS and/or because of inadequate antioxidant defenses), a condition of oxidative stress can occur. Oxidative stress has been widely associated with an increased risk of many acute and chronic diseases, mainly because of its role in altering the molecular structure and function of DNA, proteins and lipids. In addition, these oxidative products may accumulate over the time.

As skin is the most exposed organ to environmental sunlight and pathogens, it represents the major protective interface between the body and the environment. Therefore, it is exposed to many sources of oxidative stress including pollutants, infrared irradiation, xenobiotics and most of all UV radiation. Many mechanisms are involved in UV-induced damage, including up-regulation of gene expression through intracellular signal transduction pathways, suppression of immune reaction and induction of tolerance to antigens. Moreover, UV radiation seems to form a complex interaction with mitochondria, where it may contribute to a vicious circle of increasing damage.

3.2.1. Oxidative Damage to DNA

Exposure to UVA and ultraviolet B (UVB) radiation may lead to the oxidation of DNA, proteins and lipids. As a result, several products of oxidation may originate. The main classes of products directly deriving from DNA oxidation are cis-syn cyclobutane pyrimidine dimers (CPDs), followed by pyrimidine-pyrimidone photoproducts [74].

Regarding the DNA products of oxidative DNA damage due to ROS, these mainly consist of a large group of compounds deriving from the DNA bases such as the guanine. One of the main products of DNA oxidation is the 8-hydroxydeoxyguanosine (8-OHdG), a pre-mutagenic lesion in mammalian cells that is considered a ubiquitous marker of oxidative stress. 8-OHdG is generated by hydroxyl radical, singlet oxygen, or direct electron transfer which does not involve any ROS. 8-OHdG may cause mutation (G:C to T:A) at DNA replication. In addition to 8-OHdG, UV radiation may produce many other products of DNA damage, such as protein-DNA crosslinks and single-strand breaks.

To evaluate the appropriateness of oxidative damage to DNA as an outcome variable for the protection of the skin against oxidative damage, database 13 was generated (see Table 1).

Solar UV radiation is one of the most important causes of skin lesions and related diseases. In fact, UV radiation induces a variety of photoproducts in DNA, including CPDs, pyrimidine-pyrimidone photoproducts, thymine glycols, cytosine damage, purine damage, DNA strand breaks, and DNA-protein crosslinks. If unrepaired damage occurs to regulatory genes (e.g., tumor suppressor genes), this may promote the process of carcinogenesis. In this context, gene mutation and activation may be important [75]. Other responses resulting from UV ray exposure of cells include increased cellular proliferation, which could have a tumor-promoting effect on genetically altered cells, as well as changes in components of the immune system present in the skin.

It is well documented that, in contrast to UVB radiation, the less energetic UVA photons may indirectly affect membranes, proteins, and DNA, by producing ROS. Among the most representative DNA oxidation products, 8-OHdG is commonly used as an indirect biomarker of oxidative DNA stress, although several factors (e.g., artifacts during isolation of DNA and its preparation for analysis) should be carefully considered, as they can affect its measurement [76].

To gain a better understanding of the mutagenic and carcinogenic features of UVA radiation, the identification of other products of oxidatively-generated DNA damage requires further investigations. These products include DNA–protein crosslinks and adducts, which may be issued from the covalent binding of reactive aldehydes arising from the decomposition of lipid hydroperoxides to nucleobases.

In conclusion, direct measures of oxidative damage to DNA, such as CPDs, are appropriate to be used for the substantiation of health claims in the context of protection of the skin against oxidative (including UV-induced) damage. Conversely, indirect products of DNA oxidation such as 8-OHdG are not appropriate for the substantiation of health claims in the context of protection against oxidative damage to DNA when measured alone, but they could be used as supporting evidence.

Skin Biopsy and High Performance Liquid Chromatography

The in vivo evaluation of direct markers of oxidative damage to DNA must be assessed directly on the target tissue, which should be correctly harvested, treated and stored, prior to being analyzed. Skin biopsy is the procedure used to sample the outer layer of the derma, and may be performed using different techniques, according to the type of analysis, the size and the location of the part which should be sampled. Shave biopsy, performed with a scalpel or a razor blade, allows the harvest of a tangential part of the skin across the target place. Punch biopsy, performed with a circular blade, allows the harvest of a round or ellipsoidal part of the epidermis, dermis and subcutaneous fat close to the target place of the skin. Excisional biopsy is an incisional biopsy where the harvested sample includes the target place with the lesion or the mutation [77]. A particular skin collection may be performed by using stripes that allow the sampling of the lonely dead keratinocytes on the outer layer, or by using cotton pads to collect sebum or skin lipids.

Skin samples collected by biopsy can be used for the evaluation of products of oxidative damage to DNA, such as CPDs, detected by using several methods, including high performance liquid chromatography with electrospray ionization-tandem mass spectrometry, which represents the reference method. In vitro UVR radiation of standard nucleosides is performed to obtain a calibration curve useful for quantifying the products of oxidation, such as cis-syn and trans-syn CPDs, cyclobutane thymine dimers, as well as oxidized nucleosides, i.e., 1,3 dimethyluracile [78].

In conclusion, skin biopsy followed by high performance liquid chromatography is an appropriate method for the measurement of direct markers of oxidative DNA damage like CPDs.

Skin Biopsy and Immunohistochemical Techniques

The in vivo evaluation of direct marker of oxidative damage to lipids must be assessed directly on the target tissue, and skin biopsy is the most accurate procedure, as described in "Skin Biopsy and High Performance Liquid Chromatography" in Section 3.2.1.

In alternative to chromatographic techniques, oxidative damage to DNA can be measured by semiquantitative immunohistochemical ones.

After the biopsy is assessed, skin samples are washed in saline solutions and fixed in opportune buffers (i.e., formalin, formaldehyde, paraformaldehyde) and included in paraffin. Samples are then sectioned and stained with non-human primary monoclonal or polyclonal antibodies anti-CPD by using a direct or a sandwich enzyme-linked immunosorbent assay (ELISA) technique. In this last case, a secondary antibody, which may be bound to a biotin-streptavidin complex, is required to increase the signal of CPD detection. Alternatively, primary cells harvested from the biopsy samples may be cultured and allowed to grow in vitro. In this way, it is possible to harvest cells from the culture medium, and process them for immunohistochemical analysis with primary or secondary antibodies anti-CPD [79]. It has been demonstrated that cells containing CPDs have a shorter survival and tend to die quicker than non-damaged cells.

Indirect products of oxidation, such as 8-OHdG, are also assayed with immunohistochemical techniques. As described previously, the included skin cells are processed for staining with anti-8-OHdG antibodies. Further washing allows the elimination of the remaining sample, and then a secondary anti-primary antibody is added to the well. An enzyme catalyzing the production of a colored substrate is bound to the same secondary antibody. The quantification of the analyte is carried out by measuring the intensity of the immunostaining, and by subtracting the value of the background at a cell-free area of the slice. Immunostaining is measured by using microscopes or cameras equipped with computer presenting image analysis software [80].

The method results are more sensitive to both CPD and 8-OHdG than the chromatographic ones, because even very small amounts of antigen are stained with the antibodies. Nevertheless, its results are less specific, particularly when polyclonal antibodies are used, as cross-link phenomena may occur between molecules having similar structure.

In conclusion, based on these considerations, skin biopsy followed by immunohistochemical detection of CPD and 8-OHdG is an appropriate method for measurement of markers of oxidative DNA damage at skin level.

3.2.2. Oxidative Damage to Lipids

Lipids are fundamental components of the skin surface and are present as both sebaceous and epidermal lipids. Although the lipid profile is characterized by a large inter-individual variation, squalene, sebaleic acid, linoleic acid, and cholesterol are the most represented.

Skin lipids are susceptible to oxidation through three different mechanisms: free radical chain oxidation, enzymatic oxidation, and non-radical, non-enzymatic oxidation [81].

Skin photo-oxidation, which is a consequence of exposure to UVA and UVB, may result in the production of many oxidation products, including squalene monohydroperoxyde and hydroperoxycholesterol. In addition, lipid peroxidation products such as hydroxyeicosatetraenoic acids (HETEs) and isoprostanes have been found to increase in human skin following UV exposure.

Lipid peroxidation (LPO) products tend to accumulate in the cellular membranes proportionally with the cumulative oxidative stress of the skin. High concentrations of LPO products perturb the integrity of the membranes, and thus of the cells involved. Lipid peroxides can be further decomposed to many reactive aldehydic species, such as malondialdehyde, 4-hydroxynonenal, hexanal, as well as other saturated and unsaturated aldehydes and ketones [82].

To evaluate the appropriateness of oxidative damage to lipids as an outcome variable for the protection of the skin against oxidative damage, database 13 was generated (see Table 1).

UV radiation induces many indirect photo-chemical effects in the skin. In this context, LPO is one of the major pathways by which photo-oxidative stress disturbs cell signaling, and promotes photo-carcinogenesis and photo-aging. Studies have shown a significant linear relation between UVB exposure recorded by the dosimeters and colorimetry parameters of the skin reaction.

An established marker of oxidative damage to cell membranes, which is reliably measured by immunohistochemistry, is represented by F2-isoprostanes. F2-isoprostanes are a series of prostaglandin F2-like compounds produced in vivo independently of cyclo-oxygenase as products of radical catalyzed LPO. Among these F2-isoprostanes, 8-epi-prostaglandin 2a (8-isoprostane) is the most representative. A linear relation was found between the generation of 8-isoprostane in the skin and the dosimeter readouts [83]. 8-Isoprostane has been validated as a marker for oxidative stress in various conditions and in the skin.

In conclusion, products of oxidative damage to lipids, such as isoprostanes, are appropriate outcome variables to be used for the substantiation of health claims in the context of protection of the skin against oxidative (including UV-induced) damage.

Skin Biopsy and Liquid or Gas Chromatography-Mass Technique

The in vivo evaluation of direct markers of oxidative damage to lipids must be assessed directly on the target tissue, and skin biopsy is the most accurate procedure, as described in "Skin Biopsy and High Performance Liquid Chromatography" in Section 3.2.1.

The most common method for detecting and quantifying hydroxyperoxides, such as squalene monohydroperoxide and cholesterol, is based on the liquid or gas chromatography technique [84]. After the collection of the skin, samples are extracted with organic solvents, e.g., acetone or 1-butanol, and prepared for the injection into chromatographic instruments. Chromatographic detection and quantification of target compounds may be performed by analyzing their mass, and/or that of their main fragments. Gas chromatography is more frequently used than liquid chromatography, as the mobile phase is cheaper, and because of the volatility of the sampling compounds.

Liquid chromatography techniques can be also used for the detection and quantification of isoprostanes (i.e., 8-Isoprostaglandin F2α), leukotrienes (i.e., HETE), hydroperoxyeicosatetraenoic acid (HpETEs) and lipoxin (i.e., lipoxin A4 (LXA4) and B4 (LXB4)) [85]. This is the preferred method, as it is simple, cheap, and very sensitive, as the concentration of these analytes in tissues are very scarce.

In conclusion, liquid or gas chromatography-mass techniques following skin biopsy are appropriate methods to be used for the measurement of markers of lipid oxidation like isoprostanes at skin level.

Skin Biopsy and Immunohistochemical Techniques

The in vivo evaluation of direct markers of oxidative damage to lipids must be assessed directly on the target tissue, and skin biopsy is the most accurate procedure, as described in "Skin Biopsy and High Performance Liquid Chromatography" in Section 3.2.1.

The detection and quantification of isoprostanes (i.e., 8-Isoprostaglandin F2α), leukotrienes (i.e., HETE, HpETEs and lipoxin (i.e., LXA4 and LXB4) can be performed by using immunohistochemical techniques, such as ELISA assays [83]. After the biopsy is assessed, skin samples are washed in saline solutions and fixed in opportune buffers and included in paraffin. Subsequently, samples are sectioned and stained with non-human primary antibodies specific for the marker (i.e., polyclonal goat anti-8-epiPGF-2α antibody). As described in "Skin Biopsy and Immunohistochemical Techniques"in Section 3.2.1, further washing allows the elimination of the remaining sample before a secondary anti-primary antibody is added in the well and an enzyme catalyzing the production of a colored substrates is bound to the same secondary antibody. The quantification of the analyte is carried out by measuring the intensity of immunostaining by subtracting the value of the background at a cell-free area of the slice. Immunostaining is measured by using microscopes or cameras equipped with a computer running image analysis software.

The principal limitation of immunohistochemistry is the need for high-resolution image analysis to obtain reliable results. Furthermore, the technique is more specific when monoclonal antibodies are used for the precise marker compared to polyclonal ones, which may recognize similar epitopes of different isoprostanes. However, monoclonal antibodies are expensive and request long times of production.

In conclusion, skin biopsy, followed by immunohistochemical detection of lipids, is an appropriate method for the measurement of markers of oxidative damage to lipid like isoprostanes in the skin.

3.2.3. Oxidative Damage to Proteins

UV radiation can interact with cellular photosensitizers to generate ROS and ROS-mediated oxidative damage to DNA, proteins and lipids. It is well known that UVB rays induce a direct formation of DNA-photoproducts that are generally removed by the nucleotide excision repair system. UVA represents more than 95% of the incident solar radiation. The effects of UVA reflect the induction of oxidative stress that causes extensive protein oxidation.

Moreover, sustained UV-exposure can lead to a high extent of protein oxidation, which is generally increased in aged tissue [86]. ROS-induced oxidative damage to the structural dermal proteins collagen and elastin can result in changes in the protein conformation and unfolding, leading to modifications in the mechanical properties of skin. Collagen degradation and abnormal elastin accumulation are visible in photo-aged skin. Proteins undergo modifications and subsequent conformational changes when certain amino acids are converted to their oxidized forms.

Several biomarkers have been used to assess the extent of oxidative damage to protein in the skin. Reactive oxygen species (ROS) can lead to protein modifications occurring at the backbone, at amino acid side chains, as well as by the formation of protein carbonyls. Oxidative damage to proteins results in a multitude of products, arising from modification of a wide range of amino acids [87]. The various amino acid residues do not have the same susceptibility to oxidative modifications. For instance, histidine, leucine, methionine, and cysteine, as well as phenylalanine, tyrosine, and tryptophan, are more susceptible than others to the presence of thiols or hydroxyl moieties, which are more sensitive to oxidation processes [75].

Conversely, oxidation of proteins containing proline, arginine, lysine and threonine results in the formation of irreversible carbonyl groups. If compared to the deeper layers of the epidermis, these carbonyls have been found to be more concentrated in the SC.

To evaluate the appropriateness of oxidative damage to proteins as an outcome variable for the protection of the skin against oxidative damage, database 13 was generated (see Table 1).

Despite the presence of antioxidant defensive-systems, UV radiations cause extensive protein modification, which seems to be involved in aging processes and disease development [88].

ROS generated from UV exposure is the most important triggering agent of protein oxidation. Hydroxyl-, peroxyl-, nitro-, etc. radicals are able to modify both the carbon skeleton and the R group of the protein in order to create more unstable products. In detail, cysteine or methionine sulfenic/sulfonic acids, hydroxytyrosine, nitrotryptophan are produced inside the cell, causing the loss of the function of the relative proteins which they constitute. Due to their instability, the next step is the generation of protein carbonyl groups which are usually the resulting marker of protein oxidation, as they represent an irreversible form of protein modification [75].

In conclusion, products of oxidative damage to proteins such as oxidative changes in amino acids are appropriate outcome variables to be used for the substantiation of health claims in the context of protection of the skin against oxidative (including UV-induced) damage.

Conversely, protein carbonyls should be used in combination with direct markers of oxidative damage to proteins in vivo.

Skin Biopsy and Liquid Chromatography-Mass Technique

The in vivo evaluation of direct markers of oxidative damage to proteins must be assessed directly on the target tissue, and skin biopsy is the most accurate procedure, as described in "Skin Biopsy and High Performance Liquid Chromatography" in Section 3.2.1.

A sensitive and specific method for detection of the direct products of protein oxidation is based on the liquid chromatography technique [89]. After the collection of the SC samples by using strips, they are washed and treated to avoid contaminations. Then, the sample is treated to avoid artefacts, and is digested with proteases, i.e., pepsin, trypsin and chymotrypsin, in acid conditions in order to avoid the formation of polymers. Samples are injected into chromatography instruments, and the detection and quantification of target compounds may be performed by analyzing the mass of the target compounds and/or their main fragments.

In conclusion, based on these considerations, skin biopsy followed by liquid or gas chromatography techniques is an appropriate method for the measurement of markers of oxidative damage to proteins at skin level.

3.3. Protection of the Skin from UV-Induced (Other Than Oxidative) Damage

3.3.1. DNA Damage after UV Radiation Exposure

Exposure of skin to UV radiation has been shown to have a number of deleterious effects, including photo-aging, photo-immunosuppression and photo-induced DNA damage, which can lead to the development of skin cancer [90]. DNA has been shown to be a skin chromophore, and absorption of UV radiation by DNA can result in the formation of thymine dimers.

To evaluate the appropriateness of DNA damage after UV radiation exposure as OV for the protection of the skin from UV-induced damage, database 14 was generated (see Table 1).

DNA, in vitro and in vivo, is susceptible to being damaged when exposed to high-energy radiation. This damage can be a breaking of one or both of the strands in the DNA helix, a fusing of the two strands to each other, to themselves (dimers), or other types of molecular damage to the nucleotides. Usually, the majority of DNA damage is repaired. However, incomplete or deficient repair may lead to skin cancer, which is a multistep process involving tumor initiation, tumor promotion, and tumor progression, ultimately resulting in visible skin cancer [91]. Based on these considerations, the measurement of DNA damage after UV radiation exposure is an appropriate outcome variable to be used for the substantiation of health claims in the context of protection of skin from UV-induced (other than oxidative) damage.

Immunohistochemical Techniques

Methods for quantifying photoproducts in human skin include DNA extraction analysis and immunohistochemical analysis. In vitro fragmented DNA can be observed directly using conventional techniques such as capillary electrophoresis and the comet assay. The measurement of internal damage typically requires analysis such as high performance liquid chromatographic-mass spectrometry, hydrolysis of DNA followed by chromatographic separation, electrochemical measurements, or the enzymatic conversion of photoproducts into strand breaks [92]. However, in vivo quantification is more appropriate for evaluating UV-induced DNA damage in humans. There are some advantages to using immunohistochemical quantification, compared to DNA extraction. Histology is able to identify the skin compartment in which DNA damage has occurred, to which depth cells are affected, and which subpopulations of cells are damaged. Immunohistochemistry is based on the quantification of the thymine cyclobutane dimer (TT-CPD), the main DNA lesion induced by both UVB and UVA radiations. The level of TT-CPD in DNA may be determined by, immunohistochemical staining of photoproduct positive nuclei of keratinocytes in the epidermis. Manual counting of photoproduct-positive immunohistochemically stained nuclei in the epidermis is a frequently used method for quantification of DNA damage [93].

In conclusion, immunohistochemical analysis is an appropriate method for the measurement of DNA damage after UV radiation exposure.

3.3.2. Depletion of Langerhans Cells after UV Light Exposure

Langerhans cells (LCs) are effective antigen-presenting cells that function as "custodians" of the skin, altering the immune system to pathogen entry, but also the tolerance to self-antigen and commensal microbes [94]. LCs are also recognized to play a key role in the induction and maintenance of the immune response against skin cancer. Exposure of human skin to solar UV light induces local and systemic immune suppression. It is known that alterations of numbers and immune functions of LCs mediate this phenomenon [95]. The effect of UV on epidermal LCs has been studied for many years, since the first reports in the 1980s focusing on the deleterious effects of UV on epidermal LCs in humans. Exposure to UV induces a decrease in LCs within the human skin, and this depletion is probably due to both cell death and enhanced migration to regional lymph nodes.

To evaluate the appropriateness of depletion of Langerhans cells after UV-light exposure as OV for the protection of the skin from UV-induced damage, database 15 was generated (see Table 1).

It has been shown that UV radiation induces epidermal LCs to emigrate to draining lymph nodes starting a few hours or a few days after UV exposure. This leads to a decrease in the number of Langerhans cells, which can persist for up to four weeks before recovery of a normal epidermal pool. The consequence is direct damage to the immunological function of the skin. Therefore, decreasing the depletion of Langerhans cells after UV light exposure is beneficial. It has been shown that the protection afforded by sunscreens against photo-immunosuppression must be broad-spectrum with an adequate UVA protection. Based on these considerations, the evaluation of depletion of Langerhans cells after UV light exposure, measured with appropriate techniques, is appropriate for the substantiation of health claims in the context of protection of skin from UV-induced (other than oxidative) damage.

Histochemical and Immunological Techniques

The measurement of the number of LCs necessarily requires skin samples. The simplest way to obtain a skin sample is a punch skin biopsy, which is generally performed in UV-unexposed skin such as buttock skin or the inner forearm after local anesthesia. This is an easy, minimally invasive and low-cost procedure, which provides the substratum for the subsequent measurement [77].

Langerhans cells cannot be identified in routinely prepared histologic testing, but they can be visualized at the light microscope by histochemical and immunological techniques. Appropriate methods for LC detection in the human skin include histo-enzymatic methods of adenosintriphosphatases, acid phosphatase, alpha-naphthylacetate esterase and the peroxidase-antiperoxidase immunochemistry method with S-100 protein antibody [96]. Based on these considerations, skin biopsy, if followed by a histochemical or immunological technique, is an appropriate method for the measurement of the number of LCs after UV-light exposure.

3.3.3. UV-Induced Erythema and Erythema Grade (Reddening)

Erythema or skin reddening is an inflammatory response of the skin to UV-induced molecular and cellular damage [97]. If severe, i.e., sunburn, it may lead to blisters and loss of the several skin functions. Erythema and subsequent pigmentation are immediate responses of normal human skin exposure to UV radiation. Even if it is an indicator of direct UV-induced skin damage, there is no direct evidence of correlation with skin cancer and photo aging [98].

To evaluate the appropriateness of UV-induced erythema as OV for the protection of the skin from UV-induced damage, database 16 was generated (see Table 1).

A reduction in UV-induced erythema (e.g., measured as change in minimal erythema dose (MED) or erythema grade (reddening)) may indicate less UV-induced damage to the skin. However, it can also reflect a reduction in the capacity of the skin to react to molecular and cellular damage, so it does not represent a univocal measure of UV-induced damage at skin level. Moreover, erythema is a poor indicator of immunosuppression [99]. On the basis of these considerations, UV-induced erythema cannot be used alone as an outcome measure for the substantiation of health claims on protection of the skin from UV-induced damage. However, it can be used as supporting evidence when appropriate outcome variables are also used.

Minimal Erythemal Dose Test

The MED test allows the determination of the amount of UV radiation producing minimal erythema (sunburn or redness caused by engorgement of capillaries) of the skin within a few hours following exposure. The individual MED is determined by irradiating small areas of skin (usually sun un-exposed skin) with increasing UV doses. Results are read at 24 h post-exposure and the lowest dose in the series that only just produced erythema is considered to be the MED [100]. The increasing UV doses are determined in consideration of the specific skin phototype, since this strictly influences the intensity of the resulting erythema. This procedure is simple to perform, and requires only a few minutes. The only possible drawback is that an appropriate evaluation of phototype is fundamental to avoid excessive UV exposure time with consequent burning.

In conclusion, the MED test is an appropriate, simple and low-cost procedure for the measurement of UV-erythema.

3.3.4. Delayed-Type Hypersensitivity Immune Response to Recall Antigens in the Skin

The delayed-type hypersensitivity (DTH) reaction is a cell-mediated reaction to several antigens injected in the skin. The DTH skin test is used to evaluate whether prior exposure to an antigen has occurred, and reflects the cell-mediated immunity that provides the main mechanism against fungi, viruses and other hosts. Following the injection of small amounts of antigen, a typical response occurs, including induration, swelling and monocytic infiltration into the site of the lesion within 24 to 72 h. This reaction has been considered a surrogate for immune response to tumor antigens [101]. Three types of DTH reactions have been described: contact hypersensitivity (e.g., caused by metal ions), tuberculin-type reaction and granulomatous hypersensitivity.

To evaluate the appropriateness of DTH immune response as an outcome variable for the protection of the skin from UV-induced damage, database 17 was generated (see Table 1).

Solar UV radiation has been demonstrated to have suppressive effects on the immune system. UV radiation inhibits antigen presentation and induces the release of immunosuppressive cytokines. This specific immunosuppression is mediated by antigen specific suppressor/regulatory T cells, which mediates UV-induced inhibition of DTH response in human skin.

However, DTH immune responses to recall antigens in the skin is more a marker of systemic UV-induced damage on the immune system rather than a marker of UV-damage at skin level.

Therefore, based on these considerations, DTH immune responses to recall antigens in the skin cannot be used alone as an outcome measure for the substantiation of health claims on protection of the skin from UV-induced damage. However, it can be used as supporting evidence in combination with appropriate outcome variables.

Multitest Kit Merieux and Mantoux Testing

Most of the methods for determining the UV-induced immunosuppression are sunburn protection factor-based measures of UVB induced erythema response. The main drawback is the inability of these methods to provide an accurate evaluation of the immune protection. In this scenario, inhibition of DTH response has been suggested as a test for evaluating UV-induced immunosuppression, but the lack of appropriate techniques for evaluating immunosuppression still remains a challenge.

The DTH skin test is used to test if prior exposure to an antigen has occurred. So far, two procedures have been used successfully: Multitest Kit Merieux and Mantoux testing [102]. The Multitest Kit Merieux is a DTH to seven antigens (e.g., *Candida albicans*, *Streptococcus antigens*) and provides comprehensive information on the immune status of the human volunteers. Mantoux testing with tuberculin purified protein derivatives provides a possible alternative model of DTH to recall antigen.

Overall, the DTH response is not easy to assess; it requires several weeks, and it is invasive. However, it represents an interesting tool for evaluating photoimmunosuppression in subjects within RCTs.

In conclusion, Multitest Kit Merieux and Mantoux testing are appropriate methods for the measurement of DTH immune response to recall antigens in the skin.

4. Conclusions

Insufficient scientific substantiation for a health claim represents the most common reason for a negative response to a request for the authorization of a health claim. In this context, RCTs should be well-designed and well-performed, taking into account many parameters affecting the quality of a RCT, such as adequate sample size, proper study design (including an adequate duration of the intervention), adequate statistical analysis, and choice of appropriate OVs and related MMs. The present report provides a critical analysis of all the OVs and MMs that have been proposed so far in the context of maintenance of skin function, compliant with the European Regulation. This critical analysis could represent a useful tool for applicants during the design or selection of human intervention studies aimed to substantiate health claims related to skin function. Moreover, this information could serve as a basis for EFSA to develop and update the Guidance on the scientific requirements for health claims related to skin health.

Acknowledgments: This project has received financial support from the European Food Safety Authority (EFSA), Grant GP/EFSA/NUTRI/2014/01. The present article, however, is under the sole responsibility of the authors. The positions and opinions presented in this article are those of the authors alone and do not necessarily represent the views/any official position or scientific works of EFSA. To know about EFSA guidance documents and other scientific outputs of EFSA, please consult its website at: http://www.efsa.europa.eu.

Author Contributions: D.M. was the project developer and wrote the manuscript together with D.A., M.B.D.F., C.C. and S.D.N.; G.B. generated the literature databases and helped with the evaluation of the appropriateness and the validity of the statistics found in the literature studies taken into account; I.Z., M.M., C.P., G.P., M.V., D.G., P.M., M.V., A.D.C., R.C.B. and S.D.N. were expert members of the project team, helped secure the funding, and critically read and revised the manuscript; D.D.R. was the Principal Investigator of the project, critically revised the manuscript and had primary responsibility for final content.

Abbreviations

CPDs	cyclobutane pyrimidine dimers
DTH	delayed type hypersensitivity
EFSA	european food safety authority
ELISA	enzyme-linked immunosorbent assay
HETE	hydroxyeicosatetraenoic acids
HpETEs	hydroperoxyeicosatetraenoic acid
HPLC	high performance liquid chromatography
LCs	langerhans cells
LPO	lipid peroxidation
LXA4	lipoxin a4
LXB4	lipoxin b4
MED	minimal erythemal dose
MM	method of measurement
OV	outcome variable
RCT	randomized controlled trial
ROS	reactive oxygen species
SC	stratum corneum
SELS	surface evaluation of the living skin
TEWL	transepidermal water loss
TT-CPD	thymine cyclobutane dimer
UV	ultraviolet
UVA	ultraviolet A
UVB	ultraviolet B
VAS	visual analog scales
VP	vapor pressure
8-OHdG	8-hydroxydeoxyguanosine

References

1. Proksch, E.; Brandner, J.M.; Jensen, J.-M. The skin: An indispensable barrier. *Exp. Dermatol.* **2008**, *17*, 1063–1072. [CrossRef] [PubMed]
2. Madison, K.C. Barrier function of the skin: "La raison d'etre" of the epidermis. *J. Investig. Dermatol.* **2003**, *121*, 231–241. [CrossRef] [PubMed]
3. Stucker, M.; Struk, A.; Altmeyer, P.; Herde, M.; Baumgartl, H.; Lubbers, D.W. The cutaneous uptake of atmospheric oxygen contributes significantly to the oxygen supply of human dermis and epidermis. *J. Physiol.* **2002**, *538*, 985–994. [CrossRef] [PubMed]
4. Maru, G.B.; Gandhi, K.; Ramchandani, A.; Kumar, G. The role of inflammation in skin cancer. *Adv. Exp. Med. Biol.* **2014**, *816*, 437–469. [PubMed]
5. Gawkrodger, D.; Ardern-Jones, M. *Dermatology*, 6th ed.; Elsevier: London, UK, 2016.

6. Hay, R.J.; Johns, N.E.; Williams, H.C.; Bolliger, I.W.; Dellavalle, R.P.; Margolis, D.J.; Marks, R.; Naldi, L.; Weinstock, M.A.; Wulf, S.K.; et al. The global burden of skin disease in 2010: An analysis of the prevalence and impact of skin conditions. *J. Investig. Dermatol.* **2014**, *134*, 1527–1534. [CrossRef] [PubMed]
7. Lozano, R.; Naghavi, M.; Foreman, K.; Lim, S.; Shibuya, K.; Aboyans, V.; Abraham, J.; Adair, T.; Aggarwal, R.; Ahn, S.Y.; et al. Global and regional mortality from 235 causes of death for 20 age groups in 1990 and 2010: A systematic analysis for the global burden of disease study 2010. *Lancet* **2012**, *380*, 2095–2128. [CrossRef]
8. Naldi, L.; Conti, A.; Cazzaniga, S.; Patrizi, A.; Pazzaglia, M.; Lanzoni, A.; Veneziano, L.; Pellacani, G. Diet and physical exercise in psoriasis: A randomized controlled trial. *Br. J. Dermatol.* **2014**, *170*, 634–642. [CrossRef] [PubMed]
9. Jensen, P.; Zachariae, C.; Christensen, R.; Geiker, N.R.W.; Schaadt, B.K.; Stender, S.; Hansen, P.R.; Astrup, A.; Skov, L. Effect of weight loss on the severity of psoriasis. *JAMA Dermatol.* **2013**, *149*, 795–801. [CrossRef] [PubMed]
10. Smith, R.N.; Braue, A.; Varigos, G.A.; Mann, N.J. The effect of a low glycemic load diet on acne vulgaris and the fatty acid composition of skin surface triglycerides. *J. Dermatol. Sci.* **2008**, *50*, 41–52. [CrossRef] [PubMed]
11. Stahl, W.; Heinrich, U.; Wiseman, S.; Eichler, O.; Sies, H.; Tronnier, H. Dietary tomato paste protects against ultraviolet light-induced erythema in humans. *J. Nutr.* **2001**, *131*, 1449–1451. [PubMed]
12. Heinrich, U.; Neukam, K.; Tronnier, H.; Sies, H.; Stahl, W. Long-term ingestion of high flavanol cocoa provides photoprotection against UV-induced erythema and improves skin condition in women. *J. Nutr.* **2006**, *136*, 1565–1569. [PubMed]
13. Heinrich, U.; Moore, C.E.; De Spirt, S.; Tronnier, H.; Stahl, W. Green tea polyphenols provide photoprotection, increase microcirculation, and modulate skin properties of women. *J. Nutr.* **2011**, *141*, 1202–1208. [CrossRef] [PubMed]
14. Martini, D.; Biasini, B.; Rossi, S.; Zavaroni, I.; Bedogni, G.; Musci, M.; Pruneti, C.; Passeri, G.; Ventura, M.; Galli, D.; et al. Claimed effects, outcome variables and methods of measurement for health claims on foods proposed under european community regulation 1924/2006 in the area of appetite ratings and weight management. *Int. J. Food Sci. Nutr.* **2017**. [CrossRef] [PubMed]
15. Martini, D.; Rossi, S.; Biasini, B.; Zavaroni, I.; Bedogni, G.; Musci, M.; Pruneti, C.; Passeri, G.; Ventura, M.; Di Nuzzo, S.; et al. Claimed effects, outcome variables and methods of measurement for health claims proposed under european community regulation 1924/2006 in the framework of protection against oxidative damage and cardiovascular health. *Nutr. Metab. Cardiovasc. Dis.* **2017**, *27*, 473–503. [CrossRef] [PubMed]
16. Fitzpatrick, R.; Davey, C.; Buxton, M.J.; Jones, D.R. Evaluating patient-based outcome measures for use in clinical trials. *Health Technol. Assess.* **1998**, *2*, 1–74. [PubMed]
17. Rogiers, V. Eemco guidance for the assessment of transepidermal water loss in cosmetic sciences. *Skin Pharmacol. Appl. Skin Physiol.* **2001**, *14*, 117–128. [CrossRef] [PubMed]
18. Du Plessis, J.; Stefaniak, A.; Eloff, F.; John, S.; Agner, T.; Chou, T.-C.; Nixon, R.; Steiner, M.; Franken, A.; Kudla, I.; et al. International guidelines for the in vivo assessment of skin properties in non-clinical settings: Part 2. Transepidermal water loss and skin hydration. *Skin Res. Technol.* **2013**, *19*, 265–278. [CrossRef] [PubMed]
19. Pinnagoda, J.; Tupker, R.A.; Agner, T.; Serup, J. Guidelines for transepidermal water loss (TEWL) measurement. A report from the standardization group of the european society of contact dermatitis. *Contact Dermat.* **1990**, *22*, 164–178. [CrossRef]
20. Ezerskaia, A.; Pereira, S.F.; Urbach, H.P.; Verhagen, R.; Varghese, B. Quantitative and simultaneous non-invasive measurement of skin hydration and sebum levels. *Biomed. Opt. Express* **2016**, *7*, 2311–2320. [CrossRef] [PubMed]
21. Harding, C.R.; Watkinson, A.; Rawlings, A.V.; Scott, I.R. Dry skin, moisturization and corneodesmolysis. *Int. J. Cosmet. Sci.* **2000**, *22*, 21–52. [CrossRef] [PubMed]
22. Verdier-Sevrain, S.; Bonte, F. Skin hydration: A review on its molecular mechanisms. *J. Cosmet. Dermatol.* **2007**, *6*, 75–82. [CrossRef] [PubMed]
23. Berardesca, E. Eemco guidance for the assessment of stratum corneum hydration: Electrical methods. *Skin Res. Technol.* **1997**, *3*, 126–132. [CrossRef] [PubMed]

24. Heinrich, U.; Koop, U.; Leneveu-Duchemin, M.C.; Osterrieder, K.; Bielfeldt, S.; Chkarnat, C.; Degwert, J.; Hantschel, D.; Jaspers, S.; Nissen, H.P.; et al. Multicentre comparison of skin hydration in terms of physical-, physiological- and product-dependent parameters by the capacitive method (Corneometer CM 825). *Int. J. Cosmet. Sci.* **2003**, *25*, 45–53. [CrossRef] [PubMed]
25. Constantin, M.-M.; Poenaru, E.; Poenaru, C.; Constantin, T. Skin hydration assessment through modern non-invasive bioengineering technologies. *Maedica (Buchar)* **2014**, *9*, 33–38. [PubMed]
26. Khazaka, G. Assessment of stratum corneum hydration: Corneometer CM 825. In *Bioengineering of the Skin: Water and the Stratum Corneum*; Fluhr, J.W., Elsner, P., Berardesca, E., Maibach, H.I., Eds.; CRC Press: Boca Raton, FL, USA, 2005; pp. 249–261.
27. Rudikoff, D. The effect of dryness on the skin. *Clin. Dermatol.* **1998**, *16*, 99–107. [CrossRef]
28. Serup, J. Eemco guidance for the assessment of dry skin (xerosis) and ichthyosis: Clinical scoring systems. *Skin Res. Technol.* **1995**, *1*, 109–114. [CrossRef] [PubMed]
29. Chopra, R.; Vakharia, P.P.; Sacotte, R.; Patel, N.; Immaneni, S.; White, T.; Kantor, R.; Hsu, D.Y.; Silverberg, J.I. Severity strata for EASI, mEASI, oSCORAD, sCORAD, ADSI and BSA in adolescents and adults with atopic dermatitis. *Br. J. Dermatol.* **2017**. [CrossRef]
30. Rodrigues, L. Eemco guidance to the in vivo assessment of tensile functional properties of the skin. Part 2: Instrumentation and test modes. *Skin Pharmacol. Appl. Skin Physiol.* **2001**, *14*, 52–67. [CrossRef] [PubMed]
31. Chung, J.; Cho, S.; Kang, S. Why does the skin age? Intrinsic aging, photoaging, and their pathophysiology. In *Photoaging*; Rigel, D.S., Weiss, R.A., Lim, H.W., Dover, J.S., Eds.; Marcel Dekker Inc.: New York, NY, USA, 2004.
32. Pierard, G.E.; Grp, E. Eemco guidance to the in vivo assessment of tensile functional properties of the skin—Part 1: Relevance to the structures and ageing of the skin and subcutaneous tissues. *Skin Pharmacol. Appl.* **1999**, *12*, 352–362. [CrossRef] [PubMed]
33. Wilhelm, K.P.; Cua, A.B.; Maibach, H.I. In vivo study on age-related elastic properties of human skin. In *Noninvasive Methods for the Quantification of Skin Functions*; Frosch, P.J., Kligman, A.M., Eds.; Springer: Berlin, Germany, 1993; pp. 190–203.
34. Ohshima, H.; Kinoshita, S.; Oyobikawa, M.; Futagawa, M.; Takiwaki, H.; Ishiko, A.; Kanto, H. Use of cutometer area parameters in evaluating age-related changes in the skin elasticity of the cheek. *Skin Res. Technol.* **2013**, *19*, E238–E242. [CrossRef] [PubMed]
35. Qu, D.; Seehra, G.P. Improving the accuracy of skin elasticity measurement by using q-parameters in cutometer. *J. Cosmet. Sci.* **2016**, *67*, 37–44. [PubMed]
36. Ryu, H.S.; Joo, Y.H.; Kim, S.O.; Park, K.C.; Youn, S.W. Influence of age and regional differences on skin elasticity as measured by the cutometer. *Skin Res. Technol.* **2008**, *14*, 354–358. [CrossRef] [PubMed]
37. Proksch, E.; Jensen, J.-M. Skin as an Organ of Protection. In *Fitzpatrick's Dermatology in General Medicine*, 8th ed.; Goldsmith, L.A., Katz, S.I., Gilchrest, B.A., Paller, A.S., Leffell, D.J., Wolff, K., Eds.; Mc Graw Hill: New York, NY, USA, 2012.
38. Ishida-Yamamoto, A.; Igawa, S.; Kishibe, M. Order and disorder in corneocyte adhesion. *J. Dermatol.* **2011**, *38*, 645–654. [CrossRef] [PubMed]
39. Piérard, G.E.; Hermanns-Lê, T.; Piérard-Franchimont, C. Stratum corneum desquamation. In *Agache's Measuring the Skin*; Humbert, P., Maibach, H., Fanian, F., Agache, P., Eds.; Springer International Publishing: Cham, Switzerland, 2016; pp. 1–5.
40. Candi, E.; Knight, R.; Melino, G. Cornification of the skin: A non-apoptotic cell death mechanism. In *Cell Death*; Melino, G., Vaux, D., Eds.; John Wiley & Sons, Ltd.: Chichester, UK, 2009.
41. Wilhelm, K.P.; Kaspar, K.; Schumann, F.; Articus, K. Development and validation of a semiautomatic image analysis system for measuring skin desquamation with d-squames. *Skin Res. Technol.* **2002**, *8*, 98–105. [CrossRef] [PubMed]
42. Pierard, G.E. EEMCO guidance for the assessment of dry skin (xerosis) and ichthyosis: Evaluation by stratum corneum shippings. *Skin Res. Technol.* **1996**, *2*, 3–11. [CrossRef] [PubMed]
43. Gao, Y.R.; Wang, X.M.; Chen, S.Y.; Li, S.Y.; Liu, X.P. Acute skin barrier disruption with repeated tape stripping: An in vivo model for damage skin barrier. *Skin Res. Technol.* **2013**, *19*, 162–168. [CrossRef] [PubMed]
44. Jackson, S.M.; Williams, M.L.; Feingold, K.R.; Elias, P.M. Pathobiology of the stratum corneum. *West. J. Med.* **1993**, *158*, 279–285. [PubMed]

45. Masukawa, Y.; Narita, H.; Sato, H.; Naoe, A.; Kondo, N.; Sugai, Y.; Oba, T.; Homma, R.; Ishikawa, J.; Takagi, Y.; et al. Comprehensive quantification of ceramide species in human stratum corneum. *J. Lipid Res.* **2009**, *50*, 1708–1719. [CrossRef] [PubMed]
46. Cremesti, A.E.; Fischl, A.S. Current methods for the identification and quantitation of ceramides: An overview. *Lipids* **2000**, *35*, 937–945. [CrossRef] [PubMed]
47. Gołębiowski, M.; Paszkiewicz, M.; Haliński, Ł.; Stepnowski, P. Hplc of plant lipids. In *High Performance Liquid Chromatography in Phytochemical Analysis*; Waksmundzka-Hajnos, M., Sherma, J., Eds.; CRC Press: Boca Raton, FL, USA, 2010; pp. 425–452.
48. Tivoli, Y.A.; Rubenstein, R.M. Pruritus: An updated look at an old problem. *J. Clin. Aesthet. Dermatol.* **2009**, *2*, 30–36. [PubMed]
49. Zachariae, R.; Lei, U.; Haedersdal, M.; Zachariae, C. Itch severity and quality of life in patients with pruritus: Preliminary validity of a danish adaptation of the itch severity scale. *Acta Derm. Venereol.* **2012**, *92*, 508–514. [CrossRef] [PubMed]
50. Garibyan, L.; Chiou, A.S.; Elmariah, S.B. Advanced aging skin and itch: Addressing an unmet need. *Dermatol. Ther.* **2013**, *26*, 92–103. [CrossRef] [PubMed]
51. Reich, A.; Heisig, M.; Phan, N.Q.; Taneda, K.; Takamori, K.; Takeuchi, S.; Furue, M.; Blome, C.; Augustin, M.; Stander, S.; et al. Visual analogue scale: Evaluation of the instrument for the assessment of pruritus. *Acta Derm. Venereol.* **2012**, *92*, 497–501. [CrossRef] [PubMed]
52. Stander, S.; Augustin, M.; Reich, A.; Blome, C.; Ebata, T.; Phan, N.Q.; Szepietowski, J.C. Pruritus assessment in clinical trials: Consensus recommendations from the international forum for the study of itch (IFSI) special interest group scoring itch in clinical trials. *Acta Derm. Venereol.* **2013**, *93*, 509–514. [CrossRef] [PubMed]
53. Elman, S.; Hynan, L.S.; Gabriel, V.; Mayo, M.J. The 5-D itch scale: A new measure of pruritus. *Br. J. Dermatol.* **2010**, *162*, 587–593. [CrossRef] [PubMed]
54. Di Nuzzo, S.; Ercolini, E.; Carrozzo, E.; Fante, C.; Casanova, D.; Pruneti, C. Personality, alexithymic and autonomic aspects in psoriatic patients: A preliminary study. *Clin. Drug Investig.* **2013**, *33*, S88–S90.
55. Rigopoulos, D.; Tiligada, E. Stratum corneum lipids and water-holding capacity. In *Dermatoanthropology of Ethnic Skin and Hair*; Vashi, N., Maibach, H., Eds.; Springer: Cham, Switzerland, 2017.
56. Crowther, J.M.; Matts, P.J.; Kaczvinsky, J.R. Changes in stratum corneum thickness, water gradients and hydration by moisturizers. In *Treatment of Dry Skin Syndrom*; Lodén, M., Maibach, H., Eds.; Springer: Berlin/Heidelberg, Germany, 2012.
57. Tronnier, H.; Wiebusch, M.; Heinrich, U.; Stute, R. Surface evaluation of living skin. *Adv. Exp. Med. Biol.* **1999**, *455*, 507–516. [PubMed]
58. Callaghan, T.M.; Wilhelm, K.P. A review of ageing and an examination of clinical methods in the assessment of ageing skin. Part 2: Clinical perspectives and clinical methods in the evaluation of ageing skin. *Int. J. Cosmet. Sci.* **2008**, *30*, 323–332. [CrossRef] [PubMed]
59. Makrantonaki, E.; Zouboulis, C.C. Molecular mechanisms of skin aging—State of the art. *Ann N. Y. Acad. Sci.* **2007**, *1119*, 40–50. [CrossRef] [PubMed]
60. Piérard, G.E.; Piérard-Franchimont, C.; Piérard, S. Visioscan-driven ulev method. In *Non Invasive Diagnostic Techniques in Clinical Dermatology*; Berardesca, E., Maibach, H., Wilhelm, K.P., Eds.; Springer: Berlin, Germany, 2014.
61. Choi, J.W.; Kwon, S.H.; Huh, C.H.; Park, K.C.; Youn, S.W. The influences of skin visco-elasticity, hydration level and aging on the formation of wrinkles: A comprehensive and objective approach. *Skin Res. Technol.* **2013**, *19*, E349–E355. [CrossRef] [PubMed]
62. Menon, G.K.; Cleary, G.W.; Lane, M.E. The structure and function of the stratum corneum. *Int. J. Pharm.* **2012**, *435*, 3–9. [CrossRef] [PubMed]
63. Black, D.; Boyer, J.; Lagarde, J.M. Image analysis of skin scaling using d-squame samplers: Comparison with clinical scoring and use for assessing moisturizer efficacy. *Int. J. Cosmet. Sci.* **2006**, *28*, 35–44. [CrossRef] [PubMed]
64. Haroun, M.T. Dry skin in the elderly. *Geriatr. Aging* **2003**, *6*, 41–44.
65. Daungkum, K.; Foocharoen, C.; Mahakkanukrauh, A.; Suwannaroj, S.; Thinkhamrop, B.; Nanagara, R. Self-assessment of skin tightness severity by scleroderma patients. *Int. J. Rheum. Dis.* **2016**, *19*, 989–995. [CrossRef] [PubMed]

66. Vitiello, M.; Abuchar, A.; Santana, N.; Dehesa, L.; Kerdel, F.A. An update on the treatment of the cutaneous manifestations of systemic sclerosis: The dermatologist's point of view. *J. Clin. Aesthet. Dermatol.* **2012**, *5*, 33–43. [PubMed]
67. Clements, P.J.; Lachenbruch, P.A.; Seibold, J.R.; Zee, B.; Steen, V.D.; Brennan, P.; Silman, A.J.; Allegar, N.; Varga, J.; Massa, M.; et al. Skin thickness score in systemic sclerosis: An assessment of interobserver variability in 3 independent studies. *J. Rheumatol.* **1993**, *20*, 1892–1896. [PubMed]
68. Khanna, D.; Furst, D.E.; Clements, P.J.; Allanore, Y.; Baron, M.; Czirjak, L.; Distler, O.; Foeldvari, I.; Kuwana, M.; Matucci-Cerinic, M.; et al. Standardization of the modified rodnan skin score for use in clinical trials of systemic sclerosis. *J. Scleroderma Relat. Disord.* **2017**, *2*, 11–18. [CrossRef] [PubMed]
69. Braun-Falco, O.; Plewig, G.; Wolff, H.H.; Burgdorf, W.H.C. *Dermatology*; Springer: Berlin, Germany, 1996.
70. Habif, T. *Clinical Dermatology: A Color Guide to Diagnosis and Therapy*, 6th ed.; Saunders: Philadelphia, PA, USA, 2015.
71. Braverman, I.M. The cutaneous microcirculation. *J. Investig. Dermatol. Symp. Proc.* **2000**, *5*, 3–9. [CrossRef] [PubMed]
72. Berardesca, E.; Elsner, P.; Maibach, H.I. *Bioengineering of the Skin: Cutaneous Blood Flow and Erythema*; CRC Press: Boca Raton, FL, USA, 1994; Volume II.
73. Tsukahara, K.; Nagashima, Y.; Moriwaki, S.; Fujimura, T.; Hattori, M.; Takema, Y. Relationship between physical parameters and blood flow in human facial skin. *J. Cosmet. Sci.* **2003**, *54*, 499–511. [PubMed]
74. Kim, S.I.; Jin, S.G.; Pfeifer, G.P. Formation of cyclobutane pyrimidine dimers at dipyrimidines containing 5-hydroxymethylcytosine. *Photochem. Photobiol. Sci.* **2013**, *12*, 1409–1415. [CrossRef] [PubMed]
75. Rinnerthaler, M.; Bischof, J.; Streubel, M.K.; Trost, A.; Richter, K. Oxidative stress in aging human skin. *Biomolecules* **2015**, *5*, 545–589. [CrossRef] [PubMed]
76. Halliwell, B. Why and how should we measure oxidative DNA damage in nutritional studies? How far have we come? *Am. J. Clin. Nutr.* **2000**, *72*, 1082–1087. [PubMed]
77. Zuber, T.J. Punch biopsy of the skin. *Am. Fam. Phys.* **2002**, *65*, 1155–1158, 1161–1162, 1164.
78. Ravanat, J.L.; Douki, T.; Cadet, J. Direct and indirect effects of UV radiation on DNA and its components. *J. Photochem. Photobiol. B* **2001**, *63*, 88–102. [CrossRef]
79. Mori, T.; Nakane, M.; Hattori, T.; Matsunaga, T.; Ihara, M.; Nikaido, O. Simultaneous establishment of monoclonal-antibodies specific for either cyclobutane pyrimidine dimer or (6-4)photoproduct from the same mouse immunized with ultraviolet-irradiated DNA. *Photochem. Photobiol.* **1991**, *54*, 225–232. [CrossRef] [PubMed]
80. Ahmed, N.U.; Ueda, M.; Nikaido, O.; Osawa, T.; Ichihashi, M. High levels of 8-hydroxy-2′-deoxyguanosine appear in normal human epidermis after a single dose of ultraviolet radiation. *Br. J. Dermatol.* **1999**, *140*, 226–231. [CrossRef] [PubMed]
81. Niki, E. Lipid oxidation in the skin. *Free Radic. Res.* **2014**, *49*, 827–834. [CrossRef] [PubMed]
82. Ayala, A.; Munoz, M.F.; Arguelles, S. Lipid peroxidation: Production, metabolism, and signaling mechanisms of malondialdehyde and 4-hydroxy-2-nonenal. *Oxid. Med. Cell. Longev.* **2014**, *2014*, 360438. [CrossRef] [PubMed]
83. Schneider, L.A.; Bloch, W.; Kopp, K.; Hainzl, A.; Rettberg, P.; Wlaschek, M.; Horneck, G.; Scharffetter-Kochanek, K. 8-isoprostane is a dose-related biomarker for photo-oxidative ultraviolet (UV) B damage in vivo: A pilot study with personal UV dosimetry. *Br. J. Dermatol.* **2006**, *154*, 1147–1154. [CrossRef] [PubMed]
84. Nakagawa, K.; Ibusuki, D.; Suzuki, Y.; Yamashita, S.; Higuchi, O.; Oikawa, S.; Miyazawa, T. Ion-trap tandem mass spectrometric analysis of squalene monohydroperoxide isomers in sunlight-exposed human skin. *J. Lipid Res.* **2007**, *48*, 2779–2787. [CrossRef] [PubMed]
85. Fogh, K.; Herlin, T.; Kragballe, K. Eicosanoids in skin of patients with atopic dermatitis: Prostaglandin E2 and leukotriene B4 are present in biologically active concentrations. *J. Allergy Clin. Immunol.* **1989**, *83*, 450–455. [CrossRef]
86. Krutmann, J. Skin aging. In *Nutrition for Healthy Skin. Strategies for Clinical and Cosmetic Practice*; Krutmann, J., Humbert, P., Eds.; Springer: Berlin, Germany, 2011; pp. 15–24.
87. Davies, M.J. Protein oxidation and peroxidation. *Biochem. J.* **2016**, *473*, 805–825. [CrossRef] [PubMed]
88. Berlett, B.S.; Stadtman, E.R. Protein oxidation in aging, disease, and oxidative stress. *J. Biol. Chem.* **1997**, *272*, 20313–20316. [CrossRef] [PubMed]

89. Weber, D.; Davies, M.J.; Grune, T. Determination of protein carbonyls in plasma, cell extracts, tissue homogenates, isolated proteins: Focus on sample preparation and derivatization conditions. *Redox Biol.* **2015**, *5*, 367–380. [CrossRef] [PubMed]
90. Ichihashi, M.; Ueda, M.; Budiyanto, A.; Bito, T.; Oka, M.; Fukunaga, M.; Tsuru, K.; Horikawa, T. UV-induced skin damage. *Toxicology* **2003**, *189*, 21–39. [CrossRef]
91. Kim, Y.; He, Y.Y. Ultraviolet radiation-induced non-melanoma skin cancer: Regulation of DNA damage repair and inflammation. *Genes Dis.* **2014**, *1*, 188–198. [CrossRef] [PubMed]
92. Wiczk, J.; Miloch, J.; Rak, J. Dhplc and ms studies of a photoinduced intrastrand cross-link in DNA labeled with 5-bromo-2′-deoxyuridine. *J. Photochem. Photobiol. B* **2014**, *130*, 86–92. [CrossRef] [PubMed]
93. Cooke, M.S.; Podmore, I.D.; Mistry, N.; Evans, M.D.; Herbert, K.E.; Griffiths, H.R.; Lunec, J. Immunochemical detection of UV-induced DNA damage and repair. *J. Immunol. Methods* **2003**, *280*, 125–133. [CrossRef]
94. Teunissen, M.B. Dynamic nature and function of epidermal langerhans cells in vivo and in vitro: A review, with emphasis on human langerhans cells. *Histochem. J.* **1992**, *24*, 697–716. [CrossRef] [PubMed]
95. Simon, J.C.; Krutmann, J.; Elmets, C.A.; Bergstresser, P.R.; Cruz, P.D., Jr. Ultraviolet b-irradiated antigen-presenting cells display altered accessory signaling for T-cell activation: Relevance to immune responses initiated in skin. *J. Investig. Dermatol.* **1992**, *98*, 66S–69S. [CrossRef] [PubMed]
96. Kanitakis, J. Anatomy, histology and immunohistochemistry of normal human skin. *Eur. J. Dermatol.* **2002**, *12*, 390–399. [PubMed]
97. Soter, N.A. Acute effects of ultraviolet radiation on the skin. *Semin. Dermatol.* **1990**, *9*, 11–15. [PubMed]
98. Hruza, L.L.; Pentland, A.P. Mechanisms of UV-induced inflammation. *J. Investig. Dermatol.* **1993**, *100*, 35S–41S. [CrossRef] [PubMed]
99. Kelly, D.A.; Young, A.R.; McGregor, J.M.; Seed, P.T.; Potten, C.S.; Walker, S.L. Sensitivity to sunburn is associated with susceptibility to ultraviolet radiation-induced suppression of cutaneous cell-mediated immunity. *J. Exp. Med.* **2000**, *191*, 561–566. [CrossRef] [PubMed]
100. Heckman, C.J.; Chandler, R.; Kloss, J.D.; Benson, A.; Rooney, D.; Munshi, T.; Darlow, S.D.; Perlis, C.; Manne, S.L.; Oslin, D.W. Minimal erythema dose (MED) testing. *J. Vis. Exp.* **2013**, *75*, 50175. [CrossRef] [PubMed]
101. Moyal, D.D.; Fourtanier, A.M. Broad-spectrum sunscreens provide better protection from the suppression of the elicitation phase of delayed-type hypersensitivity response in humans. *J. Investig. Dermatol.* **2001**, *117*, 1186–1192. [CrossRef] [PubMed]
102. Fourtanier, A.; Moyal, D.; Maccario, J.; Compan, D.; Wolf, P.; Quehenberger, F.; Cooper, K.; Baron, E.; Halliday, G.; Poon, T.; et al. Measurement of sunscreen immune protection factors in humans: A consensus paper. *J. Investig. Dermatol.* **2005**, *125*, 403–409. [CrossRef] [PubMed]

10

Effect of Orally Administered Collagen Peptides from Bovine Bone on Skin Aging in Chronologically Aged Mice

Hongdong Song [1], Siqi Zhang [1], Ling Zhang [1] and Bo Li [1,2,*]

[1] Beijing Advanced Innovation Center for Food Nutrition and Human Health, College of Food Science and Nutritional Engineering, China Agricultural University, Beijing 100083, China; songhd@cau.edu.cn (H.S.); zsq199312@163.com (S.Z.); zhanglingys@outlook.com (L.Z.)

[2] Beijing Higher Institution Engineering Research Center of Animal Product, Beijing 100083, China

[*] Correspondence: libo@cau.edu.cn

Abstract: Collagen peptides (CPs) have demonstrated to exert beneficial effects on skin photoaging. However, little has been done to evaluate their effects on chronologically aged skin. Here, the effects of CPs from bovine bone on skin aging were investigated in chronologically aged mice. 13-month-old female Kunming mice were administered with CPs from bovine bone (200, 400 and 800 mg/kg body weight/day) or proline (400 mg/kg body weight/day) for 8 weeks. Mice body weight, spleen index (SI) and thymus index (TI), degree of skin laxity (DSL), skin components, skin histology and antioxidant indicators were analyzed. Ingestion of CPs or proline had no effect on mice skin moisture and hyaluronic acid content, but it significantly improved the skin laxity, repaired collagen fibers, increased collagen content and normalized the ratio of type I to type III collagen in chronologically aged skin. CPs prepared by Alcalase performed better than CPs prepared by collagenase. Furthermore, CPs intake also significantly improved the antioxidative enzyme activities in skin. These results indicate that oral administration of CPs from bovine bone or proline can improve the laxity of chronologically aged skin by changing skin collagen quantitatively and qualitatively, and highlight their potential application as functional foods to combat skin aging in chronologically aged process.

Keywords: collagen peptides; bovine bone; proline; skin aging; chronologically aged mice; antioxidative enzymes

---

1. Introduction

The impact of aging on the appearance and function of skin has received increasing attention in recent decades. It is widely accepted that skin aging is distinguished into chronological skin aging and skin photoaging [1]. Skin photoaging is caused by solar radiation and it is common in sunlight-exposed skin, especially in the face [2]. Therefore, skin photoaging could be prevented or decreased by photo-protection. The common clinical signs of photoaged skin include deep and coarse wrinkles, dryness, sallowness and laxity [2,3]. In contrast, chronological skin aging is caused by passage of time and it takes place all the time in whole-body skin, including facial skin. Chronologically aged skin is characterized by fine wrinkling and laxity [3]. Chronological skin aging accounts for a great part of skin aging and it is more common than skin photoaging in dark skinned individuals and females [2]. A youthful appearance is considered to play an important role in keeping self-esteem and social relations [4]. Therefore, there is increasing demand for anti-aging interventions to delay or even reverse signs of skin aging.

The use of diet supplements to improve the appearance and function of aged skin has received growing attention. Many dietary components, such as polyphenols [5], vitamins [6], fatty acids [7], trace minerals [8] and proteins [9], have reported to exert beneficial effects on aged skin and have been used as nutraceuticals or functional foods in many counties and regions. Recently, researchers have paid much attention to protein hydrolysates as potential dietary supplements. Collagen is the main structural protein of the different connective tissues, such as skin, bone, cartilage and tendons, and has been widely used in the medicine and food industries. Collagen peptides (CPs) are the enzymolysis product of collagen or gelatin and they are used as important active components because of their various bioactivities, high bioavailability and good biocompatibility [10–12]. Several studies have demonstrated the beneficial effects of CPs ingestion on skin photoaging. Oral administration of CPs from fish skin had obvious protective effects on photoaging skin, including improving moisture retention ability, repairing the endogenous collagen and elastin protein fibers [13–15]. In addition, clinical trials have also demonstrated that the beneficial effects of CPs intake on facial skin, including improving facial skin elasticity, reduce skin dryness and wrinkles, and increase the collagen content of the skin dermis [16,17]. However, little work was performed to evaluate the effects of CPs intake on chronologically aged skin.

Bovine bone is the main by-products in the bovine processing industry and has been widely used as raw material to obtain high-quality gelatin [18]. Although there are some concerns with mad cow disease in Europe and the United States, bovine bone is still one of the most abundant sources of gelatin and accounts for 23.1% of the gelatin production [19]. Therefore, bovine bone is an abundant and high-quality raw material used to prepare CPs. The biological effect of CPs from bovine bone is mainly concentrated on its beneficial effect on bone metabolism, including inhibition of bone loss and improvement of osteoarthritis [20,21]. However, there is limited knowledge about the effect of CPs from bovine bone on skin aging. Therefore, preparing CPs from bovine bone and further evaluating its effect on skin aging is a good way to utilize the by-products for an economical and environmental advantage.

The functional activities of protein-derived hydrolysates or peptides are greatly impacted by their molecular structure and weight, which are highly affected by their processing conditions and especially enzyme specificity [15,22]. Alcalase is a common protease and widely used to prepare protein hydrolysate or peptides. It is a typical endoprotease and preferentially cleaves sites containing hydrophobic residues, such as Ala, Leu, Val and Phe. Bacterial collagenase is a protease that hydrolysates collagen. It has a preference for X-Gly (X is usually a neutral amino acid) bond of the -Gly-Pro-X-Gly-Pro-X- repeating sequence in the collagen molecule [23,24]. Collagenase has a great promise in collagen processing industry. Considering enzyme specificity, the molecular structure or sequences of peptides produced by these two enzymes may be different, which may greatly impact their effects on chronologically aged skin.

The objective of the present study is to investigate the effects of CPs from bovine bone on skin aging based on the chronologically aged model. Bovine bone was employed as a raw material to prepare different CPs using Alcalase and collagenase. Then, the effects of CPs from bovine bone on chronologically aged skin were investigated in chronologically aged mice by analyzing the skin histology, skin components and antioxidative indicators. The results showed that oral administration of CPs from bovine bone has beneficial effects on chronologically aged skin by improving the skin laxity, but it had no on moisture retention of skin. CPs prepared by Alcalase performed better than CPs prepared by collagenase.

2. Materials and Methods

2.1. Materials and Chemicals

Alcalase was purchased from Novozymes (Beijing, China). Proline (food grade) and bacterial collagenase were purchased from Sigma-Aldrich (St. Louis, MO, USA). The bicinchoninic acid (BCA) protein assay kit was purchased from Beijing Solarbio Science and Technology Co., Ltd. (Beijing, China). Commercial kits used for determining hydroxyproline (Hyp), type I and type III collagen, hyaluronic acid (HA), superoxide dismutase (SOD), catalase (CAT), and malondialdehyde (MDA) were purchased from Jiancheng Inst. of Biotechnology (Nanjing, China). All other chemicals used in the study were of analytical grade or better.

2.2. Collagen Peptides (CPs) Preparation

Gelatin was extracted from bovine bone with hot water. Briefly, the bovine bone was treated in boiling water for 6 h, followed by removing bone using gauze filter. The filtrate was cooled, defatted and centrifuged at 4500× g for 15 min with a refrigerated centrifuge (TGL-185, Pingfan Co., Ltd., Changsha, China). After centrifugation, the upper soluble fractions were collected and freeze-dried to obtain the gelatin. The gelatin was enzymatically hydrolyzed by the Alcalase at pH 8.0 for 4.0 h to obtain collagen peptides (named ACP), and the collagenase at pH 7.5 for 3.0 h to obtain collagen peptides (named CCP). Finally, the hydrolysates were dialyzed to discard salt and free amino acids, freeze-dried and stored at −80 °C until use.

2.3. Molecular Weight Distribution

The molecular weight distribution of CPs was measured using a Shimadzu LC-15C high performance liquid chromatography (HPLC) system (Shimadzu, Tokyo, Japan) equipped with a TSK gel G2000 SWXL column (7.8 × 300 mm, Tosoh, Tokyo, Japan). Samples were loaded onto the column and eluted with 45% (v/v) acetonitrile containing 0.1% (v/v) trifluoroacetic acid at a flow rate of 0.5 mL/min and monitored at 214 nm at room temperature. A molecular weight calibration curve ($y = -0.1881x + 6.5867$, y: log MW, x: time, $R^2 = 0.9954$) was obtained from the average retention times of the following standards: Gly–Ser (146 Da), Asn–Cys–Ser (322 Da), Trp–Pro–Trp–Trp (674 Da), bacitracin (1423 Da) and aprotinin (6512 Da) [15].

2.4. Amino Acid Composition

The samples were hydrolyzed in 6.0 M HCl at 110 °C for 24 h. After phenylisothiocyanate (PITC) derivatization reaction, the amino acid composition was analyzed by a Shimadzu LC-15C high performance liquid chromatography (HPLC) system (Shimadzu, Tokyo, Japan) equipped with a reverse Zorbax SB-C18 column (4.6 × 250 mm, Agilent, Santa Clara, CA, USA). The mobile phase consisted of (A) 10 mM phosphate buffer solution (pH 6.9) and (B) 100% acetonitrile and the flow rate was 1.0 mL/min. The gradient was programmed as follows: 0–5 min, 5–10% B; 5–25 min, 10–17% B; 25–45 min, 17–35% B; 45–48 min, 35–100% B; 48–50 min, 100% B; 50–58 min, 100–5% B; and 58–60 min, 5% B. The detection wavelength was set at 254 nm [15].

2.5. Animals, Diets, and Treatments

Animal experiments were carried out under the protocols approved by the Committee for Animal Research of Peking University and followed the Guide for the Care and Use of Laboratory Animals (NIH publication No. 86-23, revised 1996). The present experiment was approved by the Animal Experimental Welfare & Ethical Inspection Committee, the Supervision, Inspection and Testing Center of Genetically Modified Organisms, Ministry of Agriculture (Beijing, China), and was performed in the Experimental Animal Center, Supervision and Testing Center for GMOs Food Safety, Ministry of Agriculture (SPF grade, Beijing, China).

Two-month-old (young mice, 28 ± 2 g, specific pathogen free (SPF) grade) and thirteen-month-old (old mice, 45 ± 5 g, SPF grade) female Kunming mice were purchased from Sibeifu (Beijing) Laboratory Animal Science and Technology Co., Ltd. (Beijing, China). The two-month-old mice were set as young controls ($n = 10$) and were given 0.2 mL normal saline. The thirteen-month-old mice were divided, based on body weight, into 6 groups ($n = 10$/group), including the model group and CPs treatment groups. The model group was given 0.2 mL normal saline; whereas the CPs treatment groups were given 0.2 mL ACP at doses of 200 (ACP-200), 400 (ACP-400) and 800 mg/kg body weight (ACP-800), respectively, and 0.2 mL CCP at a dose of 400 mg/kg body weight (ACP-400). In addition to free access to normal AIN-93M purified diet and water, each group was intragastrically administrated with 0.2 mL of normal saline or CPs once a day for eight weeks. After eight weeks, mice were sacrificed and samples were collected for further treatment and analysis.

2.6. Measurement of Degree of Skin Laxity (DSL)

During the period of this study, mice backs were epilated with 6% (w/w) sodium sulfide 2 days before measuring degree of skin laxity each time. Briefly, the dorsal skin, about 1 cm away from the tail root, was gently stretched by left hand with mice hind limbs off the table top slightly. Right hand controls mouse movement by pulling tail. The stretch length was measured immediately when mice were immobile. The DSL was defined as the following equation: DSL (mm) = stretch length of dorsal skin.

2.7. Measurement of Spleen Index (SI) and Thymus Index (TI)

The mice were weighed and sacrificed. Spleen and thymus were excised from the mice and weighed immediately. The spleen index (SI) and thymus index (TI) were calculated according to the following equation: SI or TI (mg/g) = (weight of spleen or thymus)/body weight.

2.8. Histological Analysis

After eight weeks, mice were sacrificed and dorsal skin samples were dissected out immediately. 4 skin samples (About 1 cm^2) in each group were fixed in 4% buffered neutral formalin solution for 24 h, and embedded in paraffin. Serial sections (7 μm) were put onto silane-coated slides and stained with haematoxylin–eosin (HE). The stained sections were further analyzed using an optical microscope. 1 representative image of HE-stained dorsal skin section in each group was presented in part of results.

2.9. Measurement of Moisture Content

Mice backs were epilated with 6% (w/w) sodium sulfide 2 days before sacrificing mice. Dorsal skins were collected after mice were sacrifice and skin moisture was measured immediately. The moisture content of skin sample was determined according to GB/T5009.3-2010, a national standard of China for measuring moisture content. This method was employed to measure moisture content of skin in several previous reports [13,14]. Briefly, about 0.1 g of powdered skin sample was put into weighing bottle and dried in an oven at 105 °C for 4 h. The moisture content was calculated according to the following equation:

$$\text{Moisture content} = (m_1 - m_2)/(m_1 - m_3) \times 100 \quad (1)$$

m_1, m_2 and m_3 is the weight of weighing bottle plus skin sample, weighting bottle plus dry finished skin sample and weighing bottle, respectively.

2.10. Determination of Hyaluronic Acid (HA) Content

About 0.1 g skin tissue was powdered in a liquid nitrogen bath and homogenized in pre-cooling saline. After centrifugation at 14,000× g for 15 min at 4 °C with a refrigerated centrifuge (TGL-185, Pingfan Co., Ltd., Changsha, China), the supernatant was collected to analyze the hyaluronic acid (HA) content using a commercial HA measurement kit (Nanjing Jiancheng Bio Inst., Nanjing, China).

2.11. Determination of Collagen Content

A commercial hydroxyproline assay kit (Nanjing Jiancheng Bio Inst., Nanjing, China) was used to analyze the Hyp content. Briefly, about 0.05 g skin tissue was totally hydrolyzed, oxidized and reacted with dimethyl-amino-benzaldehyde. The end product has a maximal absorption at 550 nm. The Hyp content in the skin was finally determined by comparison with the absorbance of the Hyp standard. The collagen content was calculated according to the Hyp content using a conversion factor of 8.00 [25].

2.12. *Ratio of Type I to Type III Collagen*

Commercial type I and type III collagen assay kits (Nanjing Jiancheng Bio Inst., Nanjing, China) were used to analyze the relative content of type I and type III collagen. The ratio of type I to type III collagen was calculated according to the following equation: ratio of type I to type III collagen = content of type I collagen/content of type I collagen.

2.13. *Antioxidant Indicators Analysis*

Skin tissue were powdered in a liquid nitrogen bath and homogenized with 9 weights of pre-cooling saline. Homogenate was centrifuged at 14,000× g for 15 min at 4 °C with a refrigerated centrifuge (TGL-185, Pingfan Co., Ltd., Changsha, China) to collect the supernatants. Total protein concentration was determined using a bicinchoninic acid (BCA) assay kit (Solarbio, Beijing, China). The SOD activity, CAT activity and malondialdehyde MDA content (expressed as MDA equivalents) were analyzed using the corresponding enzyme-linked immunosorbent assay (ELISA) kit (Nanjing Jiancheng Bio Inst., Nanjing, China) according to the manufacturer's instructions and the results were expressed in U/mg protein or nmol/mg protein.

2.14. *Statistical Analysis*

Results are expressed by the means ± standard deviation (SDs). Comparisons between two groups were analyzed by Student's t-test. Differences between the means of the individual groups were analyzed using the analysis of variance (ANOVA) with Duncan's multiple range tests. A difference was considered statistically significant when $p < 0.05$. All computations were performed with SPSS Statistics 19 (IBM, Chicago, IL, USA).

3. Results

3.1. *Characterization of Collagen Peptides*

Alcalase and collagenase (two optimized enzymes in our prior study) were used for producing different collagen peptides (named ACP and CCP, respectively). The molecular weight distributions of ACP and CCP are shown in Figure 1. ACP and CCP had a similar molecular weight distribution. Both ACP and CCP mainly consisted of peptides in molecular weight ranges of <500 Da (more than 50%), and the peptides of <1000 Da accounted for approximately 70% and 74%, respectively.

The amino acid compositions of ACP and CCP are shown in Table 1. ACP and CCP had similar amino acid compositions. Gly is the most dominant amino acid in ACP and CCP, which is consistent with the Gly-X-Y repeating sequence in the collagen macromolecule. In addition, ACP and CCP are also rich in Pro, Glu, Phe, Arg and Thr.

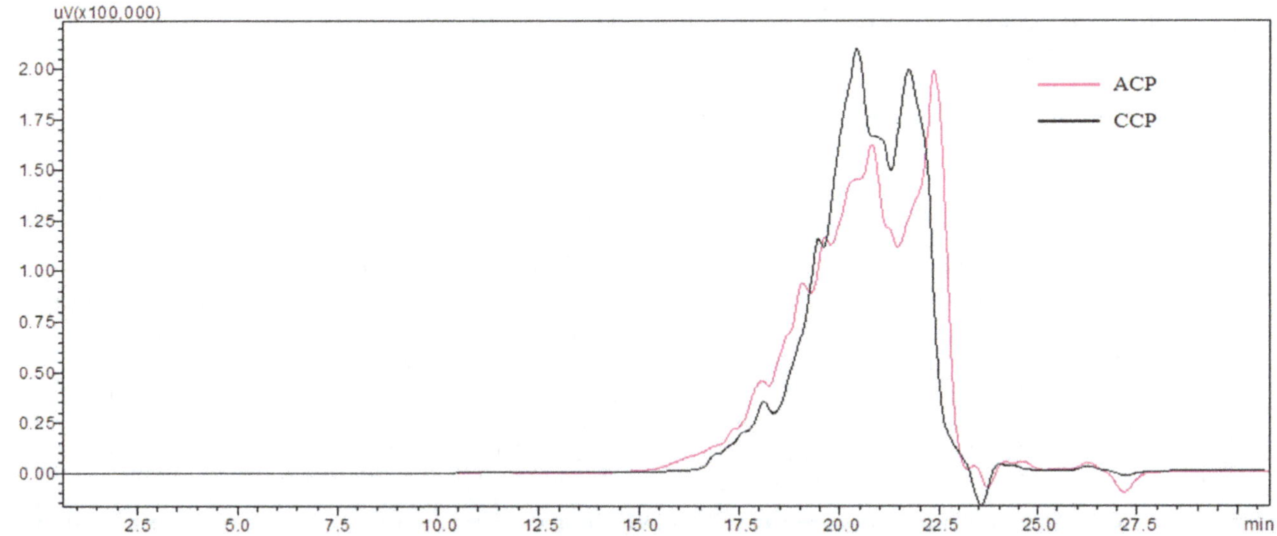

Figure 1. The molecular weight distributions of collagen peptides.

Table 1. Amino acid compositions of collagen peptides.

Amino Acid	Relative Content (g/100 g) [a,b]	
	ACP	CCP
Asp	5.68	5.17
Glu	10.51	11.53
Ser	3.38	3.17
Gly	19.84	21.28
His	3.27	2.97
Thr	7.90	8.51
Ala	4.09	4.68
Pro	12.47	12.18
Arg	8.61	8.47
Tyr	2.28	1.79
Val	3.06	2.90
Met	1.79	1.27
Cys	2.39	2.08
Ile	4.11	3.93
Leu	0.70	0.08
Phe	9.31	9.36
Lys	0.61	0.62
Total	100.00	100.00

[a] Expressed as g/100 g total amino acids; [b] ACP, collagen peptides prepared by Alcalase; CCP, collagen peptides prepared by collagenase.

3.2. Degree of Skin Laxity

As summarized in Table 2, degree of skin laxity (DSL) of young (Y) group was increased during the experiment period but significantly lower than that of model group (old mice), which indicated that skin laxity was increased in an age-dependent manner. During the 8 weeks, the DSL of mice in CPs-treated groups (ACP and CCP groups) decreased over time compared with that in week 0. Significant differences in DSL were seen between ACP-400 group and time-matched model group at week 6 ($p < 0.05$), and the DSL of ACP-400 had no significant difference with that of young group. Furthermore, when the time of oral intake of ACP was as long as 8 weeks, the DSL of all ACP-fed groups decreased to the level of young group ($p > 0.05$), and some of groups (ACP-800 and CCP-400) were even better than the young group. Similarly, oral administration of proline at a dose of

400 mg/kg body weight also reduced the DSL with a significant difference observed compared with the time-matched model group at week 8 ($p < 0.05$).

Table 2. Degree of skin laxity (DSL) of chronologically aged mice after the administration of collagen peptides for 8 weeks.

Group [a]	Degree of Skin Laxity (DSL, mm)				
	Week 0	Week 2	Week 4	Week 6	Week 8
Y	14.90 ± 2.32 *	19.15 ± 1.57 *	19.75 ± 1.03 *	19.60 ± 0.91 *	20.40 ± 1.48 *
M	22.25 ± 2.40	22.40 ± 1.67	23.80 ± 2.25	22.50 ± 1.30	23.00 ± 1.26
ACP-200	23.05 ± 0.56	23.50 ± 1.64	23.11 ± 1.26	22.00 ± 1.31	21.22 ± 1.47 *
ACP-400	22.45 ± 1.88	21.55 ± 1.78	21.65 ± 1.57	20.15 ± 1.34 *	20.25 ± 1.47 *
ACP-800	22.30 ± 1.81	22.72 ± 2.06	22.05 ± 2.26	21.60 ± 1.78	19.80 ± 0.90 *
CCP-400	22.40 ± 1.57	22.35 ± 1.41	21.25 ± 2.03	22.10 ± 1.92	19.95 ± 1.65 *
Pro-400	21.65 ± 1.23	21.30 ± 2.28	22.80 ± 0.81	21.70 ± 1.00	19.75 ± 1.44 *

[a] Y, young group; M, model group (old group); ACP, administrated by collagen peptides which was prepared by Alcalase; CCP, administrated by collagen peptides which was prepared by collagenase; Pro, proline group. 200, 400 and 800 represent administration doses of 200, 400 and 800 mg/kg body weight, respectively. The values are shown as the means ± SDs (n = 10 mice/group). A significant difference was observed at * $p < 0.05$ compared to the time-matched model group.

3.3. Body Weight, Spleen Index (SI) and Thymus Index (TI)

The body weight of young group was increased during the experiment period, whereas that of model group remained stable (Table 3). Treatment with ACP (200, 400 and 800 mg/kg body weight), CCP and proline (400 mg/kg body weight) for 8 weeks caused no statistically significant differences in the body weight compared with the untreated model group. Furthermore, the SI and TI of ACP groups, CCP and proline groups also had no significant difference compared to that of the model group. The body weight and organ indices could be measured to preliminarily determine whether a sample or sample dose had obvious toxicological effects on the animal subjects [26]. There was no obvious atrophy, hyperplasia or swelling of spleen and thymus after CPs and proline intake. Based on these results, it was concluded that oral administration of CPs from bovine bone at doses of 200–800 mg/kg body weight, or proline at 400 mg/kg body weight for 8 weeks, had no obvious toxicological effects.

Table 3. Body weight, spleen index (SI) and thymus index (TI) of chronologically aged mice after the administration of collagen peptides for 8 weeks.

Group [a]	Body Weight (g)					Spleen Index [b] (mg/g)	Thymus Index [b] (mg/g)
	Week 0	Week 2	Week 4	Week 6	Week 8		
Y	28.28 ± 0.73	30.27 ± 1.62	31.71 ± 1.30	32.63 ± 1.81	32.70 ± 1.52	3.48 ± 0.69	1.82 ± 0.39
M	47.14 ± 5.39	45.55 ± 4.67	45.55 ± 4.69	46.52 ± 3.40	46.33 ± 3.81	3.83 ± 1.14	1.55 ± 0.53
ACP-200	47.41 ± 5.47	46.28 ± 6.07	46.44 ± 4.41	47.41 ± 4.13	46.83 ± 3.34	3.72 ± 0.06	1.71 ± 0.65
ACP-400	47.50 ± 5.57	46.32 ± 4.91	46.90 ± 4.48	46.64 ± 4.90	46.35 ± 4.90	3.24 ± 1.24	2.06 ± 0.80
ACP-800	47.75 ± 5.67	46.88 ± 4.68	48.36 ± 7.42	49.40 ± 6.63	47.39 ± 6.57	3.86 ± 1.39	1.55 ± 0.62
CCP-400	47.92 ± 5.73	46.82 ± 4.61	48.13 ± 6.55	48.84 ± 4.88	47.38 ± 4.94	3.87 ± 0.94	1.62 ± 0.66
Pro-400	47.24 ± 5.39	46.96 ± 6.14	46.32 ± 5.86	47.65 ± 5.90	47.44 ± 5.69	3.64 ± 1.04	2.02 ± 0.86

[a] Y, young group; M, model group (old group); ACP, administrated by collagen peptides which was prepared by Alcalase; CCP, administrated by collagen peptides which was prepared by collagenase; Pro, proline group. 200, 400 and 800 represent administration doses of 200, 400 and 800 mg/kg body weight, respectively. The values are shown as the means ± SDs (n = 10 mice/group). No significant difference between each administration group and time-matched model group was observed ($p > 0.05$). [b] Indicates values at week 8.

3.4. Skin Histology

The results of morphological examination of mice dorsal skin are illustrated in Figure 2. Skin collagen fibers in dermis were stained a light red with haematoxylin–eosin (HE). In the model group (old mice), lighter red and more space (green arrow) were observed in the dermis tissue than were those of the young group. There were thinner dermis and less sebaceous gland (red arrow) in the model group compared with the young group. After ACP and CCP intake, the space in the dermis tissue was decreased and the fibers appeared to be denser and more organized compared with the model group. Besides, the number of sebaceous gland was increased when treated by ACP, especially at dose of 800 mg/kg body weight. These results indicated that ACP improved the aged collagen fibers in skin dermis in a dose-dependent manner. Similarly, the sparse, fragmented, and disorganized fibers were also obviously improved and the number of sebaceous gland was greatly increased by the oral administration of proline at a dose of 400 mg/kg body weight for 8 weeks.

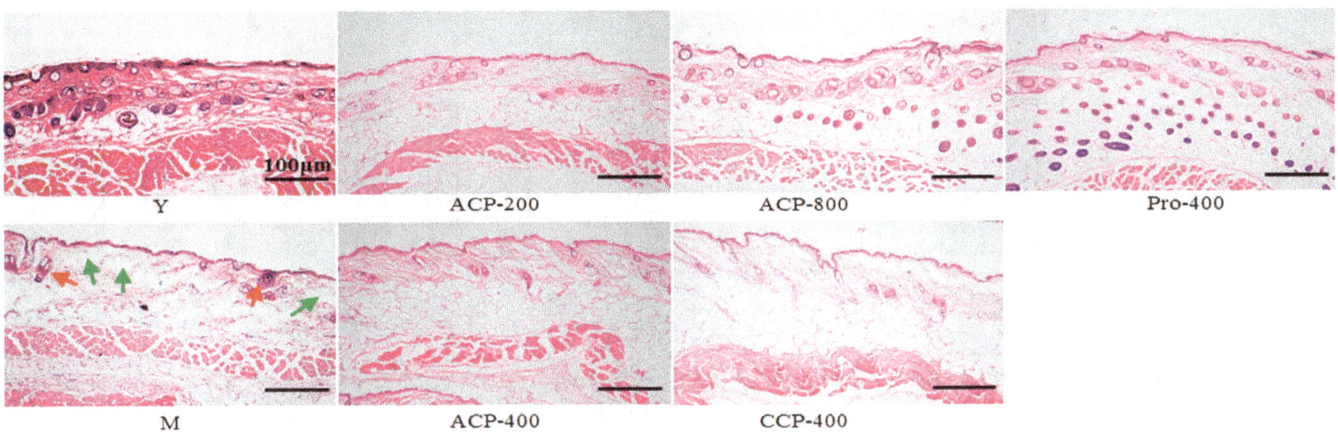

Figure 2. Representative images of haematoxylin–eosin (HE)-stained dorsal skin section from all groups, Y, young group; M, model group (old group); ACP, administrated by collagen peptides which was prepared by Alcalase; CCP, administrated by collagen peptides which was prepared by collagenase; Pro, proline group. 200, 400 and 800 represent administration doses of 200, 400 and 800 mg/kg body weight, respectively. Sebaceous glands and space in dermis tissue are shown as red arrows and green arrows, respectively. Scale bars, 100 μm.

3.5. Skin Components

The results of skin moisture, hyaluronic acid (HA), collagen content and ratio of type I to type III collagen are shown in Figure 3A–D. Skin moisture content and ratio of type I to type III collagen in the model group (old mice) were significantly lower than that in the young group (all $p < 0.05$), indicating that skin moisture content and ratio of type I to type III collagen were decreased with age. Skin HA and collagen contents were also lower than that in the young group, although there was no significant difference observed compared with the model group. Ingestion of CPs (both ACP and CCP) and proline had no significant effect on skin moisture and HA contents compared with the model group. In contrast, oral administration of ACP (200, 400 and 800 mg/kg body weight) caused a dose-dependent increase in the collagen content, and there was a significant difference in the collagen content between the group receiving 800 mg/kg of ACP and the model group ($p < 0.05$). Ingestion of CCP at a dose of 400 mg/kg body weight also increased the collagen content in skin ($p < 0.05$ vs. the model group). However, proline intake at a dose of 400 mg/kg body weight had no significant effect on collagen content compared with the model group. A dose-dependent increase was also observed for ratio of type I to type III collagen in the ACP-fed groups, and there were significant differences between the groups receiving 400 and 800 mg/kg of ACP and the model group (all $p < 0.05$); whereas CCP ingestion at a dose of 400 mg/kg body weight had no significant effect on ratio of type I to type III collagen compared to the model group. Oral administration of proline also significantly increased ratio of type I to type III collagen in skin ($p < 0.05$ vs. the model group).

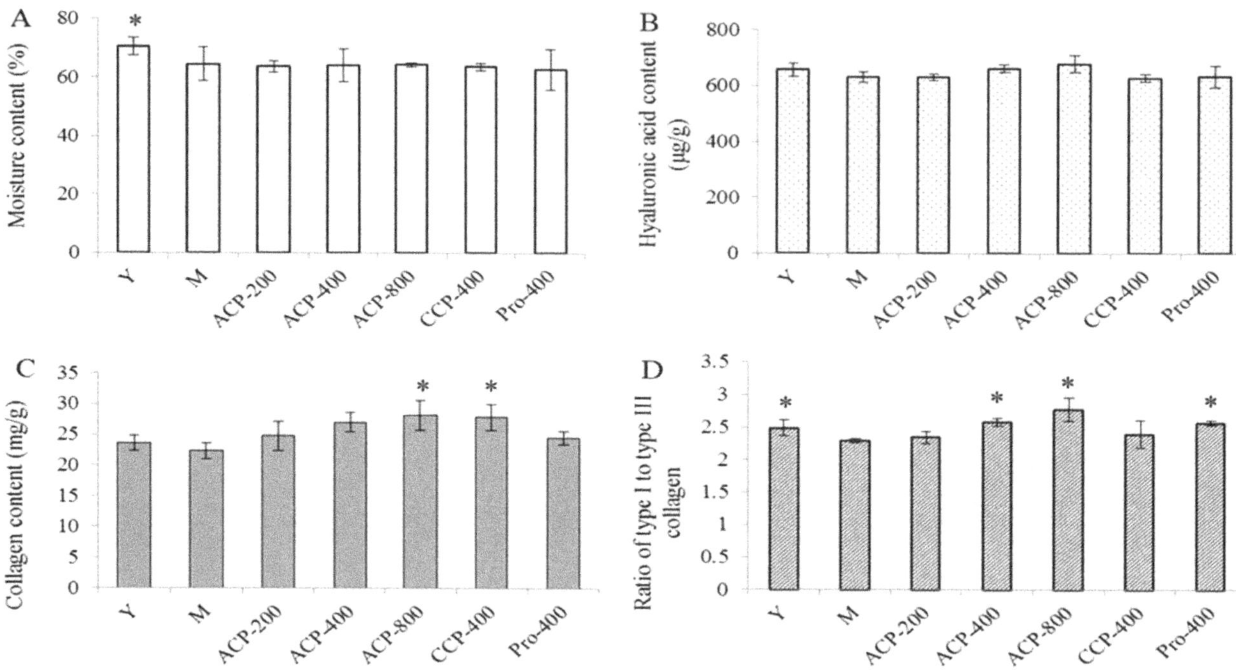

Figure 3. Moisture content (**A**), hyaluronic acid content (**B**), hydroxyproline content (**C**) and ratio of type I to type III collagen (**D**) of chronologically aged mice after the administration of collagen peptides for 8 weeks. Y, young group; M, model group (old group); ACP, administrated by collagen peptides which was prepared by Alcalase; CCP, administrated by collagen peptides which was prepared by collagenase; Pro, proline group. 200, 400 and 800 represent administration doses of 200, 400 and 800 mg/kg body weight, respectively. The values are shown as the means ± SDs (n = 10 mice/group). A significant difference was observed at * $p < 0.05$ compared to the time-matched model group.

3.6. Antioxidant Indicators

The superoxide dismutase (SOD), catalase (CAT) and malondialdehyde (MDA) content in skin are shown in Table 4. The SOD and CAT activities in the M group were significantly lower in the skin compared to the Y group ($p < 0.05$); whereas the MDA level in the model group was higher than that in the young group ($p < 0.05$). Oral administration of CPs (both ACP and CCP) significantly increased the SOD and CAT activities and reduced the MDA level (all $p < 0.05$ vs. the model group). Besides, the increase of SOD and CAT activities and the decrease of MDA level in ACP-fed groups showed a dose-dependent manner. In contrast, proline ingestion had no obvious significant effect on these three antioxidant indicators.

Table 4. SOD and CAT activities and MDA content in dorsal skin of chronologically aged mice after administration of collagen peptides for 8 weeks.

Group [a]	SOD (U/mg Protein)	CAT (U/mg Protein)	MDA Equivalents (nmol/mg Protein)
Y	36.594 ± 1.142 *	10.412 ± 1.143 *	2.209 ± 0.278 *
M	26.877 ± 3.880	4.650 ± 1.582	3.135 ± 0.302
ACP-200	38.746 ± 0.753 *	8.324 ± 0.890 *	2.347 ± 0.209 *
ACP-400	39.823 ± 3.410 *	11.327 ± 1.096 *	2.261 ± 0.107 *
ACP-800	40.036 ± 4.820 *	12.012 ± 0.752 *	2.154 ± 0.325 *
CCP-400	39.796 ± 1.211 *	9.354 ± 1.856 *	2.204 ± 0.201 *
Pro-400	32.646 ± 1.691	3.318 ± 0.665	2.456 ± 0.316

[a] Y, young group; M, model group (old group); ACP, administrated by collagen peptides which was prepared by Alcalase; CCP, administrated by collagen peptides which was prepared by collagenase.; Pro, proline group. 200, 400 and 800 represent administration doses of 200, 400 and 800 mg/kg body weight, respectively. The values are shown as the means ± SDs (n = 10 mice/group). A significant difference was observed at * $p < 0.05$ compared to the time-matched model group.

4. Discussion

Skin aging is consisted of chronological aging and photoaging. There are some difference in clinical signs and underlying mechanisms for these two processes [27,28]. Collagen peptides (CPs) have been widely reported to exert beneficial effects on photoaging skin, but few studies was carried out to evaluate their effect on chronologically aged skin. In present study, 13-month-old Kunming mice, equivalent to 45 years old of human life [29], were employed to investigate the effect of CPs on chronologically aged skin. In several previous clinical trials, a daily dose of 2.5 g or 5 g of CPs has been employed in adult subjects, and these doses were considered to be safe [16,17,30]. According to the conversion of animal doses to human equivalent dose (HED) based on the body surface area (BSA) [31], about daily dose of 500 or 1000 mg/kg body weight could be used in mice. In addition, daily doses of 50–200 mg/kg body weight have also been used in several animal experiments [13–15]. Therefore, doses of 200, 400 and 800 mg/kg body weight/day were employed in the present study.

Skin laxity is a main feature of natural skin aging and is increased with age [32]. Therefore, skin laxity was dynamically evaluated by measuring the degree of skin laxity (DSL) to observe the effect of CPs intake on chronologically aged skin. An obvious beneficial effect was observed after 8 weeks of CPs intake. Therefore, mice were sacrificed and samples were collected for further treatment and analysis after 8 weeks. Unexpectedly, proline (abundant in collagen) ingestion also significantly improved skin laxity. These results provided guidance for the application of CPs or proline against chronological skin aging. The 8-week duration of CPs ingestion might be equivalent to several years old of human life in terms of life span. But it does not mean that the beneficial effects of CPs could be observed only after several years duration of CPs intake, because several studies have reported that significant beneficial effects of CPs on aging skin could be observed after 6 to 12 weeks in both clinical trials and animal experiments [13–17].

As the main component of the skin dermis, collagen has been reported to be beneficial in improving skin laxity and decreasing the appearance of wrinkles and its reduction in the quantity and quality is a major cause of laxity and wrinkles [33,34]. In the chronologically aged skin, dermal collagen fiber became sparse, fragmented and disorganized [35,36]. However, intake of CPs (both ACP and CCP) repaired collagen fibers and the fibers appeared to be denser and more organized compared to the aged skin. Collagen in skin mainly consists of type I and type III collagen. Collagen production and the ratio of type I to type III collagen is decreased gradually with age [14,28,37,38]. Type I collagen tend to form broader bundles of fibers, while type III collagen forms narrow bundles. A decrease in the diameter and number of the collagen bundles is correlated with the decrease in load and tensile strength reported in aging skin [38]. Oral administration of CPs increased the collagen content and ratio of type I to type III collagen in a dose-dependent manner, which suggested that CPs improved skin laxity by changing skin collagen quantitatively and qualitatively. In contrast, the skin moisture and hyaluronic acid (HA) were not affected by CPs ingestion. HA is a key molecule involved in skin moisture, because it has a unique capacity to bind and retain water molecules [39]. Taken together with the results of the current study, it was concluded that oral administration of CPs had beneficial effect on chronologically aged skin by improving skin laxity, but it had no influence on moisture retention of skin.

Interestedly, ingestion of proline also had beneficial effect on chronologically aged skin in terms of skin laxity, collagen content and ratio of type I to type III collagen. This result of in vivo study was consistent with that of a previous in vitro experiment which demonstrated that proline could increase the collagen synthesis of confluent fibroblasts, but it did not stimulate the proliferation of fibroblasts [40,41]. Watanabe-Kamiyama and coworkers have reported that proline could reach the skin after proline intake [42]. Therefore, we speculated that proline intake exerted beneficial effect on chronologically aged skin by increasing the collagen synthesis of skin fibroblasts.

It has been widely accepted that oxidative stress plays a critical role in initiating and driving the signaling events that result in skin aging. Study has reported that the production of reactive oxygen species (ROS) was increased in photoaged and chronologically aged skin [43]. In addition to directly attacking macromolecules, such as proteins, lipids, DNA and RNA, the excessive ROS also initiate several signaling pathways, including mitogen-activated protein kinases (MAPKs) and nuclear factor kappa-light-chain-enhancer of activated B cells (NF-κB), and further activate transcription factor activator protein-1 (AP-1) [44]. AP-1 induces collagen degradation by upregulating collagen-degraded enzymes such as matrix metalloprotease (MMP)-1, MMP-3 and MMP-9 and downregulating the biosynthesis of collagen. These changes in the skin lead to the phenotype of aged skin [45]. Therefore, antioxidants or free radical scavengers, such as ascorbic acid and polyphenols were reported to improve skin aging by scavenging excessive ROS. Normally, endogenous antioxidant enzymes are able to scavenge the excessive ROS to protect skin tissues from oxidative injuries. SOD and CAT are two antioxidant enzymes that inactivate superoxide anions and hydrogen peroxide, respectively. MDA is a product of lipid peroxidation and is usually quantified to estimate the lipid peroxidation extent induced by ROS. The SOD and CAT activities were decreased and MDA content was increased with age. However, CPs (ACP and CCP) intake could increase SOD and CAT activities and decrease MDA content, indicating that ingestion of collagen peptides from bovine bone had the ability to decrease ROS in skin. The decreased ROS in skin might help to increase the biosynthesis of collagen and decrease the collagen degradation by reducing the MMPs production. Indeed, several previous studies have reported that collagen hydrolysate ingestion could increases skin collagen expression and suppresses MMP-1 and MMP-2 [46,47]. In vitro study had demonstrated that ACP and CCP had high antioxidant capacity base on the hydroxyl radicals and ABTS + scavenging assays (data not shown). In addition, it has been widely reported that nuclear factor E2-related factor 2 (Nrf2)-antioxidant response element (ARE) pathway plays a central role in regulating antioxidant enzymes against oxidative stress [48,49]. Therefore, we speculate that CPs exerted their antioxidant effect in a direct and/or indirect manner. It is also possible that CPs exerted their beneficial effects on chronological aged skin in other ways, as previous studies have reported that Pro–Hyp in human blood after oral ingestion of CPs stimulates fibroblast growth [41,50]. It should be noted that proline intake did not have an obvious effect on skin antioxidant capacity. These results suggested that CPs had more complex action mechanisms underlying anti-aging effect than proline.

Bovine bone is an abundant source of gelatin. The CPs from bovine bone is mainly concentrated on its beneficial effect on bone metabolism. However, the current study found that the CPs from bovine bone also had beneficial effect on skin aging. The CPs prepared in this study mainly consist of oligopeptides (<1000 Da). It was reported that small peptides, especially the di-and tripeptides, are more easily absorbed in the intestinal tract than larger molecules, and oligopeptides are more bioactive than proteins, polypeptides and free amino acids [51,52]. Therefore, we speculated that ACP and CCP are readily absorbed and might exhibit potential biological effects once they are orally administered. Another purpose of this study is to preliminary investigate whether different CPs prepared by Alcalase and collagenase have different effects on chronologically aged skin. Based on the present results, it can be drawn that the beneficial effects of ACP were slightly better than those of CCP. Therefore, Alcalase is a favorable enzyme to produce CPs with beneficial effects on skin aging in food and medical industries. The present result of molecular weight distribution provides a guide for testing and controlling the quality of CPs. Besides, CPs should be protected from oxygen and light because of its easy oxidation.

5. Conclusions

In summary, the present study demonstrated oral administration of collagen peptides from bovine bone could improve the laxity of chronologically aged skin by increasing skin collagen content and ratio of type I to type III collagen, but it had no effect on moisture retention of skin. The beneficial effects of collagen peptides prepared by Alcalase (ACP) were slightly better than those of collagen peptides prepared by collagenase (CCP). Another action mechanism underlying the beneficial effects on aged skin of collagen peptides may be involved in increasing the antioxidant properties in the body. Proline intake also improved the laxity of chronologically aged skin but it did not affect the skin antioxidant capacity. These results suggest that collagen peptides from bovine bone and proline are potential dietary supplements for use against skin aging in chronologically aged process.

Acknowledgments: This study was supported by the earmarked fund from China Agriculture Research System (CARS-46) and National Natural Science Foundation of China (NSFC, No. 31271846).

Author Contributions: Bo Li conceived and designed the experiments; Hongdong Song, Siqi Zhang and Ling Zhang performed the experiments and analyzed the data; Hongdong Song and Bo Li wrote the paper.

References

1. Rittié, L.; Fisher, G.J. Natural and sun-induced aging of human skin. *Cold Spring Harb. Perspect. Med.* **2015**, *5*, a015370. [CrossRef] [PubMed]
2. Durai, P.C.; Thappa, D.M.; Kumari, R.; Malathi, M. Aging in elderly: Chronological versus photoaging. *Indian J. Dermatol.* **2012**, *57*, 343–352. [PubMed]
3. Helfrich, Y.R.; Sachs, D.L.; Voorhees, J.J. Overview of skin aging and photoaging. *Dermatol. Nurs.* **2008**, *20*, 177–183. [PubMed]
4. Dobos, G.; Lichterfeld, A.; Blume-Peytavi, U.; Kottner, J. Evaluation of skin ageing: A systematic review of clinical scales. *Brit. J. Dermatol.* **2015**, *172*, 1249–1261. [CrossRef] [PubMed]
5. Chen, J.; Li, Y.; Zhu, Q.; Li, T.; Lu, H.; Wei, N.; Huang, Y.; Shi, R.; Ma, X.; Wang, X.; et al. Anti-skin-aging effect of epigallocatechin gallate by regulating epidermal growth factor receptor pathway on aging mouse model induced by d-Galactose. *Mech. Ageing Dev.* **2017**, *164*, 1–7. [CrossRef] [PubMed]
6. Tran, D.; Townley, J.P.; Barnes, T.M.; Greive, K.A. An antiaging skin care system containing alpha hydroxy acids and vitamins improves the biomechanical parameters of facial skin. *Clin. Cosmet. Investig. Dermatol.* **2015**, *8*, 9–17. [PubMed]
7. Latreille, J.; Kesse-Guyot, E.; Malvy, D.; Andreeva, V.; Galan, P.; Tschachler, E.; Hercberg, S.; Guinot, C.; Ezzedine, K. Association between dietary intake of *n*-3 polyunsaturated fatty acids and severity of skin photoaging in a middle-aged Caucasian population. *J. Dermatol. Sci.* **2013**, *72*, 233–239. [CrossRef] [PubMed]
8. Fanian, F.; Mac-Mary, S.; Jeudy, A.; Lihoreau, T.; Messikh, R.; Ortonne, J.P.; Sainthillier, J.M.; Elkhyat, A.; Guichard, A.; Kenari, K.H.; et al. Efficacy of micronutrient supplementation on skin aging and seasonal variation: A randomized, placebo-controlled, double-blind study. *Clin. Interv. Aging* **2013**, *8*, 1527–1537. [CrossRef] [PubMed]
9. Murata, M.; Satoh, T.; Wakabayashi, H.; Yamauchi, K.; Abe, F.; Nomura, Y. Oral administration of bovine lactoferrin attenuates ultraviolet B-induced skin photodamage in hairless mice. *J. Dairy Sci.* **2014**, *97*, 651–658. [CrossRef] [PubMed]
10. Zhuang, Y.; Hou, H.; Zhao, X.; Zhang, Z.; Li, B. Effects of collagen and collagen hydrolysate from jellyfish (*Rhopilema esculentum*) on mice skin photoaging induced by UV irradiation. *J. Food Sci.* **2009**, *74*, H183–H188. [CrossRef] [PubMed]
11. Zague, V. A new view concerning the effects of collagen hydrolysate intake on skin properties. *Arch. Dermatol. Res.* **2008**, *300*, 479–483. [CrossRef] [PubMed]
12. Oesser, S.; Adam, M.; Babel, W.; Seifert, J. Oral administration of 14C labeled gelatin hydrolysate leads to an accumulation of radioactivity in cartilage of mice (C57/BL). *J. Nutr.* **1999**, *129*, 1891–1895. [PubMed]
13. Fan, J.; Zhuang, Y.; Li, B. Effects of collagen and collagen hydrolysate from jellyfish umbrella on histological and immunity changes of mice photoaging. *Nutrients* **2013**, *5*, 223–233. [CrossRef] [PubMed]
14. Hou, H.; Li, B.; Zhang, Z.; Xue, C.; Yu, G.; Wang, J.; Bao, Y.; Bu, L.; Sun, J.; Peng, Z. Moisture absorption and retention properties, and activity in alleviating skin photodamage of collagen polypeptide from marine fish skin. *Food Chem.* **2012**, *135*, 1432–1439. [CrossRef] [PubMed]
15. Song, H.; Meng, M.; Cheng, X.; Li, B.; Wang, C. The effect of collagen hydrolysates from silver carp (*Hypophthalmichthys molitrix*) skin on UV-induced photoaging in mice: Molecular weight affects skin repair. *Food Funct.* **2017**, *8*, 1538–1546. [CrossRef] [PubMed]
16. Proksch, E.; Segger, D.; Degwert, J.; Schunck, M.; Zague, V.; Oesser, S. Oral supplementation of specific collagen peptides has beneficial effects on human skin physiology: A double-blind, placebo-controlled study. *Skin Pharmacol. Physiol.* **2014**, *27*, 47–55. [CrossRef] [PubMed]

17. Schwartz, S.R.; Park, J. Ingestion of BioCell Collagen®, a novel hydrolyzed chicken sternal cartilage extract; enhanced blood microcirculation and reduced facial aging signs. *Clin. Interv. Aging* **2012**, *7*, 267–273. [PubMed]
18. Nur, A.T.; Che, M.Y.; Rn, R.M.H.; Aina, M.A.; Amin, I. Use of principal component analysis for differentiation of gelatine sources based on polypeptide molecular weights. *Food Chem.* **2014**, *151*, 286–292.
19. Ali, M.E.; Sultana, S.; Hamid, S.B.; Hossain, M.A.; Yehya, W.A.; Kader, M.A.; Bhargava, S.K. Gelatin controversies in food, pharmaceuticals and personal care products: Authentication methods, current status and future challenges. *Crit. Rev. Food Sci. Nutr.* **2016**, *29*, 1–17. [CrossRef] [PubMed]
20. Liu, J.; Wang, Y.; Song, S.; Wang, X.; Qin, Y.; Si, S.; Guo, Y. Combined oral administration of bovine collagen peptides with calcium citrate inhibits bone loss in ovariectomized rats. *PLoS ONE* **2015**, *10*, e0135019. [CrossRef] [PubMed]
21. Kumar, S.; Sugihara, F.; Suzuki, K.; Inoue, N.; Venkateswarathirukumara, S. A double-blind, placebo-controlled, randomised, clinical study on the effectiveness of collagen peptide on osteoarthritis. *J. Sci. Food Agric.* **2015**, *95*, 702–707. [CrossRef] [PubMed]
22. Humiski, L.M.; Aluko, R.E. Physicochemical and bitterness properties of enzymatic pea protein hydrolysates. *J. Food Sci.* **2007**, *72*, S605–S611. [CrossRef] [PubMed]
23. Liang, Q.; Ren, X.; Ma, H.; Li, S.; Xu, K.; Oladejo, A.O. Effect of low-frequency ultrasonic-assisted enzymolysis on the physicochemical and antioxidant properties of corn protein hydrolysates. *J. Food Qual.* **2017**, *2017*, 1–10. [CrossRef]
24. Kanth, S.V.; Venba, R.; Madhan, B.; Chandrababu, N.K.; Sadulla, S. Studies on the influence of bacterial collagenase in leather dyeing. *Dyes Pigment.* **2008**, *76*, 338–347. [CrossRef]
25. Cheng, F.Y.; Hsu, F.W.; Chang, H.S.; Lin, L.C.; Sakata, R. Effect of different acids on the extraction of pepsin-solubilised collagen containing melanin from silky fowl feet. *Food Chem.* **2009**, *113*, 563–567. [CrossRef]
26. Zhang, X.D.; Wu, H.Y.; Wu, D.; Wang, Y.Y.; Chang, J.H.; Zhai, Z.B.; Meng, A.M.; Liu, P.X.; Zhang, L.A.; Fan, F.Y. Toxicologic effects of gold nanoparticles in vivo by different administration routes. *Int. J. Nanomed.* **2010**, *5*, 771–781. [CrossRef] [PubMed]
27. Jenkins, G. Molecular mechanisms of skin ageing. *Mech. Ageing Dev.* **2002**, *123*, 801–810. [CrossRef]
28. Chung, J.H.; Seo, J.Y.; Choi, H.R.; Lee, M.K.; Youn, C.S.; Rhie, G.; Cho, K.H.; Kim, K.H.; Park, K.C.; Eun, H.C. Modulation of skin collagen metabolism in aged and photoaged human skin in vivo. *J. Investig. Dermatol.* **2001**, *117*, 1218–1224. [CrossRef] [PubMed]
29. Song, H.; Zhang, L.; Luo, Y.; Zhang, S.; Li, B. Effects of collagen peptides intake on skin ageing and platelet release in chronologically aged mice revealed by cytokine array analysis. *J. Cell. Mol. Med.* **2017**. [CrossRef] [PubMed]
30. Ohara, H.; Ito, K.; Iida, H.; Matsumoto, H. Improvement in the moisture content of the stratum corneum following 4 weeks of collagen hydrolysate ingestion. *Nippon Shokuhin Kogaku Kaishi* **2009**, *56*, 137–145. [CrossRef]
31. Reagan-Shaw, S.; Nihal, M.; Ahmad, N. Dose translation from animal to human studies revisited. *FASEB J.* **2008**, *22*, 659–661. [CrossRef] [PubMed]
32. Quan, T.; Fisher, G.J. Role of age-associated alterations of the dermal extracellular matrix microenvironment in human skin aging: A mini-review. *Gerontology* **2015**, *61*, 427–434. [CrossRef] [PubMed]
33. Tanaka, Y.; Nakayama, J. Upregulated expression of La ribonucleoprotein domain family member 6 and collagen type I gene following water-filtered broad-spectrum near-infrared irradiation in a 3-dimensional human epidermal tissue culture model as revealed by microarray analysis. *Australas. J. Dermatol.* **2017**. [CrossRef] [PubMed]
34. Sadick, N.S.; Harth, Y. A 12-week clinical and instrumental study evaluating the efficacy of a multisource radiofrequency home-use device for wrinkle reduction and improvement in skin tone, skin elasticity, and dermal collagen content. *J. Cosmet. Laser Ther.* **2016**, *18*, 422–427. [CrossRef] [PubMed]
35. Demaria, M.; Desprez, P.Y.; Campisi, J.; Velarde, M.C. Cell autonomous and non-autonomous effects of senescent cells in the skin. *J. Investig. Dermatol.* **2015**, *135*, 1722–1726. [CrossRef] [PubMed]
36. Zouboulis, C.C.; Boschnakow, A. Chronological and photoaging of the human sebaceous gland. *Clin. Exp. Dermatol.* **2001**, *26*, 600–607. [CrossRef] [PubMed]

37. Varani, J.; Dame, M.K.; Rittie, L.; Fligiel, S.E.; Kang, S.; Fisher, G.J.; Voorhees, J.J. Decreased collagen production in chronologically aged skin: Roles of age-dependent alteration in fibroblast function and defective mechanical stimulation. *Am. J. Pathol.* **2006**, *168*, 1861–1868. [CrossRef] [PubMed]
38. Lovell, C.R.; Smolenski, K.A.; Duance, V.C.; Light, N.D.; Young, S.; Dyson, M. Type I and III collagen content and fibre distribution in normal human skin during ageing. *Br. J. Dermatol.* **1987**, *117*, 419–428. [CrossRef] [PubMed]
39. Papakonstantinou, E.; Roth, M.; Karakiulakis, G. Hyaluronic acid: A key molecule in skin aging. *Dermato-Endocrinology* **2012**, *4*, 253–258. [CrossRef] [PubMed]
40. Haratake, A.; Watase, D.; Fujita, T.; Setoguchi, S.; Matsunaga, K.; Takata, J. Effects of oral administration of collagen peptides on skin collagen content and its underlying mechanism using a newly developed low collagen skin mice model. *J. Funct. Foods* **2015**, *16*, 174–182. [CrossRef]
41. Ohara, H.; Ichikawa, S.; Matsumoto, H.; Akiyama, M.; Fujimoto, N.; Kobayashi, T.; Tajima, S. Collagen-derived dipeptide, proline-hydroxyproline, stimulates cell proliferation and hyaluronic acid synthesis in cultured human dermal fibroblasts. *J. Dermatol.* **2010**, *37*, 330–338. [CrossRef] [PubMed]
42. Watanabe-Kamiyama, M.; Shimizu, M.; Kamiyama, S.; Taguchi, Y.; Sone, H.; Morimatsu, F.; Shirakawa, H.; Furukawa, Y.; Komai, M. Absorption and effectiveness of orally administered low molecular weight collagen hydrolysate in rats. *J. Agric. Food Chem.* **2010**, *58*, 835–841. [CrossRef] [PubMed]
43. Callaghan, T.M.; Wilhelm, K.P. A review of ageing and an examination of clinical methods in the assessment of ageing skin. Part I: Cellular and molecular perspectives of skin ageing. *Int. J. Cosmet. Sci.* **2008**, *30*, 313–322. [CrossRef] [PubMed]
44. Kammeyer, A.; Luiten, R.M. Oxidation events and skin aging. *Ageing Res. Rev.* **2015**, *21*, 16–29. [CrossRef] [PubMed]
45. Xu, Y.; Fisher, G.J. Ultraviolet (UV) light irradiation induced signal transduction in skin photoaging. *J. Dermatol. Sci.* **2015**, *1*, S1–S8. [CrossRef]
46. Liang, J.; Pei, X.; Zhang, Z.; Wang, N.; Wang, J.; Li, Y. The protective effects of long-term oral administration of marine collagen hydrolysate from chum salmon on collagen matrix homeostasis in the chronological aged skin of sprague-dawley male rats. *J. Food Sci.* **2010**, *75*, H230–H238. [CrossRef] [PubMed]
47. Zague, V.; de Freitas, V.; Rosa, M.D.C.; de Castro, G.Á.; Jaeger, R.G.; Machado-Santelli, G.M. Collagen hydrolysate intake increases skin collagen expression and suppresses matrix metalloproteinase 2 activity. *J. Med. Food* **2011**, *14*, 618–624. [CrossRef] [PubMed]
48. Maltese, G.; Psefteli, P.; Rizzo, B.; Srivastava, S.; Gnudi, L.; Mann, G.E.; Siow, R.C. The anti-ageing hormone klotho induces Nrf2-mediated antioxidant defences in human aortic smooth muscle cells. *J. Cell. Mol. Med.* **2017**, *21*, 621–627. [CrossRef] [PubMed]
49. Sun, Z.; Park, S.Y.; Hwang, E.; Zhang, M.; Seo, S.A.; Lin, P.; Yi, T.H. Thymus vulgaris alleviates UVB irradiation induced skin damage via inhibition of MAPK/AP-1 and activation of Nrf2-ARE antioxidant system. *J. Cell. Mol. Med.* **2017**, *21*, 336–348. [CrossRef] [PubMed]
50. Shigemura, Y.; Iwai, K.; Morimatsu, F.; Iwamoto, T.; Mori, T.; Oda, C.; Taira, T.; Park, E.Y.; Nakamura, Y.; Sato, K. Effect of Prolyl-hydroxyproline (Pro-Hyp), a food-derived collagen peptide in human blood, on growth of fibroblasts from mouse skin. *J. Agric. Food Chem.* **2009**, *57*, 444–449. [CrossRef] [PubMed]
51. Bouglé, D.; Bouhallab, S. Dietary bioactive peptides: Human studies. *Crit. Rev. Food Sci. Nutr.* **2017**, *57*, 335–343. [CrossRef] [PubMed]
52. Jia, J.; Zhou, Y.; Lu, J.; Chen, A.; Li, Y.; Zheng, G. Enzymatic hydrolysis of Alaska pollack (*Theragra chalcogramma*) skin and antioxidant activity of the resulting hydrolysate. *J. Sci. Food Agric.* **2010**, *90*, 635–640. [CrossRef] [PubMed]

11

Capsaicin: Friend or Foe in Skin Cancer and Other Related Malignancies?

Simona-Roxana Georgescu [1], Maria-Isabela Sârbu [1], Clara Matei [1], Mihaela Adriana Ilie [2], Constantin Caruntu [3,4,*], Carolina Constantin [5], Monica Neagu [5,6] and Mircea Tampa [1]

1 Department of Dermatology, Carol DavilaUniversity of Medicine and Pharmacy, 020021 Bucharest, Romania; simonaroxanageorgescu@yahoo.com (S.-R.G.); isabela_sarbu@yahoo.com (M.-I.S.); matei_clara@yahoo.com (C.M.); tampa_mircea@yahoo.com (M.T.)
2 Department of Biochemistry, Carol Davila University of Medicine and Pharmacy, 020021 Bucharest, Romania; mihaelaadriana2005@yahoo.com
3 Department of Physiology, Carol Davila University of Medicine and Pharmacy, 050474 Bucharest, Romania
4 Department of Dermatology, Prof. N.C. Paulescu National Institute of Diabetes, Nutrition and Metabolic Diseases, 011233 Bucharest, Romania
5 Immunology Department, Victor Babes National Institute of Pathology, 050096 Bucharest, Romania; caroconstantin@gmail.com (C.C.); neagu.monica@gmail.com (M.N.)
6 Faculty of Biology, University of Bucharest, 76201 Bucharest, Romania
* Correspondence: costin.caruntu@gmail.com

Abstract: Capsaicin is the main pungent in chili peppers, one of the most commonly used spices in the world; its analgesic and anti-inflammatory properties have been proven in various cultures for centuries. It is a lipophilic substance belonging to the class of vanilloids and an agonist of the transient receptor potential vanilloid 1 receptor. Taking into consideration the complex neuro-immune impact of capsaicin and the potential link between inflammation and carcinogenesis, the effect of capsaicin on muco-cutaneous cancer has aroused a growing interest. The aim of this review is to look over the most recent data regarding the connection between capsaicin and muco-cutaneous cancers, with emphasis on melanoma and muco-cutaneous squamous cell carcinoma.

Keywords: capsaicin; skin; neurogenic inflammation; cancer; carcinogenesis; squamous cell carcinoma; melanoma

---

1. Introduction

Chili peppers belong to the genus *Capsicum* of the *Solanaceae* family and are some of the most used condiments in the world being consumed on daily basis by almost 25% of the population [1–6]. The chili extract has been long used in traditional medicine. Alcoholic hot pepper extract was used as a counterirritant analgesic and helped treat burning sensations and pruritus. In tropical countries it was administrated to induce vasodilatation and to increase heat loss [7].

The main pungent component in chili peppers is capsaicin and this plant component is probably produced as a defense mechanism against herbivores and fungi [6]. Capsaicin, an alkylamide, is the most abundant capsaicinoid found in chili peppers (69%) but dihydrocapsaicin (22%), nordihydrocapsaicin (7%), homocapsaicin (1%) and homodihydrocapsaicin (1%) are also present [1]. The history of capsaicin goes back to the 19thcentury. In 1816, Bucholtz managed for the first time the extraction as a solution of the pungent component from the chili pepper [8]. In 1846, Thresh named this component capsaicin and achieved for the first time its isolation in pure, crystalline form [9]. Another important moment is the identification of the exact structure of capsaicin, which was communicated in 1919 by Nelson [10]. There are still recent studies that try to improve the isolation and purification of capsaicin from the capsaicinoid extract [11] reinforced by studies that reveal that there are clear regulations of the composition during fruit ripening [12]. In 1930, Späth and Darling synthesized capsaicin for the first time [13]. The 20th century has thus established capsaicin as a compound with various actions besides being a natural food additive [14,15].

2. Capsaicin and Neurogenic Inflammation

Capsaicin (*trans*-8-methyl-N-vanillyl-6-noneamide) is a lipophilic substance, belonging to the class of vanilloids [16]; its molecular formula is $C_{18}H_{27}NO_3$ and its molecular weight is 305.4 Da. Capsaicin is an agonist of the transient receptor potential vanilloid 1 receptor (TRPV1) which is a member of the transient receptor potential (TRP) family of cation channels [17].

Besides capsaicin, TRPV1 can be activated by temperatures of 43 °C or higher, by acidity (pH<6), endocanabinoids such as anandamide, metabolites of polyunsaturated fatty acids or other vanilloids [18]. Its function can also be modulated by inflammatory mediators, such as bradykinin and prostaglandin E2 with a facilitatory effect induced probably by protein kinases (PKC or PKA) -mediated receptor phosphorylation [19–21]. Other agents like nerve growth factor (NGF), catecholamines, histamine can also increase TRPV1 responses [22–24].

TRPV1 receptors are expressed in the central nervous system and in sensory neurons of the dorsal root ganglion, but also in non-neuronal tissues [25]. In the skin, TRPV1 is present in the unmyelinated type C and thin myelinated A-delta sensory nerve fibres, keratinocytes, mast cells, dermal blood vessels, fibroblasts, hair follicles, vascular smooth muscle cells, sebocytes and eccrine sweat glands [26–28]. TRPV1 might therefore play the role of extraneuronal receptor [29]. To date, it has been suggested that TRPV1 might play a role in mastocyte activation [30], release of proinflammatory mediators from keratinocytes [31] and modulation of proliferation, differentiation and apoptosis of keratinocytes from the outer root sheath [32].

Applied on the skin or oral mucosa, capsaicin induces initially a local burning sensation [26], followed by allodynia and hyperesthesia to mechanical and heat stimulation [33]. These nociceptive effects are associated with a transient local wheal and flare response known as neurogenic inflammation, triggered by the release of neuropeptides from the cutaneous sensory nerve endings (see Figure 1) [34,35]. Substance P (SP) and calcitonin-gene related peptide (CGRP) are recognized as the most important neuropeptides within neurogenic inflammation [36]. SP acts upon micro vascularization through its neurokinin-1 receptor (NK-1R) and has vasodilatory effects, increases vascular permeability and favors the release of pro-inflammatory cytokines [37], whilst CGRP induces microvascular dilatation resulting in increased blood flow [38]. Besides the neuropeptides release from nerve fibers, activation of mast cells has an important role in the capsaicin-induced inflammatory reaction [39]. Neuropeptides, with SP having the most significant effects, induce mast cell degranulation and synthesis of pro-inflammatory cytokines [40,41]. Mast cell mediators in turn activate nociceptors and further amplify the release of neuropeptides from the sensory nerves [39].

On the other hand, capsaicin blocks the axoplasmic transport of substance P and somatostatin in sensory neurons, thus depleting the neuropeptides [6,42,43] and progressively reducing the initial local inflammatory effect, explaining the potential use of capsaicin in the treatment of chronic inflammatory skin diseases [28].

Moreover, subsequent applications of capsaicin lead to desensitization which is responsible for the analgesic effect of topical capsaicin [6,44] and its wide use in the treatment of neuropathic pain [45], post-herpetic neuralgia, diabetic neuropathy, post-surgical neuralgia, post-traumatic neuropathy and musculoskeletal pain [6,46].

Capsaicin can also have neurotoxic effects and can induce a gradual degeneration of cutaneous nerve fibers when used in high concentrations or for a long period of time [47–49].

Thus, capsaicin, depending on the duration and intensity of stimulation, can induce opposite effects, and the study of capsaicin-induced reactions has aroused the interest of both researchers and clinicians from a broad range of specialties.

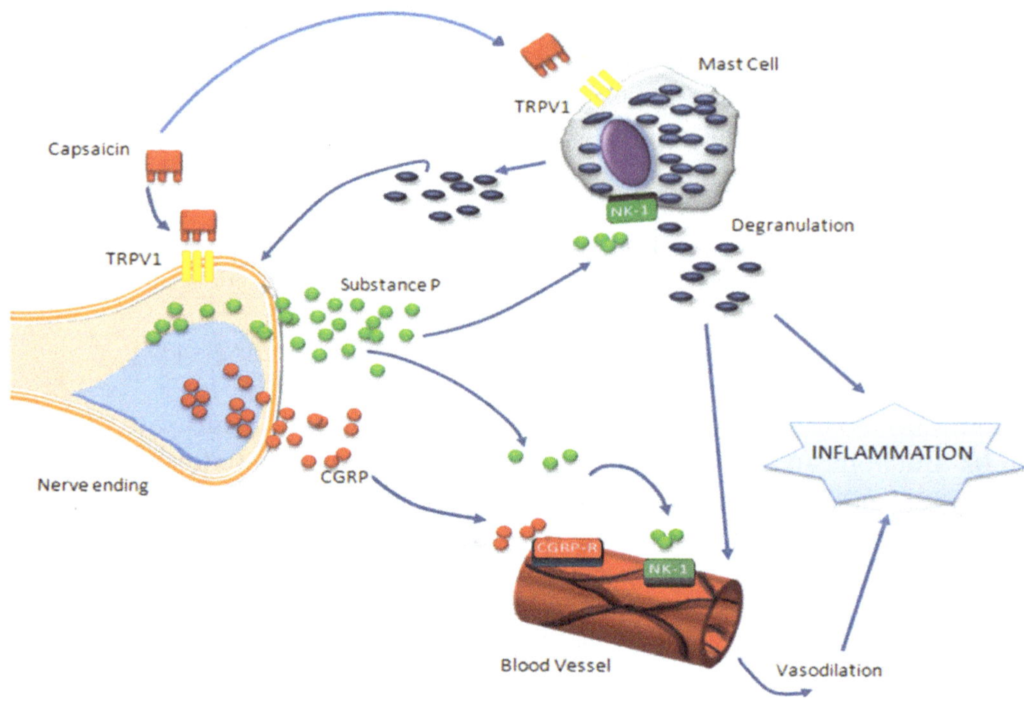

Figure 1. Capsaicin-induced inflammatory response is initiated by activation of transient receptor potential vanilloid 1 receptor(TRPV1) followed by the release of pro-inflammatory neuropeptides from nerve endings. Substance P(SP)and calcitonin-gene related peptide(CGRP), by activation of neurokinin-1 receptor (NK-1) and CGRP receptors, induce vasodilation, increased vascular permeability and release of pro-inflammatory cytokines. The released neuropeptides can induce degranulation of mast cells that play an important role in amplification of capsaicin-induced neurogenic inflammation.

3. Capsaicin and Cancer

Various studies have suggested a potential pro-carcinogenic role of capsaicin use [3] further supported by the potential connection between inflammation and tumorigenesis. In some cases, pro-inflammatory cytokines/chemokines can trigger malignant transformation and tumor associated inflammation in turn can promote proliferation and survival of malignant cells [50,51].

However, other recent studies indicate more to a protective effect against various types of cancer via different pathways, mostly unrelated to TRPV1 [3,52–60]. Thus, we will elaborate further on the capsaicin involvement in muco-cutaneous squamous cell carcinoma and melanoma, as the main malignancies where capsaicin has proven its involvement (see Table 1).

Table 1. Summarizing the carcinogenic and anti-carcinogenic effects of capsaicin, the primary pathway through which the effect is occurring, and the experimental model used to demonstrate the effect.

Effect of Capsaicin	Primary Pathway through Which the Effect Is Occurring	Model Used to Demonstrate the Effect	References
Anticarcinogenic	Mitochondrial pathway-dependent apoptosis: ↓Bcl-2 ↑Bax, ↑Bad	human pharyngeal SCC cells (FaDu)	Le et al. [61]
	Induction of reactive oxygen species; apoptosis independent oftransient receptor potential vanilloid 1 receptor (TRPV1)	oral squamous cell carcinoma (OSCC) cell lines	Gonzales et al. [62]
	Nuclear factor kappaB (NF-kB), activator protein 1 (AP-1)	ICR mouse model; humanpromyelocytic leukemiaHL-60 cells	Han et al. [63]

Table 1. *Cont.*

Effect of Capsaicin	Primary Pathway through Which the Effect Is Occurring	Model Used to Demonstrate the Effect	References
	Inhibition of the cytochrome P-450 IIE1 isoform	ICR mouse model	Surh et al. [64]
	↓nicotinamide adenine dinucleotide (NADH) oxidase activity; ↑apoptosis	A375, SK-MEL-28 human melanoma cell lines; B16 murine melanoma cell line	Morré et al. [65]
	↓nicotinamide adenine dinucleotide phosphate-reduced(NAD(P)H): quinone oxidoreductase ; ↓NF-κB	CRL 1585 and CRL 1619 human melanoma cell lines	Brar et al. [66]
	↓activation of constitutive and IL-1beta-induced NF-κB	Human melanoma cells	Patel et al. [67]
	↑p53, induces apoptosis via Bcl-2, Bax, caspases 3,8,9	A375 human melanoma cell line	Kim [68]
	Down-regulation of PI3-K/Akt pathway	B16-F10 mouse melanoma cells	Shin et al. [69]
	Downregulation of Bcl-2; induction of apoptosis	B16-F10 mouse melanoma cells	Jun et al. [60]
	↓caspase-activated DNase inhibitor(ICAD)expression; induction of apoptosis	human melanoma A375-S2 cell line	Gong et al. [70]
	Induction of apoptosis	melanocytes and HBL, A375SM, C8161 melanoma cell lines	Marques et al. [71]
	Delays tumor growth	melanoma B16-F10; mouse model	Schwartz et al. [72]
Cocarcinogenic	Epidermal growth factor receptor(EGFR) pathway	DMBA/TPA mouse model	Bode et al. [73]
	EGFR pathway; ↑cyclo-oxygenase-2 (COX-2)	DMBA/TPA mouse model	Hwang et al. [25]
	EGFR/Akt/mTOR signaling pathway	DMBA/TPA mouse model	Li et al. [74]
	Erk/p38 signaling pathway	DMBA/TPA mouse model	Liu et al. [75]

3.1. The Impact of Capsaicin on Muco-Cutaneous Squamous Cell Carcinoma

Muco-cutaneous squamous cell carcinoma is one of the most frequent malignancies among Caucasians and its incidence has increased in the last decades, probably due to lifestyle changes and the increased proportion of aged populations [76–79]. Muco-cutaneous squamous cell carcinoma is responsible for most deaths associated with non-melanoma muco-cutaneous cancer. It may generate major defects both aesthetically and functionally and require a complex therapeutic approach, depending on the stage of the disease and the general status of the patient [76–81]. For that reason, muco-cutaneous squamous cell carcinoma is an important public health problem and new therapeutic approaches are necessary [82–90].

The most important risk factors for the development of muco-cutaneous squamous cell carcinoma are fair skin type, chronic exposure to ultraviolet radiation (UVR), exposure to ionizing radiation, smoking, exposure to chemical carcinogens, human papillomavirus (HPV) infections and genetic predisposition [80,81,87–89,91–93].

Moreover, various studies have shown that neuroendocrine factors might play a role in the development of muco-cutaneous squamous cell carcinoma [94]. The release of CGRP and substance P, as well as other neuropeptides, from unmyelinated c-fibres and myelinated A delta-fibres of sensory nerves, a well-known effect triggered by capsaicin is also induced by UVR exposure and may contribute to induction of carcinogenesis [94,95]. CGRP has important vasodilatory effects on small and large vessels, potentiates microvascular permeability and edema caused by SP, enhances in vitro keratinocyte and melanocyte proliferation and is a potent immunomodulator [94–97]. By impairing the function of cutaneous macrophages and Langerhans cells, CGRP is a potent inhibitor of acute and delayed type hypersensitivity reactions [95] but also interferes with anti-tumoral immune response initiation [94].

SP is a member of the tachykinin family which has vasodilatory effects, induces protein extravasation, lymphocyte proliferation, chemotaxis, activates macrophages and promotes the secretion of interleukin 1 (IL-1), IL-6and TNF-α [94,95,98]. It has been associated with stress induced mast cell activation [41]. The effects of SP are mediated through NK-1R, which is widely expressed in the brain, skin, intestine, lung and immune cells [94,95]. There is some evidence that SP and NK1-R might be involved in the development and progression of cancer. Thus, SP has been associated with cell proliferation and migration in esophageal squamous cell carcinoma (SCC) [99], melanoma [100,101], retinoblastoma [102], neuroblastoma and glioma [103]. Brener et al. investigated the presence of SP and NK-1R in 93 oral SCC from 73 patients and concluded that the SP/NK-1R system might have a role in tumor development and progression [104]. Other authors studied the distribution of SP and NK-1R in esophageal SCC and found a higher density of SP positive nerve fibres and NK-1R expression in carcinoma cells, thus concluding that SP and NK-1R promote growth and migration of esophageal SCC cells [99]. Considering the evidence regarding the role of SP in the development of the disease some authors suggested that NK-1R antagonists might be useful in the treatment of oral cancer [104].

Taking into consideration the complex neuro-immune impact of capsaicin and the potential link between inflammation and carcinogenesis, the effect of capsaicin on muco-cutaneous cancer has aroused a growing interest. Since several reports indicated that the consumption of chili peppers might be associated with an increased risk of cancer [105], some authors studied the effect of long term capsaicin treatment. Toth and Gannett found that, after a lifelong diet with capsaicin, 22% of female mice and 14% of male mice had tumors of the cecum. In the control group only 8% of mice had cecum tumors [106]. Chanda et al. assessed the oncogenic potential of topical trans-capsaicin applied for 26 weeks in Tg.AC mice. The Tg.AC mice received trans-capsaicin dissolved in diethylene glycol monoethyl ether (DGME). Mice from the positive control group received tetradecanoylphorbol-13-acetate (TPA) dissolved in DGME and controls received lidocaine. The authors found that topical capsaicin was not associated with an increased incidence of preneoplastic and neoplastic lesions as compared to the concurrent vehicle or lidocaine while the TPA treated mice had multiple skin papillomas. The authors therefore concluded that trans-capsaicin, lidocaine and DGME should be considered non-oncogenic [107].

Le et al. studied the effect of capsaicin on human pharyngeal SCC cells (FaDu) and found that capsaicin inhibits growth and proliferation in a time and dose dependent manner and induces apoptosis via mitochondrial pathways [61]. The authors also analyzed the expression of the anti-apoptotic Bcl-2 gene and the pro-apoptotic Bax and Bad genes and found a reduction of Bcl-2 gene and enhanced expression of Bax and Bad genes [61]. Gonzales et al. studied the anti-tumor effect of capsaicin, a TRPV1 agonist, and capsazepine, a TRPV1 antagonist, on oral squamous cell carcinoma (OSCC) cell lines; the authors found that capsaicin alone reduced cell viability [62]. The association of capsazepine and capsaicin not only did not reverse the effect of capsaicin but capsazepine alone was also cytotoxic to tumor cells; the authors therefore concluded that the antiapoptotic effect of vanilloids is independent of TRPV1 and suggested that the induction of reactive oxygen species is responsible for apoptosis [62].

Han et al. showed in a study published in 2002 that topical application of capsaicin on the skin of female ICR mice suppresses phorbol ester-induced activation of nuclear factor kappaB (NF-κB) and activator protein 1 (AP-1) and concluded that this might be responsible for the chemopreventive effects of capsaicin [63]. These results are congruent with findings previously reported by another group of authors [108–111]. Surh et al. studied the chemoprotective effect of capsaicin against tumorigenesis and mutagenesis produced by vinyl carbamate (VC) and *N*-nitrosodimethylamine(NDMA) also on female ICR mice [64]. The authors found that topical capsaicin pre-treatment lowered the number of VC-induced tumors by 60% and hypothesized that capsaicin suppresses tumorigenesis and mutagenesis by inhibiting cytochrome P-450 IIE1 isoform [64].

3.2. The Effect of Capsaicin on Melanoma

Melanoma is a malignant tumor that arises from melanocytes; melanocytes are melanin-producing cells situated in the basal layer of epidermis, in uveal structures of the eye and in the meninges; of all possible sites, skin is the most frequent location of melanoma [87,88]. Even though melanoma is less frequent than most malignant cutaneous tumors (i.e., basal cell carcinoma, squamous cell carcinoma), it has the most aggressive course, accounting for more than 75% of all skin cancer deaths. Melanoma can occur at any age but it is more frequent between 30 and 70 years; females are more frequently affected than males (male:female ratio 1:1.5) [88,89]. The incidence of melanoma has been on the rise worldwide in the last decades. Excessive ultraviolet radiation exposure (from both sun and artificial sources—e.g., tanning beds) especially under the age of 20, skin phototypes I and II (light skin pigmentation), genetic predisposition, increased number of melanocytic nevi and the presence of atypical nevi are the main risk factors for developing melanoma. Most melanomas occur de novo [90,112,113].

The treatment of melanoma varies depending on the stage of the disease. Surgical excision is the mainstay treatment for primary melanoma. Metastatic melanomas however require chemotherapy, immunotherapy or palliative treatment. These are usually associated with severe adverse reactions and low response rates [87,88]. Therefore, new drugs as well as new ways of investigating their efficacy have been elaborated [114]. The prognosis of patients with metastatic melanoma was improved after the introduction of BRAF(B-Rafenzyme) inhibitors (vemurafenib, dabrafenib), mitogen-activated protein/extracellular signal-regulated kinase kinase(MEK) inhibitors (trametinib) and immune checkpoint inhibitors (nivolumab, ipilimumab) [113,115].These therapies however are very expensive and are not available for all the patients [113,115].

Under these circumstances, there is a real need to identify new therapeutic targets in order to develop cheaper, but efficient, treatment options. Hence, the mechanisms behind the development and progression of melanoma were intensely studied and recent reports showed that neuro-endocrine factors might be involved [100,101,116,117]. Several studies have investigated the potential role of NK-1R and SP, one of the main neuropeptides involved in capsaicin-induced inflammatory reaction. A recent study performed on canine melanoma tissues and cell lines found that 11 of 15 tumors revealed NK-1R immunoreactivity [118]. The expression of SP in malignant melanoma and melanoma precursors was also studied and the authors showed that 68% of primary invasive melanomas, 40% of metastatic melanomas, 60% of in situ melanomas and 58% of dysplastic nevi express the neuropeptide [119]. SP and NK-1R are also involved in melanogenesis [120]. B16-F10 melanoma cells treatment with SP results in activation of NK-1R, phosphorylation of p70 S6K1, inhibition of p38mitogen-activated protein kinase(MAPK), down-regulation in tyrosinase activity and suppression of melanogenesis [121]. There is increasing evidence regarding the involvement of SP and NK-1R in melanoma cells proliferation [100,101,122,123]. For that reason, NK-1R is now regarded as a target in melanoma treatment and NK-1R antagonists are being intensely studied [100,101,122,123].

The direct role of capsaicin in the treatment of melanoma was investigated in several studies, as explained further [65–72,124–129]. Morré et al. studied the effect of capsaicin on nicotinamide adenine dinucleotide(NADH) oxidase activity of plasma membranes and cell growth of human primary melanocytes and melanoma cells (A-375 and SK-MEL-28 cell cultures) [65]. The authors found that capsaicin inhibits plasma membrane NADH oxidase activity preferentially in melanoma cells thus inhibiting growth and increasing apoptosis [65]. Brar et al. also showed in a study performed on human melanoma cell lines that reactive oxygen species produced endogenously from nicotinamide adenine dinucleotide phosphate-reduced(NAD(P)H):quinone oxidoreductase activate NF-κB in melanoma cells in an autocrine fashion and that capsaicin significantly reduces proliferation of melanoma cells [66].

Patel et al. showed in a study published in 2002 that the NF-κB activation regulates the expression of IL-8 in melanoma cells and that the addition of capsaicin determines the inhibition of constitutive and IL1-beta and TNF-α induced IL-8 expression in melanoma cells [67]. In melanoma, IL-8 over-expression is associated with the transition from radial growth phase to vertical growth phase and with the development of metastases [124,125]. Capsaicin is a potent inhibitor of NF-κB. It suppresses the activation of NF-κB by inhibiting IκBα (nuclear factor of kappa light polypeptide gene enhancer in B-cells inhibitor, alpha) degradation and blocking the translocation of p65 in human promyelocytic leukaemia HL-60 cells [63,126].

In a study published in 2012, Kim aimed to explain the mechanism by which capsaicin induces apoptosis in melanoma cells [68]. The author therefore studied the role of nitric oxide (NO) during apoptosis induced by capsaicin and resveratrol on A375 human melanoma cells and found that NO stimulates p53 and induces conformational changes in Bax and Bcl-2 and activates caspases 3, 8 and 9. The authors concluded that capsaicin and resveratrol activate the mitochondrial and death receptor pathways [68].

In a study published in 2008, Shin et al. evaluated the effects of capsaicin on highly metastatic B16-F10 mouse melanoma cells and found that capsaicin inhibits migration of melanoma cells in a dose-dependent manner [69]. The authors also found that capsaicin decreases the phosphorylation of the p85 regulatory subunit of phosphatidylinositol 3-kinase (PI3-K) and Akt and concluded that capsaicin down-regulates the PI3-K/Akt pathway. Furthermore, the authors found that capsaicin inhibits the Rac1 activity [69]. The PI3-K/Akt pathway is one of the main signaling networks in cancer and plays an important role in melanoma initiation and in therapeutic resistance [127,128]. Rac1 is involved in cell migration and metastasis [129]. Jun et al. also studied the effect of capsaicin on B16-F10 murine melanoma cells. The authors found that capsaicin determines release of mitochondrial cytochrome c, activation of caspase-3 and cleavage of poly (ADP-ribose) polymerase and finally induces apoptosis of melanoma cells through down regulation of Bcl-2 [60]. Other studies have observed induction of apoptosis by capsaicin in melanoma cells, as well: Gong et al. showed, in a study performed on human melanoma A375-S2 cells, that capsaicin induces melanoma cell death in a time and dose dependent manner by reducing the expression of inhibitor of caspase activated DNase (ICAD); ICAD expression was decreased over the lapse of time, as cell treated with capsaicin progressed into apoptotic stages [70]. Some authors studied the combined effect of capsaicin and other agents on melanoma cells [71,72]. Marques et al. investigated the apoptotic effect of capsaicin and HA14-1, a small molecular compound that inhibits the anti-apoptotic effect of Bcl-2, on melanoma cells, melanocytes and fibroblasts [71]. The authors found that capsaicin induces apoptosis in melanocytes and HBL, A375SM and C8161 melanoma cell lines at lower concentrations than in fibroblasts and that the capsaicin and HA14-1 combination shows additive inhibitory effect on melanoma and melanocyte viability, inducing apoptosis in two of the three studied melanoma cell lines [71]. The authors concluded that capsaicin can be associated with other organic compounds as a pro-apoptotic agent to reduce toxicity and adverse reactions [71]. Schwartz et al. studied the combined effect of hydroxycitrate, lipoic acid and capsaicin on lung cancer cells, bladder cancer cells and melanoma cells and found that the association of these drugs is effective in inducing tumor regression and lacks toxicity [72].

Taking into account the increasing evidence regarding its anti-carcinogenic role, expanding the research on capsaicin actions may lead to identification of potential new therapeutic pathways.

3.3. *Capsaicin's Involvement in Carcinogenesis*

A potential co-carcinogenic role of capsaicin has aroused the interest of various researchers. A study published in 2009, showed that TRPV1 interacts with the epidermal growth factor receptor (EGFR) and determines its degradation though the lysosomal pathway [73]. EGFR is a receptor tyrosine kinase with an important role in the development of the epidermis, which is overexpressed in many epithelial cancers. Using a skin carcinogenesis model with 7,12-dimethyl benz(a)anthracene (DMBA) and TPA in TRPV1$^{-/-}$ (knockout) and TRPV1$^{+/+}$ (wild type) mice, authors have shown that TRPV1$^{-/-}$ mice developed significantly more skin tumors than TRPV1$^{+/+}$ mice [73]. Moreover, to assess to role of EGFR in skin carcinogenesis, the authors performed the same experiment, except that some of the mice received an EGFR inhibitor; the scientists discovered that carcinogenesis was substantially more suppressed in TRPV1$^{-/-}$ mice, after EGFR inhibitor was administered [73].

Another study published in 2010 showed that topical application of capsaicin on the skin of TRPV1 wildtype mice and TRPV1 knockout mice, which were previously subjected to the two-stage skin carcinogenesis experiment with DMBA (9,10-Dimethyl-1,2-benzanthracene) and TPA, was associated with significantly more and larger tumors than TPA treatment alone [25]. TRPV1 knockout mice were more affected than TRPV1 wildtype mice. Mice treated with capsaicin alone however have not developed any tumors. These findings suggest that carcinogenesis has a TRPV1 independent mechanism. Further research revealed higher levels of COX-2(cyclo-oxygenase-2) in mice treated with capsaicin and TPA than in mice treated with TPA alone thus suggesting that capsaicin induces an increased COX-2 expression in the presence of TPA. COX-2 expression was increased in EGFR wildtype cells but not in EGFR knockout cells. The authors therefore suggest that capsaicin acts as a co-carcinogen through EGFR dependent mechanisms/pathways [25].

The link between capsaicin receptor and skin tumorigenesis was the subject of an experimental in vivo research which found that topical application of TRPV1-antagonist AMG9810[(E)-3-(4-t-Butylphenyl)-N-(2,3-dihydrobenzo[b][1,4] dioxin-6-yl)acrylamide]promotes tumor development in mice previously treated with DMBA. The levels of EGFR were also higher in these mice as compared to the control group. Moreover, the phosphorylation level of EGFR was significantly increased in AMG9810 treated mice compared to the control groups. EGFR phosphorylation activates the Akt/mTOR-signaling pathway which has an important role in tumorigenesis. It was therefore concluded that the TRPV1 antagonist induces carcinogenesis by activating the EGFR/Akt/mTOR signaling pathway [74].

Liu et al. also studied the effect of topical applications of capsaicin on the dorsal skin of mice in which carcinogenesis was induced by DMBA/TPA. The authors showed that capsaicin led to the appearance of more numerous and larger skin tumors as compared to the control group and suggested that Erk, p38 and inflammation may play an important role in the cancer-promoting effect of capsaicin [75].

All these findings suggest that, even though capsaicin itself is not a carcinogen, long-term application of capsaicin for pain relief might increase the risk of carcinogenesis when it is associated with a tumor promoter [73].

4. Conclusions

Capsaicin is one of the most commonly used spices in the world and its analgesic and anti-inflammatory properties have been known for centuries. Short term administration of capsaicin has the ability to trigger the release of neuropeptides like SP and CGRP which might play a role in tumorigenesis. However, chronic administration of capsaicin progressively reduces the initial inflammatory reaction, leading to desensitization or even to neurotoxic effects, depending on the duration and intensity of applications.

In recent years various studies have focused on the potential impact of capsaicin on tumorigenesis, investigating both the anti-carcinogenic and carcinogenic actions of capsaicin. Data available so far regarding the effect of capsaicin on various types of skin cancers suggests that capsaicin has a chemopreventive role. Sinceseveral authors showed that under certain circumstances capsaicin can have a pro-tumorgenic potential, caution is mandatory when capsaicin is administered in conditions that favor tumorigenesis as it might have a co-carcinogenic effect.

Acknowledgments: This paper was partially supported by grant COP A 1.2.3., ID: P_40_197/2016, grant of the Romanian National Authority for Scientific Research and Innovation and by Young Researchers Grants from the Carol Davila University of Medicine and Pharmacy, No. 33884/11.11.2014 and 33897/11.11.2014.

Author Contributions: All authors have equally contributed in the design and preparation of the manuscript.

References

1. Barceloux, D.G. Pepper and capsaicin (*Capsicum* and *Piper* species). *Dis. Mon.* **2009**, *55*, 380–390. [CrossRef] [PubMed]
2. Kiple, K.F. *The Cambridge World History of Food.(2-Volume Set)*; Cambridge University Press: Cambridge, UK, 2001; Volume 2.
3. Bode, A.M.; Dong, Z. The two faces of capsaicin. *Cancer Res.* **2011**, *71*, 2809–2814. [CrossRef] [PubMed]
4. Srivastava, S.K. *Role of Capsaicin in Oxidative Stress and Cancer*; Springer Science & Business Media: Berlin/Heidelberg, Germany, 2013; Volume 3.
5. Dasgupta, P.; Fowler, C.J. Chillies: From antiquity to urology. *BJU Int.* **1997**, *80*, 845–852. [CrossRef]
6. Sharma, S.K.; Vij, A.S.; Sharma, M. Mechanisms and clinical uses of capsaicin. *Eur. J. Pharmacol.* **2013**, *720*, 55–62. [CrossRef] [PubMed]
7. Abdel-Salam, O.M. *Capsaicin as a Therapeutic Molecule*; Springer Science & Business Media: Berlin/Heidelberg, Germany, 2014; Volume 68.
8. Papoiu, A.D.; Yosipovitch, G. Topical capsaicin. The fire of a 'hot' medicine is reignited. *Expert Opin. Pharmacother.* **2010**, *11*, 1359–1371. [CrossRef] [PubMed]
9. Thresh, L.T. Isolation of capsaicin. *Pharm. J.* **1846**, *6*, 941–942.
10. Nelson, E.K. The constitution of capsaicin, the pungent principle of capsicum. *J. Am. Chem. Soc.* **1919**, *41*, 1115–1121. [CrossRef]
11. Fan, Y.; Lu, Y.M.; Yu, B.; Tan, C.P.; Cui, B. Extraction and purification of capsaicin from capsicum oleoresin using an aqueous two-phase system combined with chromatography. *J. Chromatogr. B.* **2017**, *1063*, 11–17. [CrossRef] [PubMed]
12. Fayos, O.; De Aguiar, A.C.; Jiménez-Cantizano, A.; Ferreiro-González, M.; Garcés-Claver, A.; Martínez, J.; Mallor, C.; Ruiz-Rodríguez, A.; Palma, M.; Barroso, C.G.; et al. Ontogenetic Variation of Individual and Total Capsaicinoids in Malagueta Peppers (*Capsicum frutescens*) during Fruit Maturation. *Molecules* **2017**, *22*, 736. [CrossRef] [PubMed]
13. Späth, E.; Darling, S.F. Synthese des capsaicins. *Eur. J. Inorg. Chem.* **1930**, *63*, 737–743. [CrossRef]
14. Zheng, J.; Zhou, Y.; Li, Y.; Xu, D.P.; Li, S.; Li, H.B. Spices for Prevention and Treatment of Cancers. *Nutrients* **2016**, *8*, 495. [CrossRef] [PubMed]
15. Qin, Y.; Ran, L.; Wang, J.; Yu, L.; Lang, H.D.; Wang, X.L.; Mi, M.T.; Zhu, J.D. Capsaicin Supplementation Improved Risk Factors of Coronary Heart Disease in Individuals with Low HDL-C Levels. *Nutrients* **2017**, *9*, 1037. [CrossRef] [PubMed]
16. Reyes-Escogido, M.D.L.; Gonzalez-Mondragon, E.G.; Vazquez-Tzompantzi, E. Chemical and pharmacological aspects of capsaicin. *Molecules* **2011**, *16*, 1253–1270. [CrossRef] [PubMed]
17. Caterina, M.J.; Schumacher, M.A.; Tominaga, M.; Rosen, T.A.; Levine, J.D.; Julius, D. The capsaicin receptor: A heat-activated ion channel in the pain pathway. *Nature* **1997**, *389*, 816–824. [PubMed]
18. Tominaga, M.; Tominaga, T. Structure and function of TRPV1. *Pflügers. Arch.* **2005**, *451*, 143–150. [CrossRef] [PubMed]
19. Premkumar, L.S.; Ahern, G.P. Induction of vanilloid receptor channel activity by protein kinase C. *Nature* **2000**, *408*, 985–990. [CrossRef] [PubMed]
20. Sugiura, T.; Tominaga, M.; Katsuya, H.; Mizumura, K. Bradykinin lowers the threshold temperature for heat activation of vanilloid receptor 1. *J. Neurophysiol.* **2002**, *88*, 544–548. [PubMed]
21. Schnizler, K.; Shutov, L.P.; Van Kanegan, M.J.; Merrill, M.A.; Nichols, B.; McKnight, G.S.; Usachev, Y.M. Protein kinase A anchoring via AKAP150 is essential for TRPV1 modulation by forskolin and prostaglandin E2 in mouse sensory neurons. *J. Neurosci.* **2008**, *28*, 4904–4917. [CrossRef] [PubMed]
22. Filippi, A.; Caruntu, C.; Gheorghe, R.O.; Deftu, A.; Amuzescu, B.; Ristoiu, V. Catecholamines reduce transient receptor potential vanilloid type 1 desensitization in cultured dorsal root ganglia neurons. *J. Physiol. Pharmacol.* **2016**, *67*, 843–850. [PubMed]
23. Shu, X.; Mendell, L.M. Nerve growth factor acutely sensitizes the response of adult rat sensory neurons to capsaicin. *Neurosci. Lett.* **1999**, *274*, 159–162. [CrossRef]
24. Kajihara, Y.; Murakami, M.; Imagawa, T.; Otsuguro, K.; Ito, S.; Ohta, T. Histamine potentiates acid-induced responses mediating transient receptor potential V1 in mouse primary sensory neurons. *Neuroscience* **2010**, *166*, 292–304. [CrossRef] [PubMed]

25. Hwang, M.K.; Bode, A.M.; Byun, S.; Song, N.R.; Lee, H.J.; Lee, K.W.; Dong, Z. Cocarcinogenic effect of capsaicin involves activation of EGFR signaling but not TRPV1. *Cancer Res.* **2010**, *70*, 6859–6869. [CrossRef] [PubMed]
26. Căruntu, C.; Negrei, C.; Ghiţă, M.A.; Căruntu, A.; Bădărău, A.I.; Buraga, I.; Brănişteanu, D. Capsaicin, a hot topic in skin pharmacology and physiology. *Farmacia* **2015**, *63*, 487–491.
27. Inoue, K.; Koizumi, S.; Fuziwara, S.; Denda, S.; Inoue, K.; Denda, M. Functional vanilloid receptors in cultured normal human epidermal keratinocytes. *Biochem. Biophys. Res. Commun.* **2002**, *291*, 124–129. [CrossRef] [PubMed]
28. Ständer, S.; Moormann, C.; Schumacher, M.; Buddenkotte, J.; Artuc, M.; Shpacovitch, V.; Metze, D. Expression of vanilloid receptor subtype 1 in cutaneous sensory nerve fibers, mast cells, and epithelial cells of appendage structures. *Exp. Dermatol.* **2004**, *13*, 129–139. [CrossRef] [PubMed]
29. Roosterman, D.; Goerge, T.; Schneider, S.W.; Bunnett, N.W.; Steinhoff, M. VI. Role of Capsaicin and transient receptor potential ion channels in the skin. *Physiol. Rev.* **2006**, *86*, 1338–1380.
30. Bíró, T.; Maurer, M.; Modarres, S.; Lewin, N.E.; Brodie, C.; Ács, G.; Blumberg, P.M. Characterization of functional vanilloid receptors expressed by mast cells. *Blood* **1998**, *91*, 1332–1340. [PubMed]
31. Southall, M.D.; Li, T.; Gharibova, L.S.; Pei, Y.; Nicol, G.D.; Travers, J.B. Activation of epidermal vanilloid receptor-1 induces release of proinflammatory mediators in human keratinocytes. *J. Pharmacol. Exp. Ther.* **2003**, *304*, 217–222. [CrossRef] [PubMed]
32. Bodó, E.; Bíró, T.; Telek, A.; Czifra, G.; Griger, Z.; Tóth, B.I.; Paus, R. A hot new twist to hair biology: Involvement of vanilloid receptor-1 (VR1/TRPV1) signaling in human hair growth control. *Am. J. Pathol.* **2005**, *166*, 985–998.
33. Geppetti, P.; Nassini, R.; Materazzi, S.; Benemei, S. The concept of neurogenic inflammation. *BJU Int.* **2008**, *101*, 2–6. [CrossRef] [PubMed]
34. Căruntu, C.; Boda, D. Evaluation through in vivo reflectance confocal microscopy of the cutaneous neurogenic inflammatory reaction induced by capsaicin in human subjects. *J. Biomed. Opt.* **2012**, *17*, 0850031–0850037. [CrossRef] [PubMed]
35. Ghita, M.A.; Caruntu, C.; Lixandru, D.; Pitea, A.; Batani, A.; Boda, D. The Quest for Novel Biomarkers in Early Diagnosis of Diabetic Neuropathy. *Curr. Proteom.* **2017**, *14*, 86–99. [CrossRef]
36. Holzer, P. Local effector functions of capsaicin-sensitive sensory nerve endings: Involvement of tachykinins, calcitonin gene-related peptide and other neuropeptides. *Neuroscience* **1998**, *24*, 739–768. [CrossRef]
37. Schmelz, M.; Petersen, L.J. Neurogenic inflammation in human and rodent skin. *News Physiol. Sci.* **2001**, *16*, 33–37. [PubMed]
38. Brain, S.D.; Tippins, J.R.; Morris, H.R.; Maclntyre, I.; Williams, T.J. Potent vasodilator activity of calcitonin gene-related peptide in human skin. *J. Investig. Dermatol.* **1986**, *87*, 533–536. [CrossRef] [PubMed]
39. Ansel, J.C.; Kaynard, A.H.; Armstrong, C.A.; Olerud, J.; Bunnett, N.; Payan, D. Skin-nervous system interactions. *J. Investig. Dermatol.* **1996**, *106*, 198–204. [CrossRef] [PubMed]
40. Ansel, J.C.; Brown, J.R.; Payan, D.G.; Brown, M.A. Substance P selectively activates TNF-alpha gene expression in murine mast cells. *J. Immunol.* **1993**, *150*, 4478–4485. [PubMed]
41. Căruntu, C.; Boda, D.; Musat, S.; Căruntu, A.; Mandache, E. Stress-induced mast cell activation in glabrous and hairy skin. *Mediat. Inflamm.* **2014**, *2014*, 105950. [CrossRef] [PubMed]
42. Anand, P.; Bley, K. Topical capsaicin for pain management: Therapeutic potential and mechanisms of action of the new high-concentration capsaicin 8% patch. *Br. J. Anaesth.* **2011**, *107*, 490–502. [CrossRef] [PubMed]
43. Frias, B.; Merighi, A. Capsaicin, nociception and pain. *Molecules* **2016**, *21*, 797. [CrossRef] [PubMed]
44. Smutzer, G.; Devassy, R.K. Integrating TRPV1 receptor function with capsaicin psychophysics. *Adv. Pharmacol. Sci.* **2016**, *2016*, 1512457. [CrossRef] [PubMed]
45. Peppin, J.F.; Pappagallo, M. Capsaicinoids in the treatment of neuropathic pain: A review. *Ther. Adv. Neurol. Disord.* **2014**, *7*, 22–32. [CrossRef] [PubMed]
46. Fattori, V.; Hohmann, M.S.; Rossaneis, A.C.; Pinho-Ribeiro, F.A.; Verri, W.A. Capsaicin: Current understanding of its mechanisms and therapy of pain and other pre-clinical and clinical uses. *Molecules* **2016**, *21*, 844. [CrossRef] [PubMed]
47. Holzer, P. Capsaicin: Cellular targets, mechanisms of action, and selectivity for thin sensory neurons. *Pharmacol. Rev.* **1991**, *43*, 143–201. [PubMed]
48. Simone, D.A.; Nolano, M.; Wendelschafer-Crabb, G.; Kennedy, W.R. Intradermal injection of capsaicin in humans: Diminished pain sensation associated with rapid degeneration of intracutaneous nerve fibers. *Soc. Neurosci. Abstr.* **1996**, *22*, 1802.

49. Simone, D.A.; Nolano, M.; Johnson, T.; Wendelschafer-Crabb, G.; Kennedy, W.R. Intradermal injection of capsaicin in humans produces degeneration and subsequent reinnervation of epidermal nerve fibers: Correlation with sensory function. *J. Neurosci.* **1998**, *18*, 8947–8959. [PubMed]
50. Neagu, M.; Caruntu, C.; Constantin, C.; Boda, D.; Zurac, S.; Spandidos, D.A.; Tsatsakis, A.M. Chemically induced skin carcinogenesis: Updates in experimental models. *Oncol. Rep.* **2016**, *35*, 2516–2528. [CrossRef] [PubMed]
51. Neagu, M.; Constantin, C.; Dumitrascu, G.R.; Lupu, A.R.; Caruntu, C.; Boda, D.; Zurac, S. Inflammation markers in cutaneous melanoma-edgy biomarkers for prognosis. *Discoveries* **2015**, *3*, e38. [CrossRef]
52. Mori, A.; Lehmann, S.; O'Kelly, J.; Kumagai, T.; Desmond, J.C.; Pervan, M.; Koeffler, H.P. Capsaicin, a component of red peppers, inhibits the growth of androgen-independent, p53 mutant prostate cancer cells. *Cancer Res.* **2006**, *66*, 3222–3229. [CrossRef] [PubMed]
53. Zhang, J.H.; Lai, F.J.; Chen, H.; Luo, J.; Zhang, R.Y.; Bu, H.Q.; Lin, S.Z. Involvement of the phosphoinositide 3-kinase/Akt pathway in apoptosis induced by capsaicin in the human pancreatic cancer cell line PANC-1. *Oncol. Lett.* **2013**, *5*, 43–48. [PubMed]
54. Lee, Y.S.; Kang, Y.S.; Lee, J.S.; Nicolova, S.; Kim, J.A. Involvement of NADPH oxidase-mediated generation of reactive oxygen species in the apototic cell death by capsaicin in HepG2 human hepatoma cells. *Free Radic. Res.* **2004**, *38*, 405–412. [CrossRef] [PubMed]
55. Lu, H.F.; Chen, Y.L.; Yang, J.S.; Yang, Y.Y.; Liu, J.Y.; Hsu, S.C.; Chung, J.G. Antitumor activity of capsaicin on human colon cancer cells in vitro and colo 205 tumor xenografts in vivo. *J. Agric. Food Chem.* **2010**, *58*, 12999–13005. [CrossRef] [PubMed]
56. Chang, H.C.; Chen, S.T.; Chien, S.Y.; Kuo, S.J.; Tsai, H.T.; Chen, D.R. Capsaicin may induce breast cancer cell death through apoptosis-inducing factor involving mitochondrial dysfunction. *Hum. Exp. Toxicol.* **2011**, *30*, 1657–1665. [CrossRef] [PubMed]
57. Huh, H.C.; Lee, S.Y.; Lee, S.K.; Park, N.H.; Han, I.S. Capsaicin induces apoptosis of cisplatin-resistant stomach cancer cells by causing degradation of cisplatin-inducible Aurora-A protein. *Nutr. Cancer* **2011**, *63*, 1095–1103. [CrossRef] [PubMed]
58. Wang, H.M.; Chuang, S.M.; Su, Y.C.; Li, Y.H.; Chueh, P.J. Down-regulation of tumor-associated NADH oxidase, tNOX (ENOX2), enhances capsaicin-induced inhibition of gastric cancer cell growth. *Cell Biochem. Biophys.* **2011**, *61*, 355–366. [CrossRef] [PubMed]
59. Moon, D.O.; Kang, C.H.; Kang, S.H.; Choi, Y.H.; Hyun, J.W.; Chang, W.Y.; Kim, G.Y. Capsaicin sensitizes TRAIL-induced apoptosis through Sp1-mediated DR5 up-regulation: Involvement of Ca2+influx. *Toxicol. Appl. Pharmacol.* **2012**, *259*, 87–95. [CrossRef] [PubMed]
60. Jun, H.S.; Park, T.; Lee, C.K.; Kang, M.K.; Park, M.S.; Kang, H.I.; Kim, O.H. Capsaicin induced apoptosis of B16-F10 melanoma cells through down-regulation of Bcl-2. *Food Chem. Toxicol.* **2007**, *45*, 708–715. [CrossRef] [PubMed]
61. Le, T.D.; Jin, D.C.; Rho, S.R.; Kim, M.S.; Yu, R.; Yoo, H. Capsaicin-induced apoptosis of FaDu human pharyngeal squamous carcinoma cells. *Yonsei Med. J.* **2012**, *53*, 834–841. [CrossRef] [PubMed]
62. Gonzales, C.B.; Kirma, N.B.; Jorge, J.; Chen, R.; Henry, M.A.; Luo, S.; Hargreaves, K.M. Vanilloids induce oral cancer apoptosis independent of TRPV1. *Oral Oncol.* **2014**, *50*, 437–447. [CrossRef] [PubMed]
63. Han, S.S.; Keum, Y.S.; Chun, K.S.; Surh, Y.J. Suppression of phorbol ester-induced NF-κB activation by capsaicin in cultured human promyelocytic leukemia cells. *Arch. Pharm. Res.* **2002**, *25*, 475–479. [CrossRef] [PubMed]
64. Surh, Y.J.; Lee, R.C.J.; Park, K.K.; Mayne, S.T.; Liem, A.; Miller, J.A. Chemoprotective effects of capsaicin and diallyl sulfide against mutagenesis or tumorigenesis by vinyl carbamate and *N*-nitrosodiinethylamine. *Carcinogenesis* **1995**, *16*, 2467–2471. [CrossRef] [PubMed]
65. Morré, D.J.; Sun, E.; Geilen, C.; Wu, L.Y.; De Cabo, R.; Krasagakis, K.; Morre, D.M. Capsaicin inhibits plasma membrane NADH oxidase and growth of human and mouse melanoma lines. *Eur. J. Cancer* **1996**, *32*, 1995–2003. [CrossRef]
66. Brar, S.S.; Kennedy, T.P.; Whorton, A.R.; Sturrock, A.B.; Huecksteadt, T.P.; Ghio, A.J.; Hoidal, J.R. Reactive oxygen species from NAD(P)H: Quinone oxidoreductase constitutively activate NF-κB in malignant melanoma cells. *Am. J. Physiol Cell. Physiol.* **2001**, *280*, C659–C676. [PubMed]

67. Patel, P.S.; Varney, M.L.; Dave, B.J.; Singh, R.K. Regulation of Constitutive and Induced NF-κB Activation in Malignant Melanoma Cells by Capsaicin Modulates Interleukin-8 Production and Cell Proliferation. *J. Interferon Cytokine Res.* **2002**, *22*, 427–435. [CrossRef] [PubMed]
68. Kim, M.Y. Nitric oxide triggers apoptosis in A375 human melanoma cells treated with capsaicin and resveratrol. *Mol. Med. Rep.* **2012**, *5*, 585–591. [CrossRef] [PubMed]
69. Shin, D.H.; Kim, O.H.; Jun, H.S.; Kang, M.K. Inhibitory effect of capsaicin on B16-F10 melanoma cell migration via the phosphatidylinositol 3-kinase/Akt/Rac1 signal pathway. *Exp. Mol. Med.* **2008**, *40*, 486–494. [CrossRef] [PubMed]
70. Gong, X.F.; Wang, M.W.; Ikejima, T. Mechanisms of capsaicin-induced apoptosis of human melanoma A375-S2 cells. *Chin. J. Oncol.* **2005**, *27*, 401–403.
71. Marques, C.M.; Dibden, C.; Danson, S.; Haycock, J.W.; MacNeil, S. Combined effects of capsaicin and HA14-1 in inducing apoptosis in melanoma cells. *J. Cosmet. Dermatol. Sci. Appl.* **2013**, *3*, 175–189. [CrossRef]
72. Schwartz, L.; Guais, A.; Israël, M.; Junod, B.; Steyaert, J.M.; Crespi, E.; Abolhassani, M. Tumor regression with a combination of drugs interfering with the tumor metabolism: Efficacy of hydroxycitrate, lipoic acid and capsaicin. *Investig. New Drugs* **2013**, *31*, 256–264. [CrossRef] [PubMed]
73. Bode, A.M.; Cho, Y.Y.; Zheng, D.; Zhu, F.; Ericson, M.E.; Ma, W.Y.; Dong, Z. Transient receptor potential type vanilloid 1 suppresses skin carcinogenesis. *Cancer Res.* **2009**, *69*, 905–913. [CrossRef] [PubMed]
74. Li, S.; Bode, A.M.; Zhu, F.; Liu, K.; Zhang, J.; Kim, M.O.; Langfald, A.K. TRPV1-antagonist AMG9810 promotes mouse skin tumorigenesis through EGFR/Akt signaling. *Carcinogenesis* **2011**, *32*, 779–785. [CrossRef] [PubMed]
75. Liu, Z.; Zhu, P.; Tao, Y.; Shen, C.; Wang, S.; Zhao, L.; Zhu, Z. Cancer-promoting effect of capsaicin on DMBA/TPA-induced skin tumorigenesis by modulating inflammation, Erk and p38 in mice. *Food Chem. Toxicol.* **2015**, *81*, 1–8. [CrossRef] [PubMed]
76. Alam, M.; Ratner, D. Cutaneous squamous-cell carcinoma. *N. Engl. J. Med.* **2001**, *344*, 975–983. [CrossRef] [PubMed]
77. Rudolph, R.; Zelac, D. Squamous cell carcinoma of the skin. *Plast. Reconstr. Surg.* **2004**, *114*, 82e–94e. [CrossRef] [PubMed]
78. Weinberg, A.S.; Ogle, C.A.; Shim, E.K. Metastatic cutaneous squamous cell carcinoma: An update. *Dermatol. Surg.* **2007**, *33*, 885–899. [CrossRef] [PubMed]
79. Ferlay, J.; Shin, H.R.; Bray, F.; Forman, D.; Mathers, C.; Parkin, D.M. Estimates of worldwide burden of cancer in 2008: GLOBOCAN 2008. *Int. J. Cancer* **2008**, *127*, 2893–2917. [CrossRef] [PubMed]
80. Shah, J.P.; Gil, Z. Current concepts in management of oral cancer–surgery. *Oral Oncol.* **2009**, *45*, 394–401. [CrossRef] [PubMed]
81. Feller, L.; Lemmer, J. Oral squamous cell carcinoma: Epidemiology, clinical presentation and treatment. *J. Cancer Ther.* **2012**, *3*, 263–268. [CrossRef]
82. Matei, C.; Caruntu, C.; Ion, R.M.; Georgescu, S.R.; Dumitrascu, G.R.; Constantin, C.; Neagu, M. Protein microarray for complex apoptosis monitoring of dysplastic oral keratinocytes in experimental photodynamic therapy. *Biol. Res.* **2014**, *47*, 33. [CrossRef] [PubMed]
83. Monta, G.; Caracò, C.; Simeone, E.; Grimaldi, A.M.; Marone, U.; Marzo, M.; Mozzillo, N. Electrochemotherapy efficacy evaluation for treatment of locally advanced stage III cutaneous squamous cell carcinoma: A 22-cases retrospective analysis. *J. Transl. Med.* **2017**, *15*, 82. [CrossRef] [PubMed]
84. Tampa, M.; Matei, C.; Popescu, S.; Georgescu, S.R.; Neagu, M.; Constantin, C.; Ion, R.M. Zinc trisulphonatedphthalocyanine used in photodynamic therapy of dysplastic oral keratinocytes. *Rev. Chim.* **2013**, *64*, 639–645.
85. Matei, C.; Tampa, M.; Ion, R.M.; Neagu, M.; Constantin, C. Photodynamic properties of aluminiumsulphonatedphthalocyanines in human displazic oral keratinocytes experimental model. *Dig. J. Nanomater. Biostruct. (DJNB)* **2012**, *7*, 1535–1547.
86. Yu, C.C.; Hung, S.K.; Lin, H.Y.; Chiou, W.Y.; Lee, M.S.; Liao, H.F.; Su, Y.C. Targeting the PI3K/AKT/mTOR signaling pathway as an effectively radiosensitizing strategy for treating human oral squamous cell carcinoma in vitro and in vivo. *Oncotarget* **2017**, *8*, 68641–68653. [CrossRef] [PubMed]
87. Goldsmith, L.A.; Katz, S.I.; Gilchrest, B.A.; Paller, A.S.; Leffell, D.J.; Wolff, K. *Fitzpatrick's Dermatology in General Medicine*, 8th ed.; McGrawHill: New York, NY, USA, 2012; ISBN 978-00-7-166904-7.

88. Bolognia, J.L.; Joseph, L.J.; Schaffer, J.V. *Dermatology*, 3th ed.; Elsevier: Amsterdam, the Netherlands, 2012; ISBN 978-07-2-343571-6.
89. Burns, T.; Breathnach, S.; Cox, N.; Griffiths, C. *Rook's Textbook of Dermatology*, 8th ed.; Wiley Blackwell: Hoboken, NJ, USA, 2010.
90. Apalla, Z.; Nashan, D.; Weller, R.B.; Castellsagué, X. Skin cancer: Epidemiology, disease burden, pathophysiology, diagnosis, and therapeutic approaches. *Dermatol. Ther. (Heidelb)* **2017**, *7*, 5–19. [CrossRef] [PubMed]
91. Petti, S. Lifestyle risk factors for oral cancer. *Oral Oncol.* **2009**, *45*, 340–350. [CrossRef] [PubMed]
92. Boda, D.; Neagu, M.; Constantin, C.; Voinescu, R.N.; Caruntu, C.; Zurac, S.; Tsatsakis, A.M. HPV strain distribution in patients with genital warts in a female population sample. *Oncol. Lett.* **2016**, *12*, 1779–1782. [CrossRef] [PubMed]
93. Wang, J.; Aldabagh, B.; Yu, J.; Arron, S.T. Role of human papillomavirus in cutaneous squamous cell carcinoma: A meta-analysis. *J. Am. Acad. Dermatol.* **2014**, *70*, 621–629. [CrossRef] [PubMed]
94. Lupu, M.; Caruntu, A.; Caruntu, C.; Papagheorghe, L.M.L.; Ilie, M.A.; Voiculescu, V.; Boda, D.; Constantin, C.; Tanase, C.; Sifaki, M.; et al. Neuroendocrine factors: The missing link in non-melanoma skin cancer. *Oncol. Rep.* **2017**, *38*, 1327–1340. [CrossRef] [PubMed]
95. Scholzen, T.; Armstrong, C.A.; Bunnett, N.W.; Luger, T.A.; Olerud, J.E.; Ansel, J.C. Neuropeptides in the skin: Interactions between the neuroendocrine and the skin immune systems. *Exp. Dermatol.* **1998**, *7*, 81–96. [CrossRef] [PubMed]
96. Hara, M.; Toyoda, M.; Yaar, M.; Bhawan, J.; Avila, E.M.; Penner, I.R.; Gilchrest, B.A. Innervation of melanocytes in human skin. *J. Exp. Med.* **1996**, *184*, 1385–1395. [CrossRef] [PubMed]
97. Seiffert, K.; Granstein, R.D. Neuropeptides and neuroendocrine hormones in ultraviolet radiation-induced immunosuppression. *Methods* **2002**, *28*, 97–103. [CrossRef]
98. Weidner, C.; Klede, M.; Rukwied, R.; Lischetzki, G.; Neisius, U.; Schmelz, M.; Petersen, L.J. Acute effects of substance P and calcitonin gene-related peptide in human skin–a microdialysis study. *J. Investig. Dermatol.* **2000**, *115*, 1015–1020. [CrossRef] [PubMed]
99. Dong, J.; Feng, F.; Xu, G.; Zhang, H.; Hong, L.; Yang, J. Elevated SP/NK-1R in esophageal carcinoma promotes esophageal carcinoma cell proliferation and migration. *Gene* **2015**, *560*, 205–210. [CrossRef] [PubMed]
100. Muñoz, M.; Rosso, M.; González-Ortega, A.; Coveñas, R. The NK-1 receptor antagonist L-732,138 induces apoptosis and counteracts substance P-related mitogenesis in human melanoma cell lines. *Cancers* **2010**, *2*, 611–623. [CrossRef] [PubMed]
101. Muñoz, M.; Rosso, M.; Robles-Frias, M.J.; Salinas-Martín, M.V.; Rosso, R.; González-Ortega, A.; Coveñas, R. The NK-1 receptor is expressed in human melanoma and is involved in the antitumor action of the NK-1 receptor antagonist aprepitant on melanoma cell lines. *Lab. Investig.* **2010**, *90*, 1259–1269. [CrossRef] [PubMed]
102. Muñoz, M.; Rosso, M.; Robles-Frías, M.J.; Coveñas, R.; Salinas-Martín, M.V. Immunolocalization of the Neurokinin-1 Receptor: A new target in the treatment of the human primary retinoblastoma. In *Eye Cancer Res. Progress*; Nova Science Publishers: Hauppauge, NY, USA, 2008; pp. 157–178. ISBN 978-1-60456-045-9.
103. Muñoz, M.; Pérez, A.; Coveñas, R.; Rosso, M.; Castro, E. Antitumoural action of L-733,060 on neuroblastoma and glioma cell lines. *Arch. Italiennes Biol.* **2004**, *142*, 105–112.
104. Brener, S.; González-Moles, M.A.; Tostes, D.; Esteban, F.; Gil-Montoya, J.A.; Ruiz-Avila, I.; Munoz, M. A role for the substance P/NK-1 receptor complex in cell proliferation in oral squamous cell carcinoma. *Anticancer Res.* **2009**, *29*, 2323–2329. [PubMed]
105. Serra, I.; Yamamoto, M.; Calvo, A.; Cavada, G.; Baez, S.; Endoh, K.; Tajima, K. Association of chili pepper consumption, low socioeconomic status and longstanding gallstones with gallbladder cancer in a Chilean population. *Int. J. Cancer* **2002**, *102*, 407–411. [CrossRef] [PubMed]
106. Toth, B.; Gannett, P. Carcinogenicity of lifelong administration of capsaicin of hot pepper in mice. *In Vivo* **1992**, *6*, 59–63. [PubMed]
107. Chanda, S.; Erexson, G.; Frost, D.; Babbar, S.; Burlew, J.A.; Bley, K. 26-Week dermal oncogenicity study evaluating pure trans-capsaicin in Tg. AC hemizygous mice (FBV/N). *Int. J. Toxicol.* **2007**, *26*, 123–133. [CrossRef] [PubMed]

108. Surh, Y.J.; Lee, S.S. Capsaicin, a double-edged sword: Toxicity, metabolism, and chemopreventive potential. *Life Sci.* **1995**, *56*, 1845–1855. [CrossRef]
109. Park, K.K.; Surh, Y.J. Effects of capsaicin on chemically-induced two-stage mouse skin carcinogenesis. *Cancer Lett.* **1997**, *114*, 183–184. [CrossRef]
110. Park, K.K.; Chun, K.S.; Yook, J.I.; Surh, Y.J. Lack of tumor promoting activity of capsaicin, a principal pungent ingredient of red pepper, in mouse skin carcinogenesis. *Anticancer Res.* **1998**, *18*, 4201–4205. [PubMed]
111. Surh, Y.J.; Han, S.S.; Keum, Y.S.; Seo, H.J.; Lee, S.S. Inhibitory effects of curcumin and capsaicin on phorbol ester-induced activation of eukaryotic transcription factors, NF-kappaBand AP-1. *Biofactors* **2000**, *12*, 107–112. [CrossRef] [PubMed]
112. Braun-Falco, O.; Plewig, G.; Wolff, H.H.; Landthaler, M. *Braun-Falco's Dermatology*, 3rd ed.; Springer: Berlin/Heidelberg, Germany, 2009; ISBN 978-3-540-29312-5.
113. Sterry, W.; Paus, R.; Burgdorf, W.; Holtermann, H. *Thieme Clinical Companions Dermatology*; Thieme: Stuttgart, Germany, 2006.
114. Tampa, M.; Matei, C.; Caruntu, C.; Poteca, T.; Mihaila, D.; Paunescu, C.; Neagu, M. Cellular impedance measurement–novel method for in vitro investigation of drug efficacy. *Farmacia* **2016**, *5*, 430–434.
115. Niezgoda, A.; Niezgoda, P.; Czajkowski, R. Novel approaches to treatment of advanced melanoma: A review on targeted therapy and immunotherapy. *BioMed Res. Int.* **2015**, *2015*, 851387. [CrossRef] [PubMed]
116. Caruntu, C.; Mirica, A.; Roca, A.E.; Mirica, R.; Caruntu, A.; Matei, C.; Moraru, L. The Role of Estrogens and Estrogen Receptors in Melanoma Development and Progression. *ActaEndocrinol.* **2016**, *12*, 234–241. [CrossRef]
117. Caruntu, C.; Boda, D.; Constantin, C.; Caruntu, A.; Neagu, M. Catecholamines Increase in vitro Proliferation of Murine B16F10 Melanoma Cells. *ActaEndocrinol.* **2014**, *10*, 545–558. [CrossRef]
118. Borrego, J.F.; Huelsmeyer, M.K.; Pinkerton, M.E.; Muszynski, J.L.; Miller, S.A.K.; Kurzman, I.D.; Vail, D.M. Neurokinin-1 receptor expression and antagonism by the NK-1R antagonist maropitant in canine melanoma cell lines and primary tumour tissues. *Vet. Comp. Oncol.* **2016**, *14*, 210–224. [CrossRef] [PubMed]
119. Khare, V.K.; Albino, A.P.; Reed, J.A. The neuropeptide/mast cell secretagogue substance P is expressed in cutaneous melanocytic lesions. *J. Cutan. Pathol.* **1998**, *25*, 2–10. [CrossRef] [PubMed]
120. Zhou, J.; Geng, K.K.; Ping, F.F.; Gao, Y.Y.; Liu, L.; Feng, B.N. Cross-talk between 5-hydroxytryptamine and substance P in the melanogensis and apoptosis of B16F10 melanoma cells. *Eur. J. Pharmacol.* **2016**, *775*, 106–112. [CrossRef] [PubMed]
121. Ping, F.; Shang, J.; Zhou, J.; Song, J.; Zhang, L. Activation of neurokinin-1 receptor by substance P inhibits melanogenesis in B16-F10 melanoma cells. *Int. J. Biochem. Cell Biol.* **2012**, *44*, 2342–2348. [CrossRef] [PubMed]
122. Muñoz, M.; Bernabeu-Wittel, J.; Coveñas, R. NK-1 as a melanoma target. *Expert Opin. Ther. Targets* **2011**, *15*, 889–897. [CrossRef] [PubMed]
123. Muñoz, M.; Pérez, A.; Rosso, M.; Zamarriego, C.; Rosso, R. Antitumoral action of the neurokinin-1 receptor antagonist L-733 060 on human melanoma cell lines. *Melanoma Res.* **2004**, *14*, 183–188. [PubMed]
124. Ueda, Y.; Richmond, A. NF-κB activation in melanoma. *Pigment. Cell. Melanoma Res.* **2006**, *19*, 112–124. [CrossRef] [PubMed]
125. Neagu, M.; Constantin, C.; Longo, C. Chemokines in the melanoma metastasis biomarkers portrait. *J. Immunoass. Immunochem.* **2015**, *36*, 559–566. [CrossRef] [PubMed]
126. Oyagbemi, A.A.; Saba, A.B.; Azeez, O.I. Capsaicin: A novel chemopreventive molecule and its underlying molecular mechanisms of action. *Indian J. Cancer* **2010**, *47*, 53–58. [CrossRef] [PubMed]
127. Davies, M.A. The role of the PI3K-AKT pathway in melanoma. *Cancer J.* **2012**, *18*, 142–147. [CrossRef] [PubMed]
128. Kwong, L.N.; Davies, M.A. Navigating the therapeutic complexity of PI3K pathway inhibition in melanoma. *Clin. Cancer Res.* **2013**, *19*, 5310–5319. [CrossRef] [PubMed]
129. Price, L.S.; Collard, J.G. Regulation of the cytoskeleton by Rho-family GTPases: Implications for tumour cell invasion. *Semin. Cancer Biol.* **2001**, *11*, 167–173. [CrossRef] [PubMed]

12

Recovery Effects of Oral Administration of Glucosylceramide and Beet Extract on Skin Barrier Destruction by UVB in Hairless Mice

Yoshihiro Tokudome *, Noriomi Masutani, Shohei Uchino and Hisano Fukai

Laboratory of Dermatological Physiology, Department of Pharmaceutical Sciences, Faculty of Pharmacy and Pharmaceutical Sciences, Josai University, Saitama 350-0295, Japan

* Correspondence: tokudome@josai.ac.jp

Abstract: Purified glucosylceramide from beet extract (beet GlcCer) and beet extract containing an equal amount of GlcCer were administered orally to ultra violet B (UVB)-irradiated mice, and differences in the protective effects against skin barrier dysfunction caused by UVB irradiation were compared. In the beet GlcCer group, epidermal thickening and the decrease in stratum corneum (SC) ceramide content caused by UVB irradiation were reduced. In the group that was orally administered beet extract containing glucosylceramide, effects similar to those in the beet GlcCer group were observed. Oral administration of beet GlcCer had no obvious effects against an increase in TEWL or decrease in SC water content after UVB irradiation, but there was improvement in the beet extract group. Oral administration of beet GlcCer is effective in improving skin barrier function in UVB-irradiated mice. Beet extract contains constituents other than GlcCer that are also effective in improving skin barrier function.

Keywords: beet; oral administration; glucosylceramide; skin barrier; ultra violet

---

1. Introduction

The stratum corneum of skin plays a barrier function that protects organisms from external stimuli and prevents water loss. Intercellular lipids in the stratum corneum, including ceramides, cholesterol and fatty acids, are important for maintaining skin barrier function. Ceramides are the most abundant, accounting for about 40% of all intercellular lipids [1]. The number of ceramides in skin is decreased in patients with atopic dermatitis and senile xerosis, and increasing the number of ceramides is important to maintaining healthy skin [2,3]. Oral administration of plant extracts from maize [4], rice [4], konjac [5] and sugar beet [6] that contain glucosylceramide (GlcCer), a ceramide precursor, or purified GlcCer has recently been reported to be effective in improving skin barrier function not only in a hairless mouse model [5,7,8], but also in humans [5,9].

The mechanism by which administered GlcCer improves skin barrier function is not entirely clear. However, sphingoid bases, as in vivo metabolites of GlcCer, have recently been reported to activate ceramide synthesis [7,10] promoting the formation of a cornified envelope [8], and increasing tight-junction function by induction of claudin-1 [11] in human keratinocytes. With regard to species of shingoid base, rice and maize GlcCer consist primarily of 8-cis-unsaturated bonds, such as d18:2^{4t}, ^{8t}, d18:1^{8c} [12], while beet GlcCer consists primarily of 8-trans-unsaturated bonds, such as d18:2^{4t}, ^{8c}, d18:1^{8t}, and t18:1^{8t} [13].

While there is no doubt about the effectiveness of GlcCer, it is not clear whether the potency of such plant extracts depends on GlcCer alone. In many cases, evaluated plant extracts have very low GlcCer contents and higher contents of other constituents. Furthermore, lipid constituents other than GlcCer present in plant extracts presumably differ considerably between plant species, plant parts (e.g., root, seeds), and method of extraction and purification. Therefore, improvement of skin barrier function by plant extracts may be related to the effects of other lipid constituents.

The present study aims to identify any differences between purified beet GlcCer and beet extract containing GlcCer and in terms of improving skin barrier function. Sugar beet is a raw material used for sugar production. The fibrous component remaining after extraction of water soluble sugar from the root is sugar beet fiber. By ethanol extraction of sugar beet fibers, beet extracts containing lipid mixtures including glucosylceramides, fatty acids and sterols can be produced as functional food materials.

This study compared differences in the effectiveness between purified GlcCer from beet extract (beet GlcCer) and beet extract containing equal amounts of GlcCer (beet extract) in preventing skin barrier dysfunction, namely, epidermal thickening, decreased stratum corneum ceramide content, increased transepidermal water loss (TEWL), and decreased stratum corneum water content, caused by UVB irradiation in hairless mice.

2. Materials and Methods

2.1. Materials

Purified glucosylceramide from beet extract (certified $\geq$ 99% purity) was purchased from Nagara Science Co., Ltd. (Gifu, Japan). Beet extract was provided by Nippon Beet Sugar Manufacturing Co., Ltd. (Tokyo, Japan), and was a powdered product derived from a mixture of the ethanol extract of sugar beet fiber and modified starch, containing 1.0% glucosylceramide. Beet extract also contained free sterols, sterylglycosides and free fatty acids. The analytical data on the beet extract used in this study were as follows: 0.39% schottenol, 0.37% α-spinasterol, 0.23% β-sitosterol, and 0.08% stigmastenol on HPLC; 1.3% sterylglycosides on TLC; and 0.12% palmitic acid, 0.11% linoleic acid, 0.08% oleic acid on GC (as reported by Nippon Beet Sugar Manufacturing Co., Ltd.). Ceramide NS and AS standards were purchased from Matreya LLC (Pleasant Gap, PA, USA). Ceramide NP and AP standards were obtained from Evonik Goldschmidt GmbH (Goldschmidtstrasse, Essen, Germany). Pentobarbital sodium salt was obtained from Kyoritsu Seiyaku Co. (Tokyo, Japan). Cyanoacrylate adhesives and O.C.T. compound were purchased from Daiichi Sankyo Co., Ltd. (Tokyo, Japan) and Sakura Finetek Japan Co., Ltd. (Tokyo, Japan). Phosphate-buffered saline (PBS) powder was obtained from Sigma (St. Louis, MO, USA). Silica gel 60 (Merck, Darmstadt, Germany) was used for the HPTLC plate. All other reagents were obtained commercially and used without further purification.

2.2. Animals

Seven-week-old male HR-1 hairless mice were purchased from Japan SLC Inc., (Hamamatsu, Shizuoka, Japan). Mice were maintained in a light- (12-h light/dark cycle) and temperature-controlled (25 $\pm$ 2 °C) barrier facility throughout the study. Mice were allowed free access to feed (Labo MR Stock; Nosan Corporation, Yokohama, Japan) and water. All animal experiments and maintenance were performed under conditions approved by the Animal Research Committee of Josai University. Mice were randomly assigned to four groups (n = 6, Table 1).

Table 1. Experimental groups and test samples.

Group	UVB Irradiation (mJ/cm^2)	Composition of Test Sample (mg/Mouse/Day)		
		GlcCer	Beet Ethanol Extract	Processed Starch
Normal	None	0	0	22
Control	200	0	0	22
Beet GlcCer	200	0.3	0	22
Beet Extract	200	(0.3) [1]	8.0	22

[1] 8.0 mg of beet ethanol extract contains 0.3 mg of beet GlcCer.

2.3. *Test Sample and Schedule*

Test samples were suspended in purified water containing processed starch (starch sodium octenyl succinate) as emulsifier and 0.3 mL was orally administered to each mouse using a sonde every day for 14 days. All of the glucosylceramide samples were prepared on the day of administration.

A single dose of UVB (200 mJ/cm^2) irradiation was applied to the back skin of each mouse using a Philips UVB lamp (TL20W/12 RS; Philips, Amsterdam, The Netherlands) at day 7 after the first administration (only one time irradiation of UVB). Collection of stratum corneum and dorsal skin sections from half of the mice was performed under anesthesia at day 3 after UVB irradiation. Table 2 shows the experimental schedule of this manuscript.

Table 2. Experimental schedule (d: day).

Events/Day	−7 d	−6 d	−5 d	−4 d	−3 d	−2 d	−1 d	0 d	1 d	2 d	3 d	4 d	5 d	6 d	7 d
Sample administration	○	○	○	○	○	○	○	○	○	○	○	○	○	○	
UV irradiation								○							
Body weight	○		○		○		○	○	○	○	○	○	○	○	○
Water content, TEWL								○			○			○	
Ceramide content											○				
HE staining											○				

2.4. *Measurement of Water Contents of Stratum Corneum, and TEWL*

Water contents of stratum corneum and TEWL in the back skin of mice were measured daily for 14 days. Water contents of the stratum corneum were measured with a Corneometer (Courage & Khazaka, Cologne, Germany) and TEWL was assessed using a VAPO SCAN AS-VT100 RS (Asahi Techno Lab., Ltd., Yokohama, Kanagawa, Japan). Corneometer and VAPO SCAN data are given in terms of indicated arbitrary units (AU) and g/m^2/h, respectively.

2.5. *Collection of Mouse Stratum Corneum*

After application of anesthesia, cyanoacrylate adhesive was dropped onto slide glass, and this was adhered to the murine back skin for one minute. Slide glass was removed to collect stratum corneum sample [2].

2.6. *Extraction Method and Lipid Analysis by HPTLC*

The slide glass used to collect stratum corneum was soaked in hexane and ethanol (95:5), and was sonicated at 37 °C for 20 min. After filtering the solution, it was dried under nitrogen gas. The residue was added to 100 μL of chloroform:methanol (2:1). Briefly, stratum corneum samples were soaked in 4 mL of chloroform:methanol (2:1 *v*/*v*) and sonicated (70 W, 10 min) with a probe-type sonicator (Sonifire B-12; Branson Ultrasonics, Danbury, CT, USA). The ceramide extracted solution was dried under nitrogen gas, and was resolved in 0.4 mL of chloroform:methanol (2:1 *v*/*v*). Various ceramide extracts were separated using an HPTLC plate (Silica Gel 60; Merck, Darmstadt, Germany). HPTLC was developed twice with chloroform:methanol:acetic acid = 190:9:1 (*v*/*v*). Ceramide molecules were visualized by treatment with 10% $CuSO_4$, 8% H_3PO_4 aqueous solution, and heating to 180 °C for 10 min. The amounts of various types of ceramide (ceramide NS, NP, AS and AP) were quantitatively determined using a densitometer.

2.7. *Measurement of Stratum Corneum Mass*

The slide glass used to collect the stratum corneum was soaked in *N*, *N*, dimethylformamide, and was sonicated for 15 min. The sonicated solution was passed through a filter that was weighed beforehand. The filter was dried for one week under vacuum. After dryness, the filter weighed again, and difference between the before and after measurements was taken as the stratum corneum mass.

2.8. *Hematoxylin and Eosin Staining*

The dorsal skin of animals was detached, cut into 0.7 cm × 0.2 cm strips with a scalpel, and embedded in OCT compound under rapid chilling on dry ice in order to prepare frozen sections. Frozen sections were cut at 0.1 μm using the Leica CM 3050 S microtome (Welzlar, Germany). Sections were subsequently stained with hematoxylin and eosin, as follows. Sections were first immersed for 30 min in a 10% formalin solution for fixation. Sections were then rinsed with water and sequentially immersed in ethanol in order to achieve dehydration. Next, sections were rinsed with water and immersed in hematoxylin solution for 10 min. Sections were again rinsed with water and immersed in an eosin solution containing acetic acid. Finally, sections were immersed in and penetrated with xylene 3 times, embedded, and observed under a microscope. Epidermal thickness was defined as the distance from the top of the stratum granulosum to the bottom of the stratum basale. Thickness of stratum corneum was measured from the top of the stratum corneum to the bottom.

2.9. *Measurement of Epidermis Thickness*

Thickness of the epidermis was measured at the horizontal midpoint of each visual field. Approximately 50 individual measurements were made along the wound margin for each histological section, and mean thickness was evaluated.

2.10. *Data and Statistical Analysis*

All results are expressed as means ± standard deviation. Statistical analysis was performed using Tukey's post-hoc test (using SAS software version 9.2, SAS Institute, Cary, NC, USA).

3. Results

3.1. *Body Weight Change after Oral Administration of Beet GlcCer or Beet Extract in UVB-Irradiated Mice*

Figure 1 shows the body weight changes in UVB-irradiated mice. Body weight did not change in any groups after oral administration of beet GlcCer or beet extract.

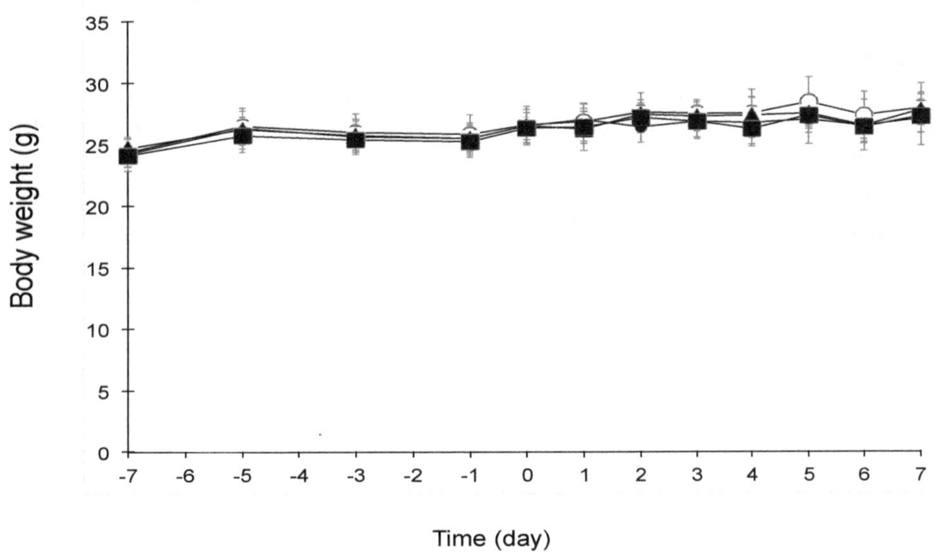

Figure 1. Body weight changes in UVB-irradiated mice after oral administration of beet GlcCer or beet extract. Symbols and bars represent means and standard deviation ($n = 6$ from day −7 to day 3, and $n = 3$ from day 4 to day 7), respectively. Symbols: Closed circles, Normal group (without UVB irradiation, vehicle administration); Open circles, Control group (200 mJ/cm^2 UVB, vehicle administration); closed triangles, beet GlcCer group (200 mJ/cm^2 UVB, beet GlcCer oral administration); closed squares, beet extract group (200 mJ/cm^2 UVB, beet extract oral administration).

3.2. Epidermal Hyperplasia Following UVB Irradiation

Frozen sections of murine dorsal skin at day 3 after UVB irradiation were prepared, and hematoxylin and eosin staining of the sections was performed (Figure 2). Skin layers were thickened by UVB irradiation (normal group, 28 ± 4 μm; control group, 119 ± 9 μm; $p < 0.01$). Interestingly, beet GlcCer reduced skin thickening induced by UVB irradiation, and a similar effect was also observed in the beet extract group (beet GlcCer group, 68 ± 11 μm; beet extract group, 69 ± 5 μm; $p < 0.01$ vs. control group).

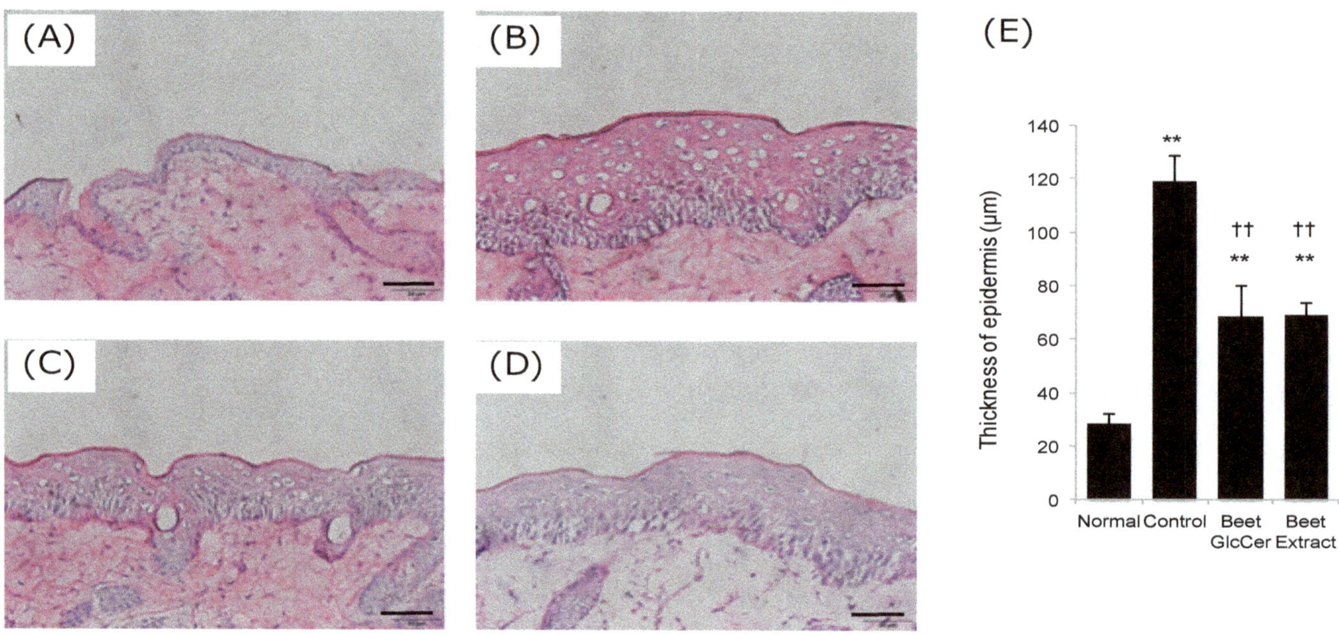

Figure 2. Hematoxylin and eosin staining, and thickness of epidermis in mouse skin. (**A**) Normal (without UVB irradiation, vehicle administration); (**B**) Control (200 mJ/cm^2 UVB irradiation, vehicle administration); (**C**) Beet GlcCer (200 mJ/cm^2 UVB irradiation, beet GlcCer oral administration); (**D**) Beet extract (200 mJ/cm^2 UVB irradiation, beet extract oral administration); and (**E**) Epidermal thickness in UVB irradiated mice ($n = 3$). Scale bar indicates 50 μm. ** $p < 0.01$ vs. normal group, †† $p < 0.01$ vs. control group, Tukey's post-hoc multiple comparison test.

3.3. Comparison of Ceramide Contents in Stratum Corneum among Mouse Groups

Quantitative analysis of ceramide contents in stratum corneum removed from the murine back skin at day 3 after UVB treatment was performed (Figure 3). UVB irradiation significantly decreased ceramide contents in stratum corneum. Remarkably, ceramide contents in UVB-irradiated mice orally given beet GlcCer were similar to those in the normal group. Similar results were observed between the beet extract group and the normal group.

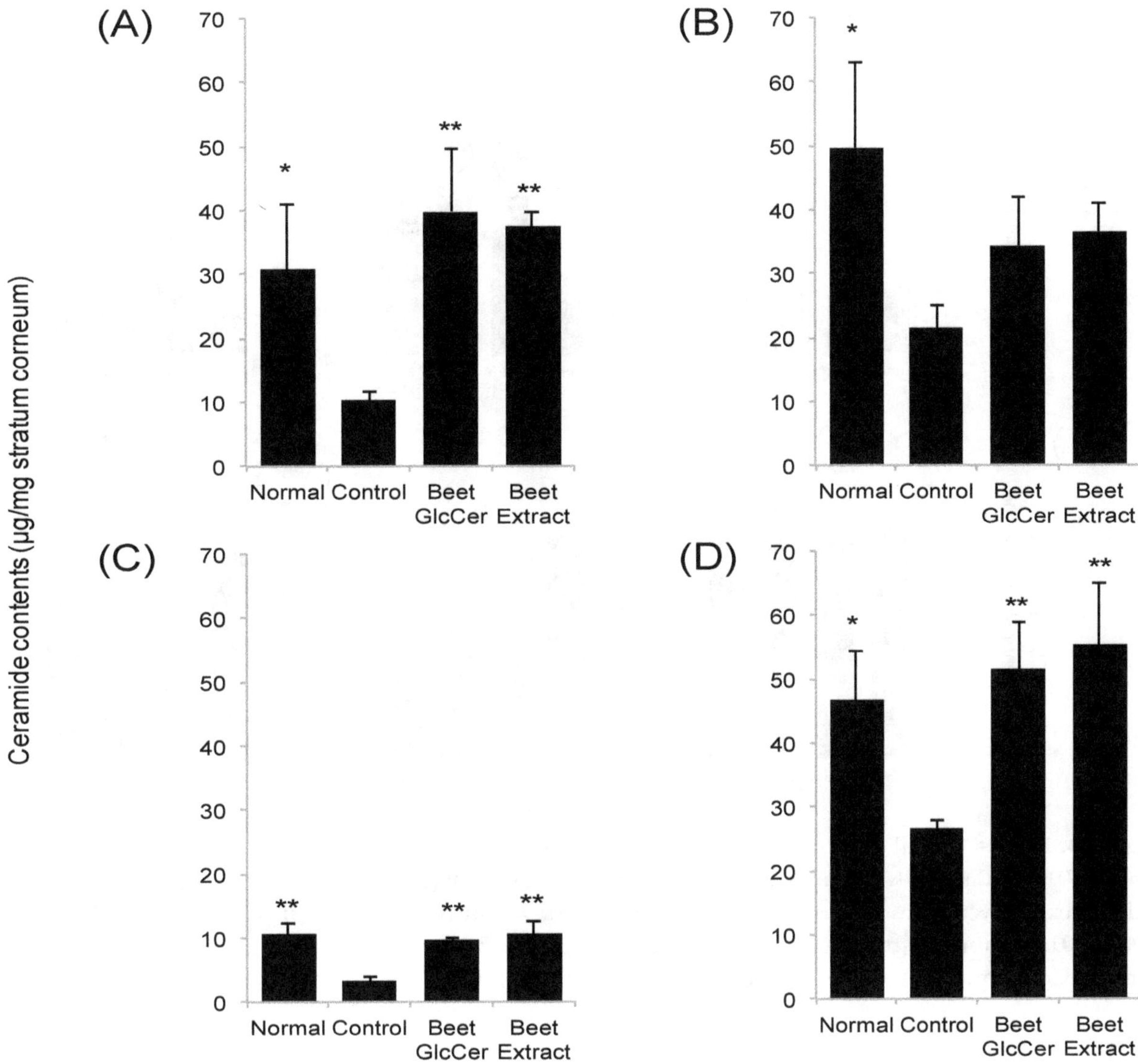

Figure 3. Ceramide contents in stratum corneum in UVB-irradiated (200 mJ/cm^2) mice after oral administration of beet GlcCer or beet extract. Ceramide NS (**A**); NP (**B**); AS (**C**) and AP (**D**); respectively. Values are given as means and standard deviation (n = 3). * $p < 0.05$, ** $p < 0.01$ vs. control group, Tukey's post-hoc multiple comparison test.

3.4. TEWL and Water Contents in Stratum Corneum

Figure 4 shows the TEWL and water contents in stratum corneum at days 0, 3 and 6 after UVB irradiation in each group. TEWL in UVB-irradiated groups temporarily increased at day 3 after UVB treatment, as compared with non-UVB-irradiated mice. Mice administered beet GlcCer showed slightly lower TEWL, but the difference was not significant, when compared with the control group at day 3. Increases in TEWL in the beet extract group after UVB irradiation were significantly lower than in the control group at days 3 and 6. UVB irradiation also decreased the water content in stratum corneum in each mouse group. Although the water content in stratum corneum from the control group remained low at day 6 when compared with the normal group, early recovery of the loss of water content in the stratum corneum was observed in the beet extract group.

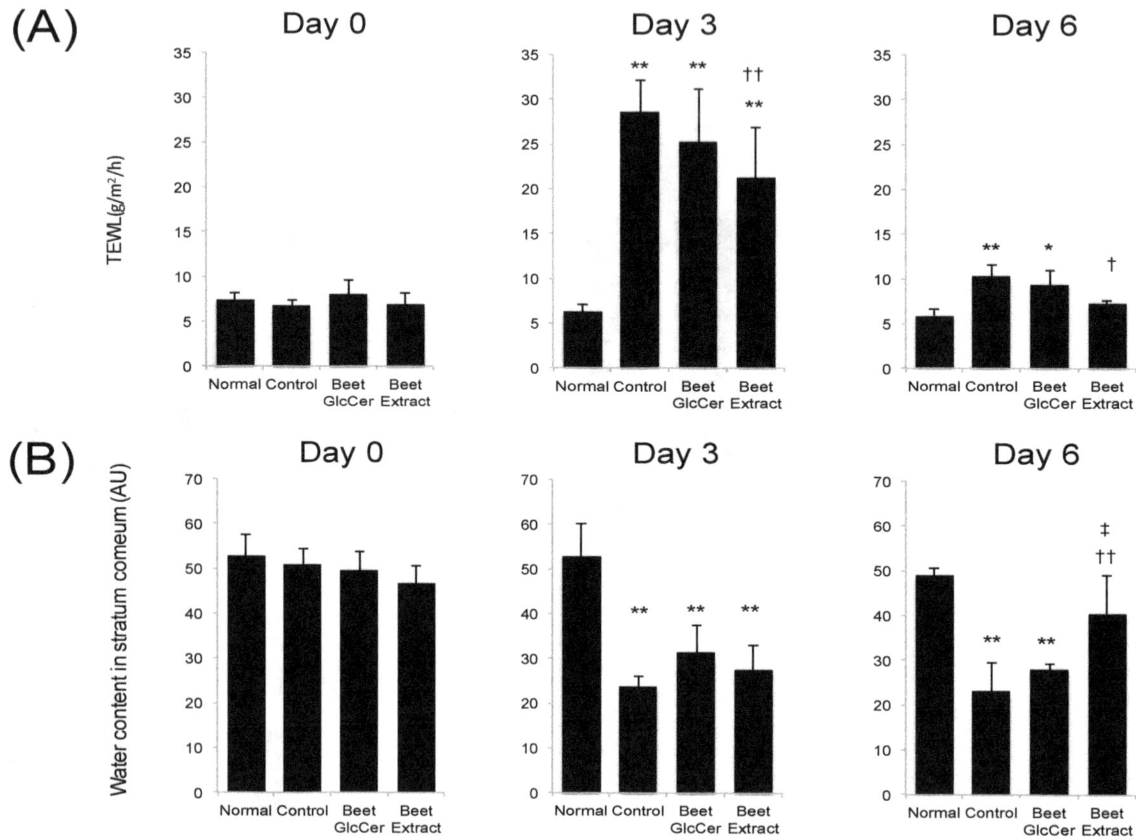

Figure 4. Effects of oral administration of beet GlcCer or beet extract on TEWL and stratum corneum after UVB irradiation. (**A**) Transepidermal water loss (TEWL); (**B**) water contents in stratum corneum. Values are shown as means $\pm$ standard deviation ($n = 6$ at day 0 and 3, $n = 3$ at day 6). * $p < 0.05$, ** $p < 0.01$ vs. normal group, † $p < 0.05$ vs. control group, †† $p < 0.01$ vs. control group, ‡ $p < 0.05$ vs. beet GlcCer group, Tukey's post-hoc multiple comparison test.

4. Discussion

This study showed that oral administration of purified GlcCer from beets was effective in preventing epidermal thickening and decreased stratum corneum ceramide content caused by UVB irradiation in hairless mice. In addition, administration of beet extract containing an equal amount of glucosyl ceramides was more effective than beet GlcCer in improving increased TEWL and decreased stratum corneum water content.

Initially, examination of skin sections on day 3 after UVB irradiation showed epidermal hyperplasia in controls. Epidermal thickness increased 4-fold when compared to the normal group. However, in the beet GlcCer group, epidermal thickness decreased to 50% when compared with controls. In the beet extract group, epidermal thickness decreased to the same degree as in the beet GlcCer group. These findings strongly suggest that inhibition of epidermal hyperplasia was due to the effects of orally administered GlcCer. Inhibition of epidermal hyperplasia by beet extract [6] and purified GlcCer from corn extract has previously been reported in a hairless mouse model of skin barrier impairment induced by an Mg-deficient HR-AD diet [7]. Our study found that beet GlcCer was also effective in preventing epidermal hyperplasia induced by UVB irradiation.

Ceramides, which account for about 40% of intercellular lipids in the stratum corneum, are important in skin barrier function [1–3]. A recent study found that UVB irradiation decreased skin ceramide content and increased ceramidase gene expression [14]. With oral administration of purified GlcCer from plant extracts to hairless mice fed an HR-AD diet, a 2-fold increase in epidermal ceramide synthase gene expression has also been reported [7]. Because of these previous findings, we decided to focus on stratum corneum ceramide content. In our study, we analyzed stratum corneum content of ceramides NS, NP, AS and AP, for which ceramide standards were available. The results showed a decrease in all measured ceramides at 3 days after UVB irradiation, but with oral administration of beet GlcCer, all of these decreases were reduced. Moreover, similar levels of stratum corneum ceramide content were seen in both the beet GlcCer group and the beet extract group, thus strongly suggesting that GlcCer in the beet extract contributed to these observed effects.

Haratake et al. reported epidermal cell hyperplasia followed by increased TEWL in UVB-irradiated hairless mice [15]. The increase in TEWL was reduced by DNA synthesis inhibitors, and they concluded that epidermal hyperproliferation was associated with the epidermal barrier disturbance [15]. TEWL reflects water loss from the body and is commonly used a parameter of skin barrier function. In our study, epidermal hyperplasia and increased TEWL were observed in the control group at 3 days after UVB irradiation. The effectiveness of purified GlcCer from plants in preventing TEWL has previously been reported in a hairless mouse model with barrier perturbation induced by single-dose UVB irradiation [8], in a hairless mouse model with sodium dodecyl sulfate-induced skin roughness [5], in a Mg-deficient diet-induced atopic dermatitis-like model [7], and in a tape-stripped injured skin mouse model with regard to GlcCer from konjac and maize [7]. However, there are few reports on GlcCer from beet. Haruta-Ono et al. reported on orally administered of sphingomyelin to the improvement of epidermal function in hairless mice [16]. TEWL and stratum corneum water content of sphingomyelin-administered mice showed better values than the control group. Ceramide also increased. From these results, oral application of GlcCer and sphingomyelin may have a good effect on epidermal function.

In our study, although TEWL was slightly lower in the beet GlcCer group when compared with the control group, the difference was not statistically significant. Interestingly, however, oral administration of beet extract containing an equal amount of GlcCer, when compared to the control group, significantly reduced the increase in TEWL caused by UVB irradiation. In addition, there was earlier recovery of decreased stratum corneum water content. These results strongly suggest that constituents other than GlcCer in beet extract help protect against or restore UVB irradiation-induced skin barrier dysfunction.

For example, beet-derived steryl glycosides, phytosterols and free fatty acids are present in beet extracts (described in Materials and Methods). Recent studies have reported that steryl glycosides and phytosterols inhibit UVB irradiation-induced inflammatory reactions (cytokines, matrix metalloproteinase production) in skin cells [17,18]. In UVB-irradiated skin tissue, inflammatory cytokines and chemokines such as IL-1α, TNFα and IL-8 are released from keratinocytes [19–21]. This is followed by activated lymphocyte infiltration into skin tissue, leading to an inflammatory reaction. Oral administration of beet extract may reduce skin barrier dysfunction after UVB irradiation more so than administration of GlcCer alone because phytosterols in beet extract prevent expansion of the inflammatory reaction in skin tissue after UVB irradiation. Confirmation of this hypothesis will require further studies.

5. Conclusions

Oral administration of beet GlcCer prevented epidermal hyperplasia and decreased stratum corneum ceramide content caused by UVB irradiation. In addition, our findings suggest that beet extract contains constituents other than GlcCer that are also effective in improving skin barrier function.

Author Contributions: Y.T. designed the research, N.M., S.U. and H.F. performed the experiments, Y.T. and N.M. analyzed the data, and Y.T. wrote the manuscript. All authors have read and approved the final manuscript.

References

1. Gray, G.M.; Yardley, H.J. Different populations of pig epidermal cells: Isolation and lipid composition. *J. Lipid Res.* **1975**, *16*, 441–447. [PubMed]
2. Imokawa, G.; Abe, A.; Jin, K.; Higaki, Y.; Kawashima, M.; Hidano, A. Decreased level of ceramides in stratum corneum of atopic dermatitis: An etiologic factor in atopic dry skin? *J. Investig. Dermatol.* **1991**, *96*, 523–526. [CrossRef] [PubMed]
3. Yamamoto, A.; Serizawa, S.; Ito, M.; Sato, Y. Stratum corneum lipid abnormalities in atopic dermatitis. *Arch. Dermatol. Res.* **1991**, *283*, 219–223. [CrossRef] [PubMed]
4. Tsuji, K.; Mitsutake, S.; Ishikawa, J.; Takagi, Y.; Akiyama, M.; Shimizu, H.; Tomiyama, T.; Igarashi, Y. Dietary glucosylceramide improves skin barrier function in hairless mice. *J. Dermatol. Sci.* **2006**, *44*, 101–107. [CrossRef] [PubMed]
5. Uchiyama, T.; Nakano, Y.; Ueda, O.; Mori, H.; Nakashima, M.; Noda, A.; Ishizaki, C.; Mizoguchi, M. Oral Intake of Glucosylceramide Improves Relatively Higher Level of Transepidermal Water Loss in Mice and Healthy Human Subjects. *J. Health Sci.* **2008**, *54*, 559–566. [CrossRef]
6. Kawano, K.-I.; Umemura, K. Oral intake of beet extract provides protection against skin barrier impairment in hairless mice. *Phytother. Res.* **2013**, *27*, 775–783. [CrossRef] [PubMed]
7. Duan, J.; Sugawara, T.; Hirose, M.; Aida, K.; Sakai, S.; Fujii, A.; Hirata, T. Dietary sphingolipids improve skin barrier functions via the upregulation of ceramide synthases in the epidermis. *Exp. Dermatol.* **2012**, *21*, 448–452. [CrossRef] [PubMed]
8. Hasegawa, T.; Shimada, H.; Uchiyama, T.; Ueda, O.; Nakashima, M.; Matsuoka, Y. Dietary glucosylceramide enhances cornified envelope formation via transglutaminase expression and involucrin production. *Lipids* **2011**, *46*, 529–535. [CrossRef] [PubMed]
9. Hori, M.; Kishimoto, S.; Tezuka, Y.; Nishigori, H.; Nomoto, K.; Hamada, U.; Yonei, Y. Double-blind study on effects of glucosyl ceramide in beet extract on skin elasticity and fibronectin production in human dermal fibroblasts. *Anti-Aging Mag.* **2010**, *7*, 129–142. [CrossRef]
10. Shirakura, Y.; Kikuchi, K.; Matsumura, K.; Mukai, K.; Mitsutake, S.; Igarashi, Y. 4,8-Sphingadienine and 4-hydroxy-8-sphingenine activate ceramide production in the skin. *Lipids Health Dis.* **2012**, *11*, 108. [CrossRef] [PubMed]
11. Kawada, C.; Hasegawa, T.; Watanabe, M.; Nomura, Y. Dietary glucosylceramide enhances tight junction function in skin epidermis via induction of claudin-1. *Biosci. Biotechnol. Biochem.* **2013**, *77*, 867–869. [CrossRef] [PubMed]
12. Aida, K.; Takakuwa, N.; Kinoshita, M.; Sugawara, H.; Imai, H.; Ono, J.; Ohnishi, M. Properties and physiological effects of plant cerebroside species as functional lipids. *Adv. Res. Plant Lipids* **2003**, 233–236. [CrossRef]
13. Takakuwa, N.; Saito, K.; Oda, Y. Content of Functional Lipid Ceramide in Crop Tissues and By-Products from Their Processing. *Atarashii Kenkyu Seika* **2005**, 173–177.
14. Ra, J.; Lee, D.E.; Kim, S.H.; Jeong, J.W.; Ku, H.K.; Kim, T.Y.; Choi, I.D.; Jeung, W.; Sim, J.H.; Ahn, Y.T. Effect of oral administration of Lactobacillus plantarum HY7714 on epidermal hydration in ultraviolet B-irradiated hairless mice. *J. Microbiol. Biotechnol.* **2014**, *24*, 1736–1743. [CrossRef] [PubMed]
15. Haratake, A.; Uchida, Y.; Schmuth, M.; Tanno, O.; Yasuda, R.; Epstein, J.H.; Elias, P.M.; Holleran, W.M. UVB-induced alterations in permeability barrier function: Roles for epidermal hyperproliferation and thymocyte-mediated response. *J. Investig. Dermatol.* **1997**, *108*, 769–775. [CrossRef] [PubMed]
16. Haruta-Ono, Y.; Ueno, H.; Ueda, N.; Kato, K.; Yoshioka, T. Investigation into the dosage of dietary sphingomyelin concentrate in relation to the improvement of epidermal function in hairless mice. *Anim. Sci. J.* **2012**, *83*, 178–183. [CrossRef] [PubMed]
17. Lee, T.H.; Lee, S.M.; Lee, D.Y.; Son, Y.; Chung, D.K.; Baek, N.I.; Kim, J. A glycosidic spinasterol from Koreana stewartia promotes procollagen production and inhibits matrix metalloproteinase-1 expression in UVB-irradiated human dermal fibroblasts. *Biol. Pharm. Bull.* **2011**, *34*, 768–773. [CrossRef] [PubMed]
18. Hwang, E.; Park, S.Y.; Sun, Z.W.; Shin, H.S.; Lee, D.G.; Yi, T.H. The protective effects of fucosterol against skin damage in UVB-irradiated human dermal fibroblasts. *Mar. Biotechnol.* **2014**, *16*, 361–370. [CrossRef] [PubMed]

19. Kupper, T.S.; Chua, A.O.; Flood, P.; McGuire, J.; Gubler, U. Interleukin 1 gene expression in cultured human keratinocytes is augmented by ultraviolet irradiation. *J. Clin. Investig.* **1987**, *80*, 430–436. [CrossRef] [PubMed]
20. Kondo, S.; Kono, T.; Sauder, D.N.; McKenzie, R.C. IL-8 gene expression and production in human keratinocytes and their modulation by UVB. *J. Investig. Dermatol.* **1993**, *101*, 690–694. [CrossRef] [PubMed]
21. Bashir, M.M.; Sharma, M.R.; Werth, V.P. UVB and proinflammatory cytokines synergistically activate TNF-alpha production in keratinocytes through enhanced gene transcription. *J. Investig. Dermatol.* **2009**, *129*, 994–1001. [CrossRef] [PubMed]

13

Dioscorea quinqueloba Ameliorates Oxazolone- and 2,4-Dinitrochlorobenzene-Induced Atopic Dermatitis Symptoms in Murine Models

Jonghwan Jegal [1,†], No-June Park [2,†], Sim-Kyu Bong [2], Hyun Jegal [2], Su-Nam Kim [2,*] and Min Hye Yang [1,*]

[1] College of Pharmacy, Pusan National University, Busan 46241, Korea; puhahaha2027@naver.com
[2] Natural Products Research Institute, Korea Institute of Science and Technology, Gangneung 25451, Korea; parknojune1@naver.com (N.-J.P.); 115044@kist.re.kr (S.-K.B.); 116524@kist.re.kr (H.J.)
* Correspondence: snkim@kist.re.kr (S.-N.K.); mhyang@pusan.ac.kr (M.H.Y.);
† These authors contributed equally to this work.

Abstract: *Dioscorea quinqueloba* has been used for food substances, as well as in herbal medicines for allergic diseases such as asthma. This study aimed to investigate the anti-atopic dermatitis (AD) effects of the total extract of *D. quinqueloba* rhizomes and active fractionson murine oxazolone- and 2,4-dinitrochlorobenzene-induced models of AD. Specific AD symptoms, such as erythema, ear swelling, and epidermis thickening, were significantly reduced in the oxazolone-mediated AD BALB/c mice upon topical application of *D. quinqueloba* rhizomes 95% EtOH extract (DQ). DQEA (*D. quinqueloba* rhizomes EtOAc fraction) was beneficial for protecting the skin barrier against AD in DNCB-sensitized SKH-1 hairless mice. Decreased total serum IgE and IL-4 levels could be observed in atopic dorsal skin samples of the DQEA-treated group. On the basis of the phytochemical analysis, DQEA was found to contain dioscin and gracillin as its main compounds. Therapeutic applications with *D. quinqueloba* might be useful in the treatment of AD and related inflammatory skin diseases.

Keywords: *Dioscorea quinqueloba*; atopic dermatitis; transepidermal water loss; skin hydration; interleukin 4; immunoglobulin E

---

1. Introduction

Atopic dermatitis (AD) is a pruritic chronic inflammatory skin disease [1]. Worldwide, AD occurs with a prevalence of 2–10% in adults, and up to 15–30% in children [2,3]. Atopic disease is triggered by a variety of allergic factors, including irritants, food, and stress factors [4]. The symptoms of AD include atopic eczema, itching, and dryskin [5]. Intense pruritus is the most common dermatologic feature of AD, thus negatively impacting the health-related quality of life in patients suffering from AD [5,6].

Atopic dermatitis can be categorized into two types, including an extrinsic type (environmental or allergic AD) and an intrinsic type (genetic or non-allergic AD) [7]. Extrinsic AD is the classical type of AD, while the incidence of intrinsic AD is approximately 20% of patients [7,8]. Extrinsic or environmental triggers enhance IgE-mediated sensitization and allergic reaction, thus further contributing to severe forms of skin inflammation in AD [9]. Diverse inflammatory cytokines orchestrate atopic skin inflammation, and the concomitant activation of IL-4 is thought to play a critical role in the pathogenesis of AD [10]. An impaired epidermal skin barrier is also a characteristic feature and causative factor of AD [10]. Skin barrier damage contributes to the high serum IgE level, reduced skin surface hydration, and enhanced transepidermal water loss in patients with extrinsic AD [8,11,12]. Therefore, improvements in skin barrier function with natural moisturizing agents show great potential as a pharmacological target in atopic diseases.

Dioscorea quinqueloba Thunb. belongs to the Dioscoreaceae family, and has been cultivated in China, Japan, and Korea as a food. The rhizomes of *D. quinqueloba* have been used in traditional Korean medicine as an alternative therapy for cardiovascular disease, as well as various medical conditions, mainly for arthrosclerosis, myocardial infarction, and asthma [12–14]. Analysis of the chemical composition of *Dioscorea* species indicates that the main metabolites are steroidal saponins such as diosin and diosgenin, which have convulsive, local anesthetic and antidiuretic effects [15,16]. Recent reports have shown that the genus *Dioscorea* exhibits various biological properties, including anti-inflammatory, antitumor, and anti-adipogenic activities [17–19]. However, studies on the *D. quinqueloba* are comparatively few in number, and furthermore, there have not been any attempts to reveal its anti-atopic effect. This study aimed to investigate the potential therapeutic effects of *D. quinqueloba* on oxazolone- and 2,4-dinitrochlorobenzene (DNCB)-induced murine AD models. Histopathological examination and blood serum analysis, including total IL-4 and IgE levels, were performed to observe anti-atopic properties of *D. quinqueloba*.

2. Material and Methods

2.1. Plant Material and Extraction

Dried rhizomes of *D. quinqueloba* were purchased from JirisanHanbang Food® (Sancheong, Gyeongnam, South Korea) and identified by Eun Ju Jeong of Department of Agronomy and Medicinal Plant Resources, Gyeongnam National University of Science and Technology. A voucher specimen (PNU-0023) has been deposited in the Medicinal Herb Garden, Pusan National University. *Dioscorea quinqueloba* sample (20 kg) was extracted with 95% EtOH and evaporated under reduced pressure to yield *D. quinqueloba* EtOH extract (DQ) (670 g). The DQ was suspended in distilled water (2 L) and partitioned with EtOAc (4 L) and *n*-BuOH (4 L) to yield *D. quinqueloba* EtOAc fraction (DQEA) (150 g) and *n*-BuOH fraction (DQB) (300 g).

2.2. Animals

Six-week-old female BALB/c and SKH-1 hairless mice were purchased from the animal facility of Orient Bio Inc. (Seongnam, Republic of Korea) and housed in an air-conditioned animal room at a temperature of 25 ± 5 °C and 55 ± 5% humidity. Mice were given access to a standard laboratory diet and water ad libitum. All animal experiments were conducted in accordance with the Guide for the Care and Use of Laboratory Animals of the National Institutes of Health (NIH publication No. 85-23, revised 1996) and were approved by the Institutional Animal Care and Use Committee of the KIST (Certification No. KIST-2016-011).

2.3. Induction of Topical AD-Like Skin Dermatitis in Mice by Oxazolone and Treatment with DQ

4-Ethoxymethylene-2-phenyl-2-oxazolin-5-one (oxazolone) (1%) dissolved in vehicle (propylene glycol:EtOH = 7:3) was used as sensitizer to induce AD in BALB/c mouse ears according to the previously described method [20]. In brief, the ears of BALB/c mice were sensitized with 20 μL of 1% oxazolone on the first day. After the first challenge, 20 μL of 0.1% oxazolone was repeatedly applied to ears for an additional 3 weeks at 2-day intervals. At the same time, the ears of the BALB/c mice were exposed to 20 μL of 1% DQ daily in the oxazolone-DQ-group for 3 weeks, and the application of 1% DQ was separated by 4 h from that of oxazolone. The normal control animals (CON) were treated with distilled water alone. No substances were applied to the skin surface on the last day of the experiment. On the last day, measurements of skin inflammation signs, including ear swelling and erythema, were carried out.

2.4. Induction of AD-Like Skin Lesions in Mice by DNCB and Treatment with DQEA

2,4-dinitrochlorobenzenedissolved in acetone was used to induce AD in SKH-1 hairless mice as previously described with small modification [21,22]. Briefly, the dorsal skin of hairless mice was sensitized by painting 100 μL of 1% DNCB daily for 7 days. After the first challenge, the mice were challenged with 100 μL of 0.1% DNCB for an additional 2 weeks at 3-day intervals. The DNCB-DQEA group animals were painted with 100 μL of 1% DQEA for 2 weeks, and the application of DQEA was separated by 4 h from that of DNCB. The normal control animals (CON) were treated with distilled water alone. No substances were applied to the skin surface on the last day of the experiment. On the last day, mice were sacrificed, and dorsal skin and blood samples were collected for further analysis.

2.5. Histology

For histologic examination, the ear or dorsal skin from mice were fixed in 10% formalin and processed for paraffin embedding. Tissue sections (2–3 mm) were then stained with hematoxylin and eosin. Histopathological changes were examined by light microscopy (Olympus CX31/BX51, Olympus Optical Co., Tokyo, Japan) and photographed (TE-2000U, Nikon Instruments Inc., Melville, NY, USA).

2.6. Measurement of Transepidermal Water Loss, Skin Hydration, and Skin Surface pH

Skin barrier repair was monitored by estimating transepidermal water loss (TEWL), skin hydration, and skin surface pH. Tewameter TM210 device (Courage and Khazaka, Cologne, Germany) and SKIN-O-MAT (Cosmomed, Ruhr, Germany) were used to evaluate the skin surface of the hairless mice according to the manufacturer's instructions. TEWL, skin hydration, and skin surface pH were measured once per week after the twice-daily application of DQEA or vehicle.

2.7. Measurement of Serum IgE and IL-4 Levels

Blood samples were centrifuged at 10,000 rpm for 15 min at 4 °C, and then serum was collected and stored at −80 °C for further investigations. Total IgE and IL-4 concentration in mouse serum were measured via enzyme-linked immunosorbent assay (eBioscience, San Diego, CA, USA) according to the manufacturer's instructions.

2.8. Measurement of IL-4 mRNA Expression in RBL-2H3 Cells

The rat basophilic leukemia cell line, RBL-2H3, was obtained from the American Type Culture Collection (CRL-2256, Bethesda, MD, USA) and grown in minimum essential medium with Eagle's salt, supplemented with 10% fetal bovine serum (FBS), 2 mM L-glutamine, 100 U/mL penicillin, and 100 μg/mL streptomycin at 37 °C in a humidified incubator with a 5% CO_2/95% air atmosphere. The RBL-2H3 cells were treated with dimethylsulfoxide (DMSO), DQ, DQEA, and DQB (10 μg/mL) 30 min before the induction of inflammation with phorbol 12-myristate 13-acetate/ionomycin (PI), which induced a state similar to AD. Controls were treated with DMSO without PMA/ionomycin (PI). After 16 h of treatment, cells were harvested to synthesize cDNA, and mRNA of IL-4 was measured with quantitative real-time PCR (qPCR). Total RNA from the treated cells was prepared with RNAiso Reagent (TaKaRa, Shiga, Japan) according to the manufacturer's protocol and stored at −80°C until use. Accumulated PCR products were detected directly by monitoring the increase in the reporter dye (SYBR). The expression levels of cytokines in the exposed cells were compared to the expression levels in control cells at each collection time point using the comparative cycle threshold (Ct) method. The sequences of the primers used in this study were: IL-4 forward: 5′-ACC TTG CTG TCA CCC TGT TC-3′; IL-4 reverse: 5′-TTG TGA GCG TGG ACTCAT TC-3′; β-actin forward: 5′-TCA TCA CCA TCG GCA ACG-3′, β-actin reverse: 5′-TTC CT GAT GTC CAC GTC GC-3′. The quantity of each transcript was calculated as described in the instrument manual and normalized to the amount of β-actin.

2.9. Chromatographic Conditions

The DQEA sample was analyzed using an Agilent 6530 Accurate-Mass Q-TOF LC/MS system (Agilent Technologies, Palo Alto, CA, USA) for phytochemical characterization. A Poroshell 120 EC-C18 column (3.0 × 100 mm, 2.7 μm, Agilent, Palo Alto, CA, USA) was used for analysis at a flow rate of 0.3 mL/min. The mobile phase consisted of acetonitrile (solvent A) and water (solvent B), using a linear gradient elution: 5–95% A (0–20 min); 10% A (20–30 min). All acquisitions were performed under positive ionization mode. Mass spectra were recorded across the range m/z = 100–1500 with accurate mass measurement of all mass peaks.

2.10. Statistical Analysis

Data are expressed as the mean ± standard deviation (S.D.). The values were expressed as percent changes from the mean value of the control experiment. Statistical analyses were performed by a one-way analysis of variance (ANOVA) using Statistical Package (SPSS, Inc., Chicago, IL, USA). p-values less than 0.05 were considered statistically significant.

3. Results

3.1. Effects of DQ on AD Symptoms Induced by Oxazolone in BALB/c Mouse Ears

Pathological reactions of AD such as increased ear thickness, erythema, and dryness were observed in the ears of oxazolone-challenged BALB/c mice (Figure 1a). According to the phenotypic observation, ear swelling and erythematic intensity caused by oxazolone were significantly reduced when ears were exposed to 1% DQ for 21 days (Figure 1b). Histologic evaluation also showed that the DQ was efficient at improving AD-like skin lesions in the oxazolone-sensitized mouse ears. Skin thickening and the number of infiltrating lymphocytes were significantly increased in AD mice compared with those in normal mice, and these changes were attenuated by DQ treatment (Figure 1c).

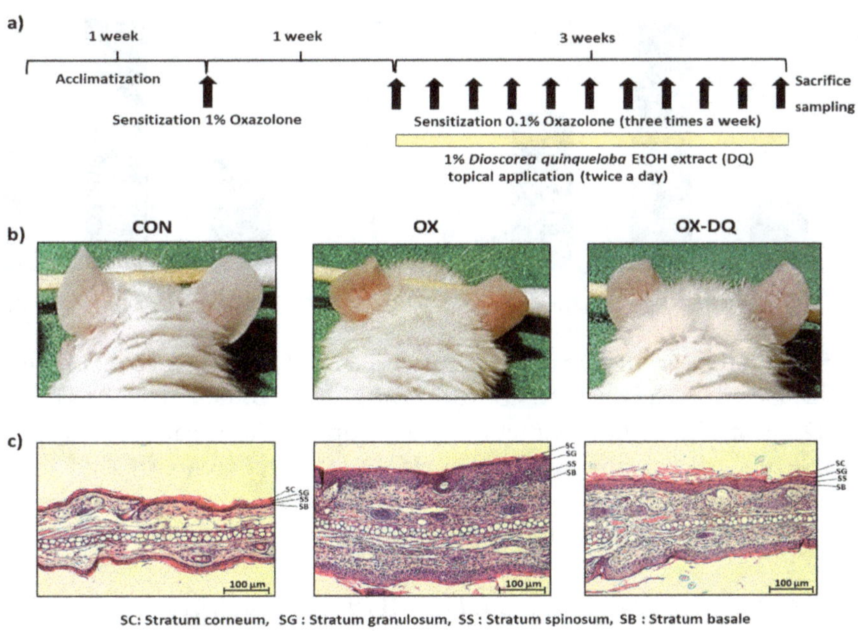

Figure 1. Effects of DQ on the development of oxazolone-induced AD-like symptoms in BALB/c mouse ears and histopathological analysis. CON: control group, OX: oxazolone-treated group, OX-DQ: oxazolone and 1% *D. quinqueloba* EtOH extract-treated group. (**a**) Schematic representation of the experiment; (**b**) Clinical features of AD-like skin lesions; (**c**) Histopathological features of skin lesions. Tissues were excised, fixed in 10% formaldehyde, embedded in paraffin, and sectioned. The sections were stained with hematoxylin and eosin (H&E) (magnification, 100× g).

3.2. Effects of DQ on Ear Thickness and Serum IgE and IL-4 Levels in Oxazolone-Induced AD BALB/c Mouse Ears

Increased ear thickness (2.3-fold) and epidermis thickness (2.5-fold) were observed after application of 1% oxazolone to the ears of mice, but these were reversed by treatment with DQ. The ear and epidermal thickness were reduced by 25% and 79%, respectively, on day 28 compared with the oxazolone-treated group (Figure 2a,b). Serum levels of IL-4 and Ig-E were markedly lower in mice of OX-DQ group as compared to the OX group. The 1% DQ application noticeably attenuated total IgE concentration (CON: 52.1 ng/mL, OX: 190.9 ng/mL, and OX-DQ: 118.5 ng/mL) (Figure 2c) and IL-4 concentration (CON: 12.6 pg/mL, OX: 28.6 pg/mL, and OX-DQ: 16.9 pg/mL) (Figure 2d).

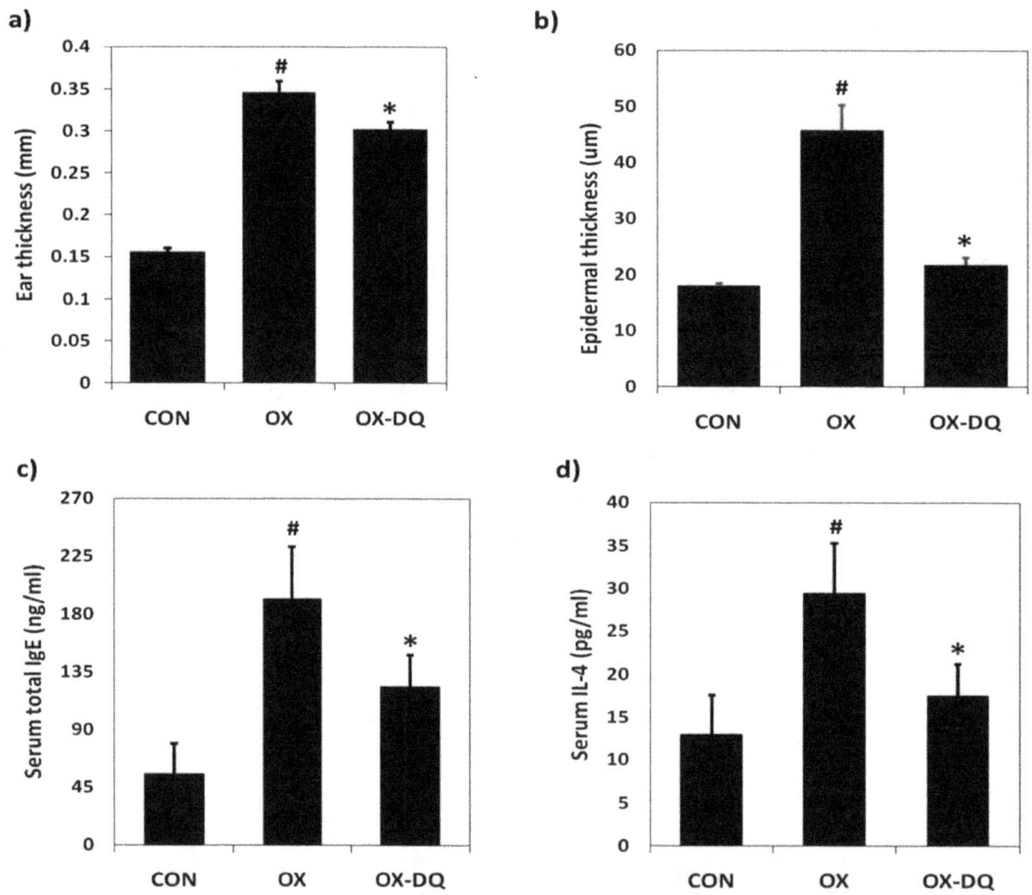

Figure 2. Effects of DQ on the ear thickness and serum IgE and IL-4 levels in oxazolone-induced AD-like symptoms in BALB/c mouse ears. CON: control group, DNCB: DNCB-treated group, DNCB-DQ: oxazolone and 1% *D. quinqueloba* EtOH extract-treated group. (**a**) Ear thickness; (**b**) epidermal thickness; (**c**) Serum total IgE levels; (**d**) Serum total IL-4 levels (D). Results are expressed as the mean ± SEM (standard error of the mean) ($n = 7$). The means ± SEM of two independent experiments are shown. $^{\#}$ $p < 0.05$ vs. control; * $p < 0.05$ vs. oxazolone-treated group.

3.3. Effects of DQEA on AD Symptoms Induced by DNCB in Hairless Mice

Out of two fractions from DQ (DQEA and DQB), the DQEA exhibited a dramatic drop in mRNA expression of IL-4 genes in RBL-2H3 cells stimulated by PMA/ionomycin (PI) A further experiment was performed to investigate anti-atopic properties of DQEA on AD skin lesions induced by DNCB. For DNCB sensitization, mice were given paintings of 1% DNCB for 3 weeks (Figure 3a). Treatment of 1% DQEA for 2 weeks markedly alleviated DNCB-induced atopy-like dermatitis such as definite erythema, papula, and vesiculation in SKH-1 hairless mice (Figure 3b). Histopathological features of the dorsal skin lesions from DQEA-treated AD hairless mice were shown in Figure 3c. Epidermal thickening by cell hyperplasia, slight spongiosis, and lymphocyte infiltration in the dermis were observed in DNCB-treated control mice, but these were reversed by treatment with DQEA.

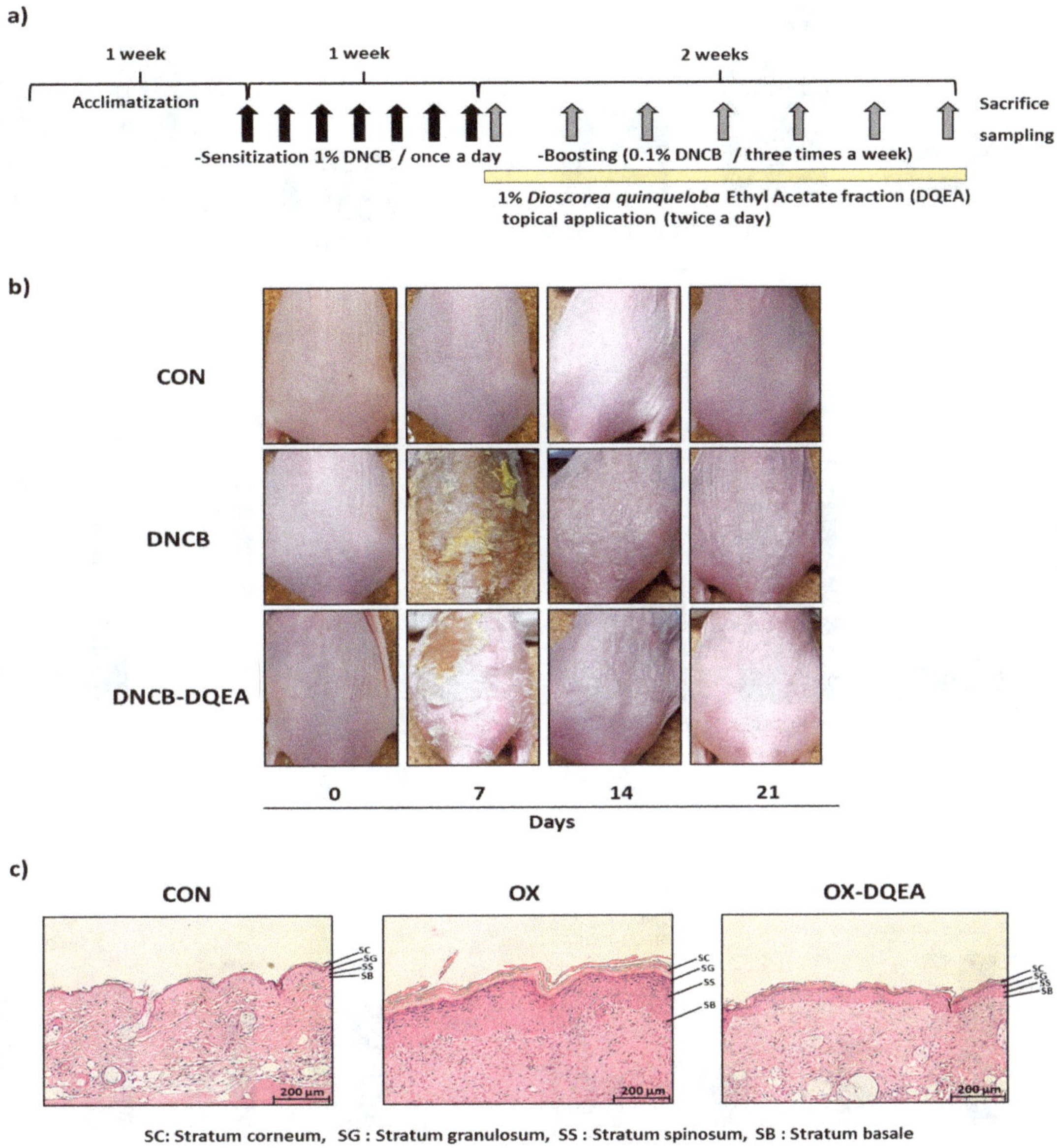

Figure 3. Effects of DQEA on the development of DNCB-induced AD-like symptoms in hairless mice and histopathological analysis. CON: control group, DNCB: DNCB-treated group, DNCB-DQEA: DNCB and 1% *D. quinqueloba* EtOAc fraction-treated group. (**a**) Schematic representation of the experiment; (**b**) Clinical features of AD-like skin lesions; (**c**) Histopathological features of skin lesions. Tissues were excised, fixed in 10% formaldehyde, embedded in paraffin, and sectioned. The sections were stained with hematoxylin and eosin (H&E) (magnification, 100× *g*).

3.4. Effects of DQEA on Ear Thickness and Serum IgE and IL-4 Levels in DNCB-Induced AD Hairless Mice

DNCB-sensitized mice showed a dramatic increase in epidermis thickness, which was significantly reduced in mice treated with DQEA (Figure 4a). DQEA inhibited the DNCB-induced epidermal hyperplasia by 67% in AD hairless mice. The results of serum testing showed that the levels of IgE and IL-4 were increased in the DNCB-stimulated group. The 1% DQEA application noticeably decreased the DNCB-induced serum IgE levels by 65% and IL-4 levels by 57% of DNCB-treated controls (Figure 4b,c).

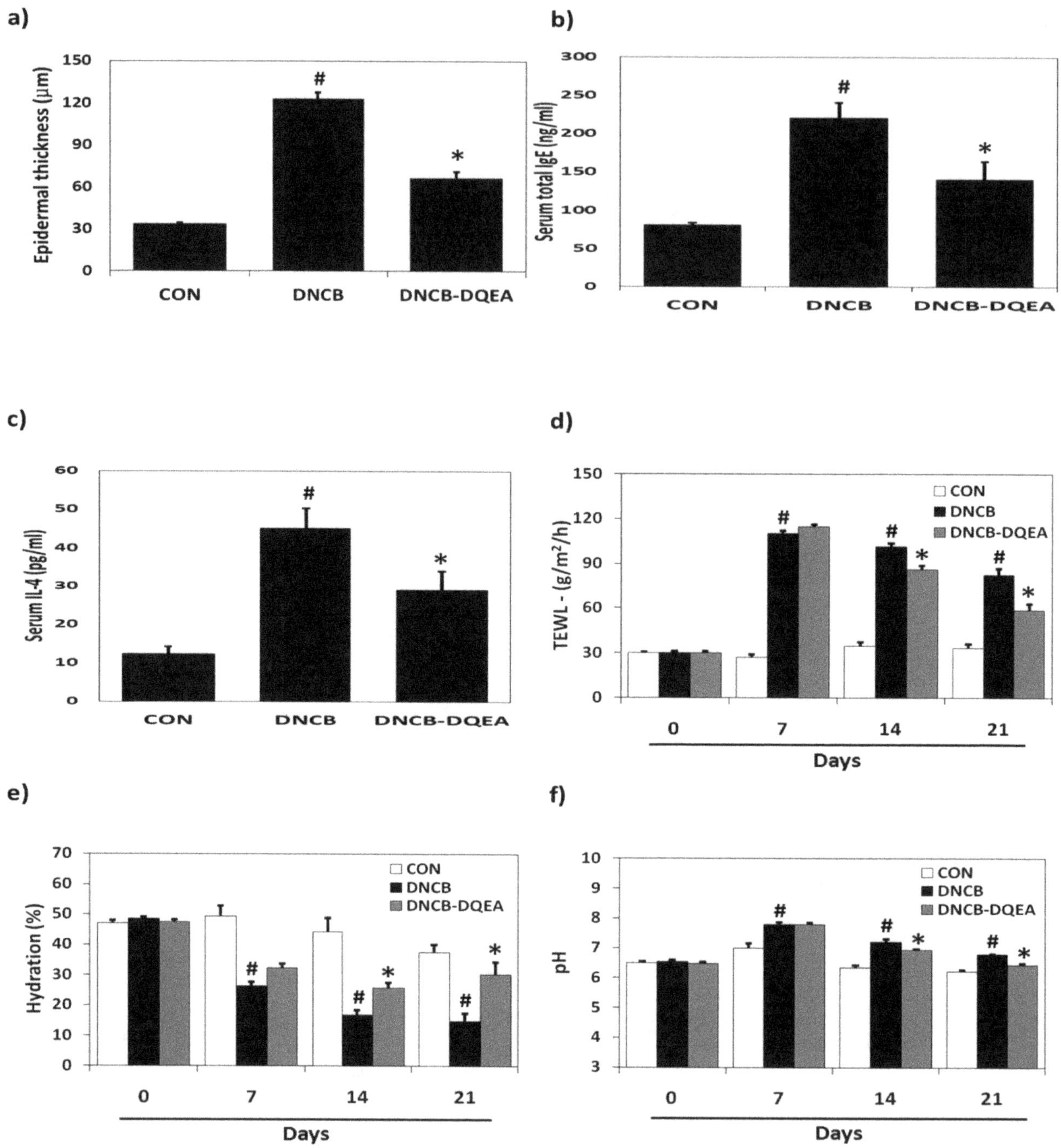

Figure 4. Effects of DQEA on the epidermal thickness, serum IgE and IL-4 levels, and skin barrier function in DNCB-induced AD-like symptoms in hairless mice. CON: control group, DNCB: DNCB-treated group, DNCB-DQEA: DNCB and 1% *D. quinqueloba* EtOAc fraction-treated group. (**a**) Epidermal thickness; (**b**) Serum total IgE levels (**c**) Serum total IL-4 levels; (**d**) TWEL; (**e**) Skin hydration; (**f**) Skin surface pH. Results are expressed as the mean ± SEM ($n = 7$). The means ± SEM of two independent experiments are shown. $^{\#}$ $p < 0.05$ vs. control; * $p < 0.05$ vs. DNCB-treated group.

3.5. Effects of DQEA on Skin Barrier Function in DNCB-Induced AD Hairless Mice

Severe skin barrier damage, such as increased TEWL and skin surface PH, and decreased epidermal hydration, was detected in the DNCB-treated control group. This AD-like skin barrier dysfuction was reversed by treatment with 1% DQEA. After 21 days of treatment, DNCB greatly increased TEWL to 79.8 J (g/(m^{2}h)), whereas it was markedly reduced to 59.5 J (g/(m^{2}h)) by the transdermal application of DQEA (Figure 4d). Consistent with this finding, skin hydration level was decreased in the DNCB-induced group (65.8% decrease) compared with the control group, whereas DQEA increased the hydration level to 68% (Figure 4e). Skin surface pH value was significantly increased in lesional skin, but not in non-lesional skin of AD. Figure 4f revealed that DQEA treatment normalized the altered pH of DNCB-sensitized hairless mouse skin.

3.6. The Standardization of DQEA Using the High-Performance Liquid Chromatography/Mass Spectrometry (HPLC/MS)

For the simultaneous determination of the major constituents of DQEA, the optimized chromatographic condition was investigated. The optimal mobile phase, which consisted of acetonitrile/water, was subsequently employed for the analysis of DQEA, and led to a good resolution and satisfactory peak shape. The presence of two compounds, 1: dioscin (*m/z* 868.08 at t_R 18.66 min) and 2: gracillin (*m/z* 884.08 at t_R 19.78 min) in DQEA was verified by comparing each retention time and UV spectrum with those of each standard compound and spiking with authentic standards (Figure 5a,b). DQEA was found to contain dioscin (319 mg/g) and gracillin (91.6 mg/g) as major compounds.

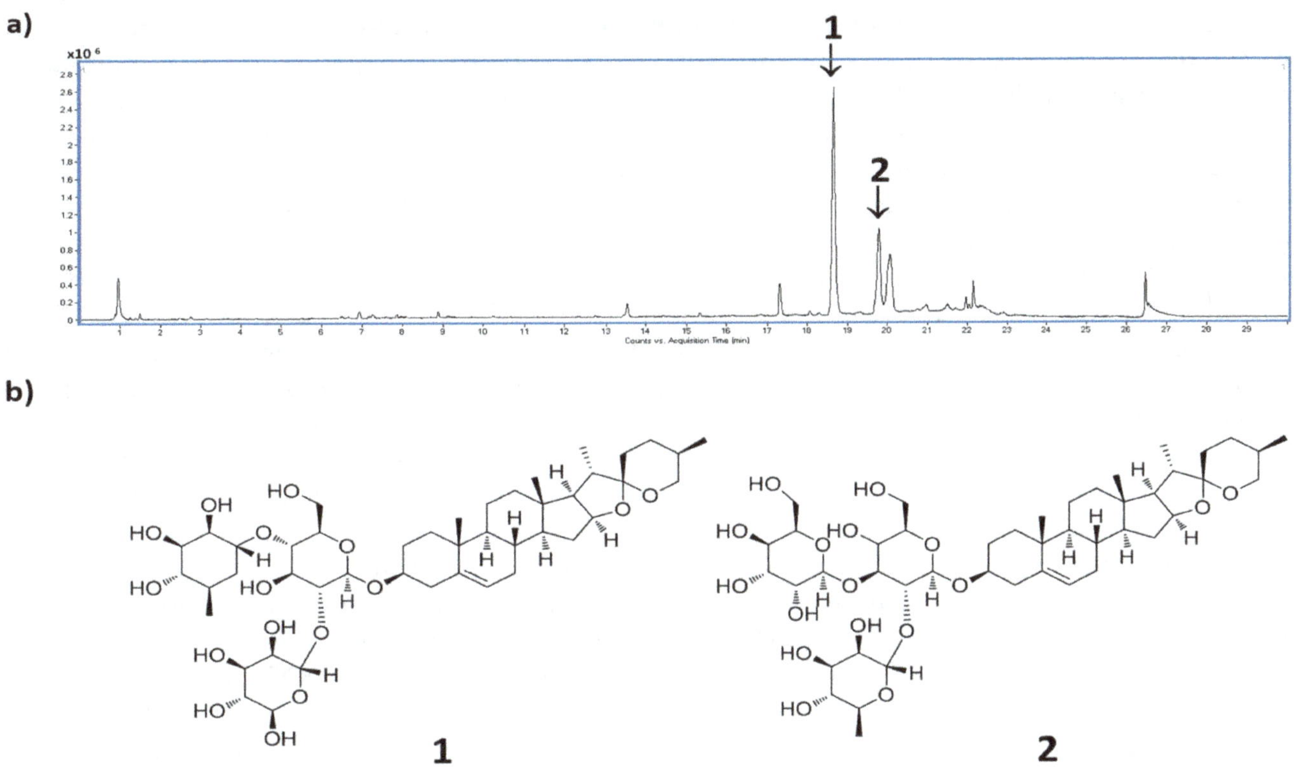

Figure 5. (**a**) HPLC chromatogram of DQEA (**a**) and chemical structures of major components (**b**). Fingerprint analysis of *D. quinqueloba* EtOAc fraction was performed in positive ion mode using HPLC/MS (high-performance liquid chromatography/mass spectrometry). **1**: dioscin, **2**: gracillin.

4. Discussion

Skin barrier dysfunction is one of the primary causes of allergic disorders, and is crucially involved in the pathogenesis of AD [23]. The skin barrier function is mainly disturbed in contact and extrinsic AD, the classical type of AD, which has high prevalence [24]. Impaired permeability barrier function of skin in AD patients enhances penetration of environmental allergens into the skin, thus triggering immunological reactions and inflammation [24,25]. Use of proper moisturizers/emollients to enhance skin hydration is likely to play a key part in management of AD [26]. Natural products are a rich source of medicinal agents, and natural product-related drugs account for over 50% of the most-prescribed drugs in the USA [27]. Substances of natural origin have been widely used for treatment of skin problems due to their therapeutic efficacies in dermatology, which include anti-inflammatory, antimicrobial, and cell-stimulating properties [28]. In addition, plants—including extracts, pure compounds, and phytochemical combinations—are commonly added to moisturizers to improve dry skin conditions in AD patients [28,29]. For this reason, naturally occurring moisturizing agents can be useful in the treatment of at allergic and atopic diseases through improvement skin barrier function [30].

In our preliminary research to find anti-inflammatory materials from plant extracts, the 95% EtOH extract of *D. quinqueloba* (DQ) showed strong IL-4 inhibition in RBL-2H3 cells. The anti-atopic property of DQ was studied using an experimental animal model of AD induced by oxazolone. BALB/c mouse ears were sensitized with oxazolone and treated with DQ subcutaneously for 2 weeks. The results indicated that the topical application of DQ could improve atopic damage in oxazolone-induced BALB/c mouse ears. This finding strongly suggested that the specific fraction from total extract of *D. quinqueloba* is responsible for the anti-atopic effect. For this reason, the DQ was fractionated in order to find the most active principles. Out of two fractions of DQ, the production of IL-4 in RBL-2H3 was only affected by the EtOAc fraction of DQ (DQEA). IL-4 has been considered one of the key proximal cytokines of type 2 inflammation in atopic disease. Impaired barrier function induced by skin sensitizers develops into a pruritic inflammatory skin disease characterized by hyperactivated cytokines of helper T cells [22]. The hyperproduction of IL-4, a key regulatory cytokine for IgE synthesis, is generally detected in various experimental animal models to study AD [31]. In addition, transgenic mice expressing epidermal IL-4 have been reported to develop skin inflammation reproducing all key features of human AD [27,32]. Broad application of DQEA to dorsal skins of DNCB-sensitized SKH-1 hairless mice attenuated severe atopic symptoms such as erythema and lichenification. Taken together, it was concluded that *D. quinqueloba* improves severe AD symptoms in both oxazolone- and DNCB-induced AD mice as a potent IL-4 inhibitor.

Stratum corneum hydration and transepidermal water loss are considered as a marker of the inside-outside skin barrier [33]. The water-holding capacity of the *D. quinqueloba* sample in atopic skin was evaluated by measuring both epidermal hydration and TEWL. Barrier repair was delayed and skin hydration was impaired in DNCB-sensitized mice. Treatment with DQEA significantly increased skin hydration and decreased TWEL and skin surface pH in DNCB-induced AD hairless mice. Atopic skin normally shows a defective skin barrier function, both in rough and in clinically healthy skin [34]. Emollient enhancement of the skin barrier from DQEA-applied AD animals was observed after 3 weeks of treatment. Therefore, DQEA might be an appropriate material for improving barrier function and dry skin as a skin therapeutic agent for AD. An elevated serum level of IgE is a main feature of AD and IL-4 acts as a key cytokine in the process of atopic inflammation [35].DQEA also attenuated IgE hyperproduction and epidermal overexpression of IL-4, resulting in the prevention and treatment of Th2-dominated inflammation in AD-like skin lesions. Based on the results, we propose that DQEA corrects skin barrier dysfunction and early inflammation in murine AD models.

Standardization of *D. quinqueloba* is necessary to provide information on quality standards of natural product-derived drug development. Phytochemical screening, using steroidal saponins as bioactive marker compounds, was performed to standardize the DQEA sample. Steroidal saponins have long attracted scientific attention, due to their structural diversity and significant biological activities [36]. Dioscin and disogenin, steroidal saponins obtained from *Dioscorea* species, are currently being considered as an important starting material for the industrial production of steroid drugs [37]. Phytochemical analysis of the DQEA resulted in the presence of dioscin and gracillin as major components.

5. Conclusions

In conclusion, topical treatment with *D. quinqueloba* total extract was protective against oxazolone-induced AD-like lesions in mice ears. Bioassay-guided fractionation of the DQ led to the finding of the most biologically active fraction, DQEA. Clinical symptoms of AD, such as pruritus, erythema, fissuring, and lichenification (skin thickening), were significantly reduced in the DQEA-treated mice. The DQEA improved skin barrier dysfunction and suppressed the overproduction of serum IgE and IL-4 in murine DNCB-sensitized atopic models. Based on the fingerprint analysis, dioscin, and gracillin were confirmed to be the major active constituents of DQEA. Further study is warranted to identify the therapeutic effects of DQEA against AD symptoms in human skin.

Acknowledgments: This study was supported by a grant from the Korea Healthcare Technology R&D Project, the Ministry of Health & Welfare, Republic of Korea. (Grant No. HI14C2687), the Korea Institute of Science and Technology, Republic of Korea (Grant No. 2Z04930 and 2Z04950), the National Research Foundation of Korea (NRF) grant funded by the Ministry of Science, ICT & Future Planning (NRF-2016R1C1B2007694 and NRF-2016K1A1A8A01938595), and the "Cooperative Research Program for Agriculture Science and Technology Development (Project No. PJ01282301)" Rural Development Administration, Republic of Korea.

Author Contributions: S.-N.K. and M.H.Y. designedthe research; J.J., N.-J.P., S.-K.B. and H.J. performed the experiments; J.J., N.-J.P., S.-N.K. and M.H.Y. analyzed the data, and interpreted the results of the experiments. J.J., S.-N.K. and M.H.Y. drafted the manuscript. All authors read and approved the final manuscript.

References

1. Williams, H.C. Is the prevalence of atopic dermatitis increasing? *Clin. Exp. Dermatol.* **1992**, *17*, 385–391. [CrossRef] [PubMed]
2. Kapoor, R.; Menon, C.; Hoffstad, O.; Bilker, W.; Leclerc, P.; Margolis, D.J. The prevalence of atopic triad in children with physician-confirmed atopic dermatitis. *J. Am. Acad. Dermatol.* **2008**, *58*, 68–73. [CrossRef] [PubMed]
3. Larsen, F.S.; Hanifin, J.M. Epidemiology of atopic dermatitis: A review. *Allergy Asthma Proc.* **2002**, *22*, 1–24. [CrossRef]
4. Morren, M.A.; Przybilla, B.; Bamelis, M.; Heykants, B.; Reynaers, A.; Degreef, H. Atopic dermatitis: Triggering factors. *J. Am. Acad. Dermatol.* **1994**, *31*, 467–473. [CrossRef]
5. Guttman-Yassky, E.; Nograles, K.E.; Krueger, J.G. Contrasting pathogenesis of atopic dermatitis and psoriasis-part I: Clinical and pathologic concepts. *J. Allergy Clin. Immunol.* **2011**, *127*, 1110–1118. [CrossRef] [PubMed]
6. Ständer, S.; Steinhoff, M. Pathophysiology of pruritus in atopic dermatitis: An overview. *Exp. Dermatol.* **2002**, *11*, 12–24. [CrossRef] [PubMed]
7. Charman, C.; Williams, H. Outcome measures of disease severity in atopic eczema. *Arch. Dermatol.* **2000**, *136*, 763–769. [CrossRef] [PubMed]
8. Tokura, Y. Extrinsic and intrinsic types of atopic dermatitis. *J. Dermatol. Sci.* **2010**, *58*, 1–7. [CrossRef] [PubMed]
9. Darlenski, R.; Kazandjieva, J.; Hristakieva, E.; Fluhr, J.W. Atopic dermatitis as a systemic disease. *Clin. Dermatol.* **2014**, *32*, 409–413. [CrossRef] [PubMed]
10. Renz, H.; Jujo, K.; Bradley, K.L.; Domenico, J.; Gelfand, E.W.; Leung, D.Y. Enhanced IL-4 production and IL-4 receptor expression in atopic dermatitis and their modulation by interferon-gamma. *J. Investig. Dermatol.* **1992**, *99*, 403–408. [CrossRef] [PubMed]
11. Mori, T.; Ishida, K.; Mukumoto, S.; Yamada, Y.; Imokawa, G.; Kabashima, K.; Kobayashi, M.; Bito, T.; Nakamura, M.; Ogasawara, K.; et al. Comparison of skin barrier function and sensory nerve electric current perception threshold between IgE-high extrinsic and IgE-normal intrinsic types of atopic dermatitis. *Br. J. Dermatol.* **2010**, *162*, 83–90. [CrossRef] [PubMed]
12. Kim, S.J.; Jung, J.Y.; Kim, H.W.; Park, T. Anti-obesity effects of *Juniperus chinensis* extract are associated with increased AMP-activated protein kinase expression and phosphorylation in the visceral adipose tissue of rats. *Biol. Pharm. Bull.* **2008**, *31*, 1415–1421. [CrossRef] [PubMed]
13. Ali, A.M.; Mackeen, M.M.; Intan-Safinar, I.; Hamid, M.; Lajis, N.H.; el-Sharkawy, S.H.; MurakoshI, M. Antitumour-promoting and antitumour activities of the crude extract from the leaves of *Juniperus chinensis*. *J. Ethnopharmacol.* **1996**, *53*, 165–169. [CrossRef]
14. Viruel, J.; Catalan, P.; Segarra-Moragues, J.G. New microsatellite loci in the dwarf yams *Dioscorea* group Epipetrum (Dioscoreaceae). *Am. J. Bot.* **2010**, *97*, e121–e123. [CrossRef] [PubMed]

15. Broadbent, J.L.; Schnieden, H. A comparison of some pharmacological properties of dioscorine and dioscine. *Br. J. Pharmacol. Chemother.* **1958**, *13*, 213–215. [CrossRef] [PubMed]
16. Karnick, C.R. Dioscorea (YAMS)-The Food of the Slaves, with Potentials for Newer Drugs: A review. *Q. J. Crude Drug Res.* **1969**, *9*, 1372–1391. [CrossRef]
17. Yang, M.H.; Yoon, K.D.; Chin, Y.W.; Park, J.H.; Kim, J. Phenolic compounds with radical scavenging and cyclooxygenase-2 (COX-2) inhibitory activities from Dioscoreaopposita. *Bioorg. Med. Chem.* **2009**, *17*, 2689–2694. [CrossRef] [PubMed]
18. Wang, J.M.; Ji, L.L.; Branford-White, C.J.; Wang, Z.Y.; Shen, K.K.; Liu, H.; Wang, Z.T. Antitumor activity of *Dioscorea bulbifera* L. rhizome in vivo. *Fitoterapia* **2012**, *83*, 388–394. [CrossRef] [PubMed]
19. Yang, M.H.; Chin, Y.W.; Chae, H.S.; Yoon, K.D.; Kim, J. Anti-adipogenic Constituents from Dioscoreaopposita in 3T3-L1 Cells. *Biol. Pharm. Bull.* **2014**, *37*, 1683–1688. [CrossRef] [PubMed]
20. Blaylock, B.L.; Newsom, K.K.; Holladay, S.D.; Shipp, B.K.; Bartow, T.A.; Mehendale, H.M. Topical exposure to chlordane reduces the contact hypersensitivity response to oxazolone in BALB/c mice. *Toxicol. Lett.* **1995**, *81*, 205–211. [CrossRef]
21. Matsumoto, K.; Mizukoshi, K.; Oyobikawa, M.; Ohshima, H.; Sakai, Y.; Tagami, H. Objective evaluation of the efficacy of daily topical applications of cosmetics bases using the hairless mouse model of atopic dermatitis. *Skin Res. Technol.* **2005**, *11*, 209–217. [CrossRef] [PubMed]
22. Matsumoto, K.; Mizukoshi, K.; Oyobikawa, M.; Ohshima, H.; Tagami, H. Establishment of an atopic dermatitis-like skin model in a hairless mouse by repeated elicitation of contact hypersensitivity that enables to conduct functional analyses of the stratum corneum with various non-invasive biophysical instruments. *Skin Res. Technol.* **2004**, *10*, 122–129. [CrossRef] [PubMed]
23. Aioi, A.; Tonogaito, H.; Suto, H.; Hamada, K.; Ra, C.; Ogawa, H.; Maibach, H.; Matsuda, H. Impairment of skin barrier function in NC/Nga Tnd mice as a possible model for atopic dermatitis. *Br. J. Dermatol.* **2001**, *144*, 12–18. [CrossRef] [PubMed]
24. Proksch, E.; Fölster-Holst, R.; Jensen, J.M. Skin barrier function, epidermal proliferation and differentiation in eczema. *J. Dermatol. Sci.* **2006**, *43*, 159–169. [CrossRef] [PubMed]
25. Boguniewicz, M.; Leung, D.Y. Atopic dermatitis: A disease of altered skin barrier and immune dysregulation. *Immunol. Rev.* **2011**, *242*, 233–246. [CrossRef] [PubMed]
26. Leung, D.Y.; Boguniewicz, M.; Howell, M.D.; Nomura, I.; Hamid, Q.A. New insights into atopic dermatitis. *J. Clin. Investig.* **2004**, *113*, 651–657. [CrossRef] [PubMed]
27. Newman, D.J.; Cragg, G.M.; Snader, K.M. The influence of natural products upon drug discovery. *Nat. Prod. Rep.* **2000**, *17*, 215–234. [CrossRef] [PubMed]
28. Bodeker, G.; Ryan, T.J.; Volk, A.; Harris, J.; Burford, G. Integrative Skin Care: Dermatology and traditional and complementary medicine. *J. Altern. Complement. Med.* **2017**, *23*, 479–486. [CrossRef] [PubMed]
29. Loden, M. The clinical benefit of moisturizers. *J. Eur. Acad. Dermatol. Venereol.* **2005**, *19*, 672–688. [CrossRef] [PubMed]
30. Loden, M.; Andersson, A.C.; Lindberg, M. Improvement in skin barrier function in patients with atopic dermatitis after treatment with a moisturizing cream (Canoderm). *Br. J. Dermatol.* **1999**, *140*, 264–267. [CrossRef] [PubMed]
31. Poulsen, L.K.; Reimert, C.M.; Bindslev-Jensen, C.; Hansen, M.B.; Bendtzen, K. Biomolecular regulation of the IgE immune response. II. In vitro IgE synthesis and spontaneous production of cytokines. *Int. Arch. Allergy Immunol.* **1995**, *106*, 55–61. [CrossRef] [PubMed]
32. Chan, L.S.; Robinson, N.; Xu, L. Expression of interleukin-4 in the epidermis of transgenic mice results in a pruritic inflammatory skin disease: An experimental animal model to study atopic dermatitis. *J. Investig. Dermatol.* **2001**, *117*, 977–983. [CrossRef] [PubMed]
33. Jensen, J.M.; Pfeiffer, S.; Witt, M.; Bräutigam, M.; Neumann, C.; Weichenthal, M.; Schwarz, T.; Fölster-Holst, R.; Proksch, E. Different effects of pimecrolimus and betamethasone on the skin barrier in patients with atopic dermatitis. *J. Allergy Clin. Immunol.* **2009**, *124*, R19–R28. [CrossRef] [PubMed]
34. Sator, P.G.; Schmidt, J.B.; Hönigsmann, H. Comparison of epidermal hydration and skin surface lipids in healthy individuals and in patients with atopic dermatitis. *J. Am. Acad. Dermatol.* **2003**, *48*, 352–358. [CrossRef] [PubMed]
35. Ricci, M. IL-4: A key cytokine in atopy. *Clin. Exp. Allergy* **1994**, *24*, 801–812. [CrossRef] [PubMed]

Permissions

All chapters in this book were first published by MDPI; hereby published with permission under the Creative Commons Attribution License or equivalent. Every chapter published in this book has been scrutinized by our experts. Their significance has been extensively debated. The topics covered herein carry significant findings which will fuel the growth of the discipline. They may even be implemented as practical applications or may be referred to as a beginning point for another development.

The contributors of this book come from diverse backgrounds, making this book a truly international effort. This book will bring forth new frontiers with its revolutionizing research information and detailed analysis of the nascent developments around the world.

We would like to thank all the contributing authors for lending their expertise to make the book truly unique. They have played a crucial role in the development of this book. Without their invaluable contributions this book wouldn't have been possible. They have made vital efforts to compile up to date information on the varied aspects of this subject to make this book a valuable addition to the collection of many professionals and students.

This book was conceptualized with the vision of imparting up-to-date information and advanced data in this field. To ensure the same, a matchless editorial board was set up. Every individual on the board went through rigorous rounds of assessment to prove their worth. After which they invested a large part of their time researching and compiling the most relevant data for our readers.

The editorial board has been involved in producing this book since its inception. They have spent rigorous hours researching and exploring the diverse topics which have resulted in the successful publishing of this book. They have passed on their knowledge of decades through this book. To expedite this challenging task, the publisher supported the team at every step. A small team of assistant editors was also appointed to further simplify the editing procedure and attain best results for the readers.

Apart from the editorial board, the designing team has also invested a significant amount of their time in understanding the subject and creating the most relevant covers. They scrutinized every image to scout for the most suitable representation of the subject and create an appropriate cover for the book.

The publishing team has been an ardent support to the editorial, designing and production team. Their endless efforts to recruit the best for this project, has resulted in the accomplishment of this book. They are a veteran in the field of academics and their pool of knowledge is as vast as their experience in printing. Their expertise and guidance has proved useful at every step. Their uncompromising quality standards have made this book an exceptional effort. Their encouragement from time to time has been an inspiration for everyone.

The publisher and the editorial board hope that this book will prove to be a valuable piece of knowledge for researchers, students, practitioners and scholars across the globe.

List of Contributors

VijayKumar Patra
Center for Medical Research, Medical University of Graz, 8010 Graz, Austria
Research Unit for Photodermatology, Department of Dermatology, Medical University of Graz, 8010 Graz, Austria

Peter Wolf
Research Unit for Photodermatology, Department of Dermatology, Medical University of Graz, 8010 Graz, Austria

Irène Gallais Sérézal
Department of Medicine, Unit of Rheumatology, Karolinska Institutet, 171 77 Solna, Sweden
Department of Dermatology, Besançon University Hospital, 25000 Besancon, France

Anna Winiarska-Mieczan
Department of Bromatology and Food Physiology, University of Life Sciences in Lublin, 20-950 Lublin, Poland

Tomasz Mieczan
Department of Hydrobiology and Protection of Ecosystems, University of Life Sciences in Lublin, 20-262 Lublin, Poland

Grzegorz Wójcik
Department of Inorganic Chemistry, Maria Curie-Sklodowska University, 20-031 Lublin, Poland

Agata Jabłońska-Trypuć, Monika Kalinowska, Grzegorz Świderski and Włodzimierz Lewandowski
Department of Chemistry, Biology and Biotechnology, Faculty of Civil Engineering and Environmental Engineering, Białystok University of Technology, Wiejska 45E Street, 15-351 Białystok, Poland

Rafał Krętowski and Marzanna Cechowska-Pasko
Department of Pharmaceutical Biochemistry, Medical University of Bialystok, 15-222 Białystok, Poland

Amitis Karrys
School of Life Sciences, Arizona State University, Tempe, AZ 85281, USA
Department of Basic Medical Sciences, University of Arizona College of Medicine–Phoenix, Phoenix, AZ 85004, USA

Mark R. Haussler and G. Kerr Whitfield
Department of Basic Medical Sciences, University of Arizona College of Medicine–Phoenix, Phoenix, AZ 85004, USA

Roxane-Cherille N. Chamcheu
Department of Dermatology, School of Medicine and Public Health, University of Wisconsin, Madison, WI 53706, USA

Islam Rady
Department of Dermatology, School of Medicine and Public Health, University of Wisconsin, Madison, WI 53706, USA
Department of Zoology, Faculty of Science, Al-Azhar University, Nazr City, Cairo, Egypt

Marya S. Sabir and Sanchita Mallick
School of Mathematical and Natural Sciences, Arizona State University, Phoenix, AZ 85306, USA

Peter W. Jurutka
Department of Basic Medical Sciences, University of Arizona College of Medicine–Phoenix, Phoenix, AZ 85004, USA
School of Mathematical and Natural Sciences, Arizona State University, Phoenix, AZ 85306, USA

Jean Christopher Chamcheu
Department of Dermatology, School of Medicine and Public Health, University of Wisconsin, Madison, WI 53706, USA
Department of Basic Pharmaceutical Sciences, School of Pharmacy, College of Health & Pharmaceutical Sciences, University of Louisiana at Monroe, 1800 Bienville Drive, Bienville 362, Monroe, LA 71201, USA

Shih-Yi Chuang
Research Center for Food and Cosmetic Safety and Research Center for Chinese Herbal Medicine, Chang Gung University of Science and Technology, Kweishan, Taoyuan 333, Taiwan

Yin-Ku Lin
Department of Traditional Chinese Medicine, Chang Gung Memorial Hospital, Keelung 204, Taiwan
School of Traditional Chinese Medicine, Chang Gung University, Kweishan, Taoyuan 333, Taiwan

Chwan-Fwu Lin
Research Center for Food and Cosmetic Safety and Research Center for Chinese Herbal Medicine, Chang Gung University of Science and Technology, Kweishan, Taoyuan 333, Taiwan
Department of Cosmetic Science, Chang Gung University of Science and Technology, Kweishan, Taoyuan 333, Taiwan

Pei-Wen Wang
Department of Medical Research, China Medical University Hospital, China Medical University, Taichung 404, Taiwan

En-Li Chen
Pharmaceutics Laboratory, Graduate Institute of Natural Products, Chang Gung University, Kweishan, Taoyuan 333, Taiwan

Jia-You Fang
Research Center for Food and Cosmetic Safety and Research Center for Chinese Herbal Medicine, Chang Gung University of Science and Technology, Kweishan, Taoyuan 333, Taiwan
Pharmaceutics Laboratory, Graduate Institute of Natural Products, Chang Gung University, Kweishan, Taoyuan 333, Taiwan
Chinese Herbal Medicine Research Team, Healthy Aging Research Center, Chang Gung University, Kweishan, Taoyuan 333, Taiwan
Department of Anesthesiology, Chang Gung Memorial Hospital, Kweishan, Taoyuan 333, Taiwan

Martina C. Meinke, Ceylan K. Nowbary, Sabine Schanzer, Jürgen Lademann and Maxim E. Darvin
Charité-Universitätsmedizin Berlin, Corporate Member of Freie Universität Berlin, Humboldt-Universität zu Berlin, and Berlin Institute of Health, Center of Experimental and Applied Cutaneous Physiology (CCP), Department of Dermatology, Charité-Universitätsmedizin Berlin, 10117 Berlin, Germany

Henning Vollert
Bioactive Food GmbH, Am Ihlsee 36a, 23795 Bad Segeberg, Germany

Montserrat Rojo de la Vega, Andrea Krajisnik, Donna D. Zhang and Georg T. Wondrak
Department of Pharmacology and Toxicology, College of Pharmacy & Arizona Cancer Center, University of Arizona, Tucson, AZ 85724, USA

Natasha Irrera, Gabriele Pizzino, Mario Vaccaro, Vincenzo Arcoraci, Francesco Squadrito and Alessandra Bitto
Department of Clinical and Experimental Medicine, University of Messina, Messina 98125, Italy

Rosario D'Anna
Department of Human Pathology, University of Messina, Messina 98125, Italy

Domenica Altavilla
Department of Biomedical Sciences, Dentistry and Morphological and Functional Images, University of Messina, Messina 98125, Italy

Daniela Martini, Donato Angelino and Daniele Del Rio
The Laboratory of Phytochemicals in Physiology, Department of Food and Drug, University of Parma, 43125 Parma, Italy

Chiara Cortelazzi, Sergio Di Nuzzo and Maria Beatrice De Felici
Department of Medicine and Surgery, Section of Dermatology, University of Parma, 43125 Parma, Italy

Ivana Zavaroni, Alessandra Dei Cas and Riccardo C. Bonadonna
Department of Medicine and Surgery, Division of Endocrinology, University of Parma, 43125 Parma, Italy
The Azienda Ospedaliera Universitaria of Parma, Division of Endocrinology, 43125 Parma, Italy

Giorgio Bedogni
Clinical Epidemiology Unit, Liver Research Center, Basovizza, 34149 Trieste, Italy

Marilena Musci
Department of Food and Drug, University of Parma, 43125 Parma, Italy

Carlo Pruneti
Department of Medicine and Surgery, Clinical Psychology Unit, University of Parma, 43125 Parma, Italy

Giovanni Passeri
Department of Medicine and Surgery, University of Parma, Building Clinica Medica Generale, 43125 Parma, Italy

Marco Ventura
Laboratory of Probiogenomics, Department of Chemistry, Life Sciences and Environmental Sustainability, University of Parma, 43125 Parma, Italy

Daniela Galli, Prisco Mirandola and Marco Vitale
Department of Medicine and Surgery, Sport and Exercise Medicine Centre (SEM), University of Parma, 43125 Parma, Italy

Hongdong Song, Siqi Zhang and Ling Zhang
Beijing Advanced Innovation Center for Food Nutrition and Human Health, College of Food Science and Nutritional Engineering, China Agricultural University, Beijing 100083, China

Bo Li
Beijing Higher Institution Engineering Research Center of Animal Product, Beijing 100083, China

Simona-Roxana Georgescu, Maria-Isabela Sârbu, Clara Matei and Mircea Tampa
Department of Dermatology, Carol Davila University of Medicine and Pharmacy, 020021 Bucharest, Romania

Mihaela Adriana Ilie
Department of Biochemistry, Carol Davila University of Medicine and Pharmacy, 020021 Bucharest, Romania

Constantin Caruntu
Department of Physiology, Carol Davila University of Medicine and Pharmacy, 050474 Bucharest, Romania
Department of Dermatology, Prof. N.C. Paulescu National Institute of Diabetes, Nutrition and Metabolic Diseases, 011233 Bucharest, Romania

Carolina Constantin
Immunology Department, Victor Babes National Institute of Pathology, 050096 Bucharest, Romania

Monica Neagu
Immunology Department, Victor Babes National Institute of Pathology, 050096 Bucharest, Romania
Faculty of Biology, University of Bucharest, 76201 Bucharest, Romania

Yoshihiro Tokudome, Noriomi Masutani, Shohei Uchino and Hisano Fukai
Laboratory of Dermatological Physiology, Department of Pharmaceutical Sciences, Faculty of Pharmacy and Pharmaceutical Sciences, Josai University, Saitama 350-0295, Japan

Jonghwan Jegal and Min Hye Yang
College of Pharmacy, Pusan National University, Busan 46241, Korea

No-June Park, Sim-Kyu Bong, Hyun Jegal and Su-Nam Kim
Natural Products Research Institute, Korea Institute of Science and Technology, Gangneung 25451, Korea

Index

www.ingramcontent.com/pod-product-compliance
Lightning Source LLC
LaVergne TN
LVHW060600210926
848485LV00005B/1350
9781639278060